EXERCISE AND HEART FAILURE

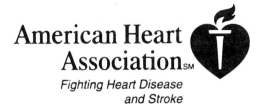

American Heart
Association℠
*Fighting Heart Disease
and Stroke*

Monograph Series

EXERCISE AND HEART FAILURE

Edited by

Gary J. Balady, MD

*Director,
Preventive Cardiology;
Associate Professor of Medicine,
Boston University School of Medicine,
Boston, MA*

and

Ileana L. Piña, MD

*Associate Professor of Medicine;
Director, Cardiomyopathy and Cardiac Rehabilitation,
Temple University School of Medicine,
Cardiomyopathy and Transplant Center,
Philadelphia, PA*

Futura Publishing
Company, Inc.
Armonk, NY

Library of Congress Cataloging-in-Publication Data

Exercise and heart failure / edited by Gary J. Balady and Ileana L. Pinã.
    p.   cm. — (American Heart Association monograph series)
    Includes bibliographical references and index.
    ISBN 0-87993-667-3
    1. Heart failure.   2. Heart failure—exercise therapy.
  3. Exercise test.   I. Balady, Gary J.   II. Pinã, Ileana L.   III. Series.
    [DNLM: 1. Cardiac Output, Low—physiopathology.   2. Cardiac
  Output, Low—therapy.   3. Exercise Tolerance.   4. Exercise Therapy.
  WG 210   E958   1997]
  RC685.C53E94   1997
  616.1´062—dc21
  DNLM/DLC
  for Library of Congress   97-6841
                                                     CIP

Copyright © 1997
Futura Publishing Company, Inc.

Published by
Futura Publishing Company
135 Bedford Road
Armonk, New York 10504

LC #: 97-6841
ISBN #: 0-87993-6673

To Rosemary, Stephen, and Andrew
for your inspiration and support,
and for sharing the joys and challenges of my life as a
physician
GJB

To Victoria
who gives up play time so that I can pursue my love of
medicine and writing
ILP

Preface

The relationship between heart failure and exercise is fascinating and can be viewed from many vantage points. Indeed, the dynamic interplay between these entities may in some ways appear to be paradoxical. Heart failure often leads to impaired exercise tolerance, incurring significant disability among patients with this condition. Objective measures of exercise capacity provide important prognostic information upon which therapeutic decisions are made, including the selection for cardiac transplantation. Although the wide variety of current and emerging medical and surgical treatments target improvement in prognosis, many are assessed and valued for their beneficial influence on exercise capacity. Thus, exercise testing has become an integral component in the management of the patient with chronic heart failure. It is not surprising that this area of exercise science has witnessed increased attention in recent years. Data derived from exercise testing with expired gas analysis have proven to be important measures in the assessment of patients with heart failure and have become a key component of the cardiac transplantation evaluation.

The application of exercise training as a therapeutic intervention in these patients has yielded exciting and important insights into the central and peripheral mechanisms of functional capacity impairment. A growing body of knowledge regarding improvement in functional capacity with exercise training in these patients has lead to the recognition of regular exercise as a valuable adjunctive treatment strategy in stable heart failure and heart transplant patients. The rapid evolution of cardiac transplantation as a separate discipline has presented a new and remarkable physiological aspect to exercise testing and training—that of the denervated heart. The extensive deconditioning in these patients offers a challenge to the rehabilitation team. This challenge continues after transplantation in the midst of rejection and infections.

This book provides unique and comprehensive overview of epidemiological, physiological, and clinical topics regarding *exercise and heart failure*. We are indebted to the many outstanding scientists and clinicians who have contributed their words to this book and their lives to this exciting field.

Gary J. Balady

Ileana L. Piña

Contributors

Carl S. Apstein, MD   Director, Cardiac Muscle Research Laboratory; Professor of Medicine, Boston University School of Medicine, Boston, MA

Michael Argenziano, MD   Research Fellow, Division of Cardiothoracic Surgery, Columbia University College of Physicians and Surgeons, New York, NY

Gary J. Balady, MD   Director, Preventive Cardiology; Associate Professor of Medicine, Boston University School of Medicine, Boston, MA

Michael R. Bristow, MD, PhD   Head, Division of Cardiology, University of Colorado Health Sciences Center, Denver, CO

Don B. Chomsky, MD   Cardiology Fellow, Vanderbilt University Medical Center, Nashville, TN

Sandra Dunbar, RN, DSN   Associate Professor, Emory University, Atlanta, GA

Brian D. Duscha, MS   Exercise Physiologist, Duke Center for Living, Duke University Medical Center, Durham, NC

Franz R. Eberli, MD   Assistant Professor of Medicine, Boston School of Medicine, Boston, MA

Victor M. Fernandez, BS   Research Associate, Mayo Clinic, Jacksonville, FL

Barbara J. Fletcher, RN, BSN, MN   Research Nurse; Consultant, Cardiovascular Diseases, Mayo Clinic, Jacksonville, FL

Gerald F. Fletcher, MD   Professor of Medicine, Mayo Medical School, Senior Associate Consultant, Mayo Clinic, Jacksonville. FL

Gary S. Francis, MD   Professor of Medicine, Cardiovascular Division, Department of Medicine, University of Minnesota Medical School, Minneapolis, MN

Michael B. Higginbotham, MB BS   Associate Professor of Medicine; Director, Heart Failure Service; Medical Director, Heart Transplant Program, Duke University Medical Center, Durham, NC

Brian E. Jaski, MD   Associate Clinical Professor, San Diego Cardiac Center, San Diego, CA

Valluvan Jeevanandam, MD   Assistant Professor of Surgery, Surgical Director Cardiomyopathy and Transplantation, Temple University School of Medicine, Philadelphia, PA

Carey D. Kimmelstiel, MD   Assistant Professor of Medicine,Tufts University School of Medicine; Associate Director, Cardiac Catheterization Lab; Director, Ambulatory Cardiology, New England Medical Center, Boston MA

Jon A. Kobashigawa, MD   Associate Clinical Professor of Medicine, Division of Cardiology, University of California at Los Angeles School of Medicine, Los Angeles, CA

Marvin A. Konstam, MD   Acting Chief of Cardiology; Director, Heart Failure and Transplant Center; Professor of Medicine and Radiology, Tufts University School of Medicine, New England Medical Center, Boston, MA

Joseph R. Libonati, PhD   Assistant Professor, Department of Cardiopulmonary Services, Bouve' College of Pharmacy and Health Sciences, Northeastern University, Boston, MA

Richard S. Maly, MS   San Diego Cardiac Center, San Diego, CA

Barry M. Massie, MD   Professor of Medicine, Cardiovascular Research Institute, University of California at San Francisco, San Francisco, CA

Jonathan Myers, PhD   Clinical Assistant Professor of Medicine, Stanford University, Veterans Affairs Palo Alto Health Care System, Palo Alto CA

Ileana L. Piña, MD   Associate Professor of Medicine; Director, Cardiomyopathy and Cardiac Rehabilitation, Temple University School of Medicine, Cardiomyopathy and Transplant Center, Philadelphia, PA

Rebecca J. Quigg, MD   Associate Professor of Medicine; Director, Heart Failure/Co-Director, Cardiac Transplant Program, Northwestern University Medical School, Chicago, IL

Eric A. Rose, MD   Department Chairman, Division of Cardiothoracic Surgery, Columbia College of Physicians and Surgeons, New York, NY

Nihir B. Shah, MD   Research Fellow, Cardiovascular Research Institute, University of California at San Francisco, San Francisco, CA.

John R. Stratton, MD   Professor of Medicine, Department of Cardiology, University of Washington School of Medicine, Seattle, WA

Martin J. Sullivan, MD   Associate Professor of Medicine, Division of Cardiology, Duke University Medical Center, Durham, NC

Niraj Varma, MD   Assistant Professor of Medicine, Boston University School of Medicine, Boston, MA

Suzanne K. White, MN, RN, FAAN, FCCM, CNAA   Senior Manager, Ernst & Young LLP, Atlanta, GA

John R. Wilson, MD   Professor of Medicine, Vanderbilt University Medical Center, Nashville, TN

Eugene E. Wolfel, MD   Associate Professor of Medicine, Division of Cardiology, University of Colorado Health Sciences Center, Denver, CO

James B. Young, MD   Head, Section of Heart Failure and Cardiac Transplant Medicine, Cleveland Clinic Foundation, Cleveland, OH

Contents

SECTION 4
Exercise Testing and Expired Gas Analysis

SECTION 5
Physiological Responses to Exercise Training

SECTION 6
The Exercise Training Program

Epidemiology of Left Ventricular Dysfunction

Chapter 1

Epidemiology of Heart Failure:
Evolving Trends

Nihir B. Shah, MD and Barry M. Massie, MD

Introduction

Although there has been a dramatic downward trend in mortality and morbidity from most cardiovascular diseases over the past several decades,[1-3] the incidence and prevalence of congestive heart failure (CHF), and the resulting mortality and morbidity, have dramatically increased. Indeed, the improved survival of patients with coronary heart disease and hypertension might be responsible, in part, for this upsurge, since heart failure appears to be a long-term consequence of these conditions.[4-7] However, from an epidemiological perspective, it is the aging of the population that is the major factor in these trends.

Incidence and Prevalence of Congestive Heart Failure

The most frequently cited estimates suggest that there are approximately 400,000 new cases of CHF each year in the United States, and as many as 4.7 million Americans and 15 million individuals worldwide have this condition.[8-10] However, it should be noted that these statistics are derived from relatively small studies and require a number of unproven assumptions. More importantly, many of these patients do

This work was supported in part by the Department of Veterans Affairs Research Service.

Parts of this manuscript have been previously published in Current Opinion in Cardiology, May-June, 1996.

From: Balady GJ, Piña I (eds). *Exercise and Heart Failure*. Armonk, NY: Futura Publishing Company, Inc.;©1997.

not have dilated cardiomyopathies, and many have normal or near normal left ventricular systolic function. Because of the heterogeneity of patients classified as having this diagnosis, these statistics provide insights into the burden that CHF puts on society as a whole, but do not provide a firm basis on which to extrapolate the results of the widely cited clinical trials in patients with reduced ejection fractions to the entire population.

Several studies in the United States and Europe have estimated the incidence and prevalence of CHF(Table 1).[11-18] Despite widely varying approaches (population-based versus case finding), diagnostic criteria, geographic regions, and population demography, and therefore reporting somewhat disparate findings, several important points are apparent. The most striking of all is the increasing incidence and prevalence with advancing age. In the Framingham Study (Figure 1), which followed cohorts of individuals over many decades, the incidence of new CHF cases doubled with each decade of age, affecting approximately 10 persons per 1000 annually in individuals ≥65 years. In the oldest individuals, 85 to 94 years of age, the incidence reached 2% to 3% each year. Men were slightly more commonly affected until the eighth decade, but then the incidence became higher in women.[19] As seen in

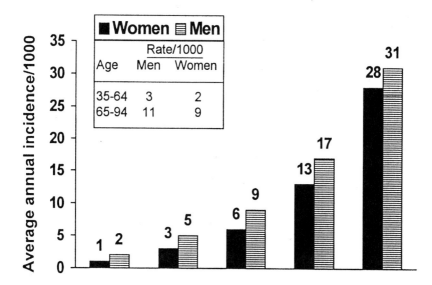

Figure 1: This figure illustrates the average annual incidence of new cases of CHF per 1000 population in the Framingham Heart Study. The incidence in women is shown by the solid bars and in men by horizontally hatched bars. The incidence approximately doubles each decade. The mean incidence for ages 35–64 years was 3/1000 and 2/1000 in men and women, respectively, and increased to 11/1000 and 9/1000 for 65–94 year olds. Modified from Reference 19 with permission from the author and publisher.

Table 1

Incidence and Prevalence of CHF in Six Epidemiological Studies

Study (Patient Subset)	Incidence per 1000 Patient-Years			Prevalence per 1000 Patients		
	Men	Women	Total	Men	Women	Total
Rochester, MN[12]						
45–54 years	0.8			0.8	1.5	
55–64 years	4.0	1.3		9.7	5.2	
65–74 years	13.2	7.2		26.8	19.4	
0–74 years	0.7	1.6	1.1	3.3	2.1	2.7
Framingham[13,14]						
45–54 years	2.0	1.0				8*
55–64 years	4.0	3.0				23*
65–74 years	8.0	5.0				49*
75–84 years	14	13				91*
45–74 years	3.7	2.5				10
Göteborg[15]						
50–54 years	1.5			21		
55–60 years	4.3			32		
61–67 years	10.2			130		
Eastern Finland[16]						
45–54 years	1.5	1.2				
55–64 years	3.8	2.5				
65–74 years	9.1	4.2				
45–74 years	4.7	2.4				
NHANES[17]						
55–64 years				45	30	37
65–74 years				48	43	45
24–75 years				19	20	20
London Practices[18]						
Under 65 years						0.6
Over 65 years						28
Total population						4

*Prevalence rates are for ages 50–59 years, 60–69 years, 70–79 years, and 80–89 years, respectively. Reproduced with permission from Reference 11.

CHF: congestive heart failure.

Table 1, similar figures for the incidence of CHF have been reported in other studies following cohorts of patients[15] or examining new cases in a specified geographic region.[12,16] Extrapolating these figures to the age-adjusted population of the United States yields an estimated annual incidence of 465,000 new CHF cases.[19]

The prevalence of CHF is also heavily dependent on age, increasing from very low levels below age 45 to 2% to 5% in the eighth decade, and nearly 10% above age 80. Of note is that the prevalence is higher in population-based studies, such as Framingham, National Health and Nutrition Examination Survey (NHANES), and Göteborg,[13–15,17] than in the studies in which cases are identified by medical records, such as in Rochester and London.[12,18] Most likely, this is due to the case ascertainment approaches. When medical records are utilized, the diagnosis may be more specific but less sensitive, since patients with mild symptoms may be less likely to seek medical attention, but alternative diagnoses would probably be excluded. Because it is a broad based community survey, NHANES may provide the best estimate of the prevalence of CHF in the United States.[17] This study found a prevalence of heart failure from 1971 to 1975, ranging from 1.1% to 2.0% of the noninstitutionalized adult population below the age of 75 years. The 1.1% represents self-reporting diagnoses, and the 2.0% is based on clinical criteria. These numbers were extrapolated to 2 to 3 million patients. Still further extrapolation to current demographic figures provides the basis for the recent estimate of 4.7 million CHF patients.[8]

Causes of Congestive Heart Failure

There is some disagreement about the etiology of heart failure. The most rigorous information comes from the Framingham Cohort Study, which includes prospective longitudinal follow-up, with careful documentation of blood pressure, blood lipids, and evidence of coronary heart disease in advance of the onset of CHF. However, because the diagnosis of heart failure is primarily clinical and is not based on measurements of left ventricular size and function, many cases probably reflect primarily diastolic dysfunction or ischemic symptoms, but such patients also comprise a significant proportion of those presenting to physicians with the clinical picture of heart failure.

In the Framingham Study, significant changes in the etiology of heart failure and the prevalence of pre-existing conditions which are thought to play a role in the development of heart failure have occurred over the 4-decade period of observation. In the initial cohort, which was identified and followed up until 1965, hypertension was the most common etiology, being the only identifiable cause in 30% of men and 20% of women, and being a co-factor in another 33% and 25%, respectively.[13] Coronary heart disease was present in 42% of men and 35% of women. In subsequent analyses which evaluated both the original cohort and their offspring,[14,19] substantial changes in these patterns were observed. The prevalence of coronary heart disease prior to the diagnosis of CHF increased by 41% per calendar decade in men and 25% per

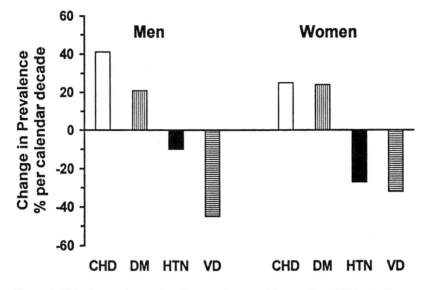

Figure 2: This figure shows the changes in causal factors for CHF in the Framingham Heart Study between 1950 and 1987. The bars indicate the percent change per decade in each underlying condition. In both men and women, coronary heart disease and diabetes mellitus became more frequent over time, while valvular heart disease and hypertension appeared to play less of a causal role. Modified, with permission, from Reference 19.

decade in women (Figure 2). Coronary disease was the primary attributable cause in 22% of patients in the 1950s, 36% in the 1960s, 53% in the 1970s, and 67% in the 1980s. The prevalence of diabetes rose by over 20% per decade, while valvular heart disease declined dramatically. Pre-existing hypertension and left ventricular hypertrophy also became less frequent over time. Although it is not certain that this evolution away from hypertension to coronary disease as the primary etiology of heart failure reflects a true change or improved diagnosis of coronary disease, the more widespread and effective treatment of hypertension and the decreasing prevalence of left ventricular hypertrophy argue for a declining role of hypertension.

The characteristics of patients entered into recent treatment trials also provide insight into the etiology of CHF, although retrospective characterization of prior conditions may not be reliable. Furthermore, the entry criteria for these studies, the populations served by the participating centers, and the approaches used to enroll them, necessarily select patients with certain characteristics. Table 2 shows the proportion of patients whose CHF was attributed to ischemic heart disease in eight large trials conducted in the United States and Europe. Factors that might serve to distort the patient populations are indicated. Overall, these fig-

Table 2

Etiology of CHF in Trials

Trial	N	Location	% Ischemic	Other Factors
CONSENSUS (26)	253	Scandinavia	74	Hospitalized patients with severe CHF
V-HeFT I (27)	642	US VA Hospitals	44	Exercise without angina pectoris required
SOLVD Rx (28)	2569	N. America	71	Active screening of post-MI patients
PROMISE (29)	1088	N. America	54	Severe CHF, angina pectoris excluded
V-HeFT II (30)	904	US VA Hospitals	53	Exercise without angina pectoris required
CIBIS (31)	641	Europe	55	β-blockers may have biased towards non-ischemic patients
PRAISE (32)	1153	United States	64	Severe CHF, angina pectoris excluded
CHF-STAT (33)	673	US VA Hospitals	71	Ventricular ectopy required

CHF = congestive heart failure; MI = myocardial infarction.

ures suggest that underlying coronary disease was present in at least 60% to 65% of these patients. The trials with the lowest proportion of patients with ischemic heart disease either required exercise to a nonanginal endpoint or excluded patients with more than rare clinical angina. Since coronary angiography was not required and not done in most patients, the presence of coronary disease was probably underestimated. However, it should be noted that the requirement for reduced left ventricular ejection fractions excluded patients with primarily diastolic dysfunction who are more likely to have hypertension and diabetes.[20]

Mortality from Congestive Heart Failure

CHF remains a highly lethal condition. In 1991, there were 39,206 deaths attributed primarily to heart failure, and approximately 250,000 deaths in which CHF was listed as a contributory cause of death. More significantly, the number of deaths due to heart failure has risen markedly over the past 4 decades, the same period during which coronary heart disease and stroke deaths have declined by 50%. Unadjusted mortality rates rose by 42% from 1979 to 1992, 3.3-fold since 1970, and 6-fold since 1955 (Figure 3).[4,8,21]

Most (92%) of CHF deaths occur in patients over age 65, and as can be seen in Figure 4, heart failure mortality rates rise dramatically in older individuals. Thus, much of the increase in CHF mortality reflects the aging population, but even after adjustment for age, mortality rates have risen in the older age groups.[21] This may reflect the delayed impact of prolonged survival in patients with longstanding hypertension and coronary artery disease.[4,22] Mortality rates have been consistently higher in men than in women, and higher in African-Americans than in whites, as reflected by the 1990 statistics shown in Figure 5.

Perhaps the one surprising statistic among this dreary litany is the progressive decline in hospital mortality rates from 10.7 per 100 discharges in 1983 to 7.2 per 100 discharges in 1993.[23–25] While this may reflect improvement in therapy, it may also reflect differences in admission and discharge practices, and in particular, a tendency toward early discharge to nursing homes and convalescent facilities.

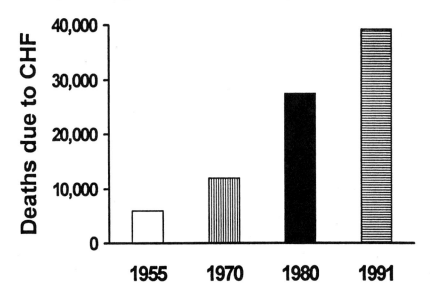

Figure 3: This figure illustrates the unadjusted mortality rates for CHF as a primary diagnosis at several time points. The numbers of deaths from CHF have risen dramatically over the period since 1955. Although much of the increase reflects the growing number of older persons in the population, it persists after age adjustment. Data derived from References 4, 8, 21.

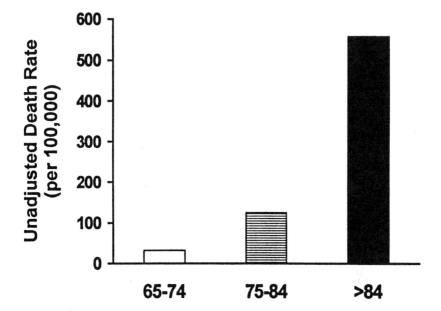

Figure 4: Overall, 92% of the CHF deaths occur in patients over age 65. This figure demonstrates how dramatically the death rates rise in the very elderly. Data derived from Reference 21.

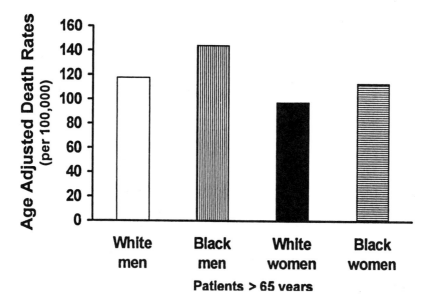

Figure 5: Death rates from CHF are higher in African-Americans and in men. These figures are from individuals over age 65, but they account for most of the CHF-related mortality. Data derived from Reference 21.

Survival Rates in Patients with Congestive Heart Failure

In population-based studies, the survival rates of patients with CHF remain very poor. In the Framingham Study, from 1948 to 1988, the median survival time after the diagnosis was 1.7 years in men and 3.2 years in women.[14] After 5 years, only 25% of men and 38% of women remained alive (Figure 6), and after 10 years these figures fell to 11% and 21%, respectively. Importantly, when these results are compared to those in clinical trials, if only patients who survive the first 90 days are considered, thus excluding patients presenting with acute myocardial infarction or shock and those requiring early surgery, these statistics improve to 35% in men and 53% in women. In Rochester, MN, the 8-year survival of patients diagnosed in 1981 was 30%,[12] but in the NHANES follow-up survey, 10-year survival of patients identified from 1971 to 1975 was somewhat better—57% in patients with self-reported heart failure and 62% in patients with survey criteria for heart failure.[17]

A number of factors were associated with a poorer prognosis in the Framingham Study,[14] and again, these need to be considered carefully in

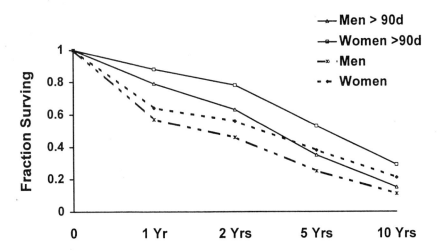

Figure 6: This figure illustrates the survival of patients following the diagnosis of CHF. The interrupted lines show the figures for men (long-short dash pattern) and women (short dashes) from the time of onset, while the solid lines represent the figures for men (open triangle symbols) and women (open square symbols) who have survived the initial 90 days after the onset of CHF. Although still poor, survival in patients with chronic CHF is substantially better, reflecting the high early-mortality rates. This is noteworthy, since clinical trials usually exclude patients with new-onset CHF. Reproduced from Reference 14 with permission from the author and publisher.

comparing these epidemiological data to the results of clinical trials. Age was the most powerful predictor of outcome, with a hazard ratio of 1.27 per decade in men, eg, a 27% higher mortality rate, and 1.61 per decade in women. Since the mean age at the onset of heart failure was 70 years, a figure somewhat higher than in most clinical trials, higher mortality rates might be expected. Valvular heart disease was associated with a 1.68 hazard ratio in men, and is an exclusion in most clinical trials. In women, diabetics had a 1.70 hazard ratio, and again the 19% prevalence of diabetes in Framingham was high compared to most treatment trials.

Hospitalizations for Congestive Heart Failure

Hospitalizations for CHF are perhaps the best marker of morbidity and the major determinant of the economic impact of this condition. In 1993, the last year for which statistics are currently available, there were 875,000 hospital discharges with CHF as the primary diagnosis, and approximately 2.5 million discharges in which CHF was listed as an associated condition.[25] As with mortality, CHF hospitalizations have risen markedly (by 70%) over the past decade (Table 3).[23-25] CHF hospitalization rates increase dramatically with age, from an average of 12 per 10,000 persons below age 65 to 328 per 10,000 above age 74, making CHF the most frequent cause of hospitalization in the Medicare (over 65 years) population. Hospitalizations are approximately 15% more frequent in women and in African-Americans (Table 4).

A better example of the tremendous economic burden produced by heart failure is the number of hospital days for this diagnosis (Table 3): 6.5 million in 1993.[25] Of note is that this figure has leveled off despite the still rising number of hospitalizations due to a sharply declining length of stay. It is perhaps a portent of the future that the number of

---

Table 3

Hospitalization for CHF (ICD code 428.0) by
Number of Discharges, Rate of Hospitalization, Hospital Days
and Length of Stay from Short Stay Hospitals.
(Data from National Hospital Discharge Survey)

	Hospital Discharges	Hospitalization Rate/ 10,000 Population	Hospital Days	Length of Stay	Hospital Mortality
1983 (23)	464,000	20/10,000	4,494,000	9.7 days	9.7%
1988 (24)	624,000	26/10,000	5,560,000	8.8 days	8.5%
1993 (25)	875,000	34/10,000	6,567,000	7.5 days	6.1%

Table 4

Number of Discharges and Rate of Discharges from Short-Stay Hospitals for Year 1993, with Regard to the First Listed Diagnosis of CHF (ICD code 428.0) by Age, Sex, and Race (From, National Hospital Discharge Survey)[25]

		Number of Discharges in Thousands	Rate of Discharges/10,000 Population
All	All	875	34.1
Age	Under 15 years	—	—
	15–44 years	21	1.8
	45–64 years	169	34.1
	65–74 years	218	116.7
	75 years and over	463	327.6
Sex	Men	394	31.6
	Women	481	36.5
Race	Whites	611	28.6
	Blacks	106	33.3

hospitalizations in the Western United States was 18.2 per 10,000 population, 50% lower than the 37.5 to 39.3 per 10,000 rate in the remainder of the country.[25] Similarly, the average length of stay in the West was 6.2 days, compared to 7.0, 7.1, and 9.5 days in the South, Midwest, and Northeast, respectively. It seems likely that these figures reflect the limited penetration of managed care and health maintenance organizations outside of the West at that point in time.

Strategies of Prevention

As with any epidemic, it is likely that only preventative measures will have a major impact on these statistics. In that regard, "primary" prevention, which might be defined as treatment strategies to prevent CHF before the onset of left ventricular dysfunction or symptoms, offers the best opportunity (Table 5). Not surprisingly, these are the areas where tested treatments which reduce the incidence of coronary heart disease and left ventricular dysfunction have been dramatically successful. Effective antihypertensive therapy, particularly directed to systolic hypertension, has reduced the incidence of CHF by 50% or more in the original VA Cooperative Study of antihypertensive therapy, the Systolic Hypertension in the Elderly (SHEP) trial, and in the Scandinavian STOP-Hypertension trial.[34–36] Aggressive lipid-lowering therapy

Table 5

Strategies to Prevent Heart Failure and its Progression

A. Primary prevention*
   1. Treat hypertension (especially systolic hypertension)
   2. Treat hyperlipidemia
B. Secondary prevention**
   1. ACE inhibitor
   2. Beta-blocker
   3. Secondary prevention post-MI
      a. Aspirin
      b. Beta-blocker
      c. Anti-hyperlipidemic therapy
      d. Anti-coagulation
      e. Coronary revascularization in appropriate patients
C. Tertiary prevention†
   1. ACE inhibitor
   2. Beta-blocker
   3. Digoxin
   4. Secondary prevention post-MI (see B-3)
   5. Intensive home monitoring and intervention

*Prior to onset of left ventricular dysfunction or cardiac disease.
**After onset of left ventricular dysfunction or CAD, but without CHF.
†After onset of heart failure, to delay progression and prevent events.
ACE = angiotensin-converting enzyme.

in patients with clinically apparent atherosclerosis has also been shown to prevent new cases of CHF (37).

Table 5 also lists several approaches to the secondary prevention of CHF, which has been defined as prevention of CHF after the onset of left ventricular dysfunction or coronary artery disease. The SOLVD prevention trial, the SAVE trial, and numerous other postmyocardial infarction angiotensin-converting (ACE) inhibitor trials have provided the most elegant indications of the efficacy of this approach.[38, 39] It also seems likely that β-blockers can prevent heart failure in this setting. Since in the patient with coronary artery disease, the onset of CHF is often heralded by new ischemic events, aggressive use of post-myocardial infarction secondary prevention strategies is also warranted. These latter approaches should not be neglected, despite the impressive data with ACE inhibitors.

Once CHF has occurred, it is not too late to employ interventions which can mitigate progression and prevent hospitalization. Data support the use of ACE inhibitors,[28] β-blockers,[31,40–42] and digoxin[43] for this objective. Intensive follow-up and early intervention have also been shown to prevent rehospitalization in selected patients, and this approach has resulted in a cost savings.[44,45]

Summary

This chapter has highlighted some of the most current information concerning the incidence and prevalence of CHF and the resulting morbidity and mortality from this condition. It is clear that CHF represents an enormous clinical problem and a major social and economic burden. The increase in the number of patients with CHF and CHF-related deaths is primarily driven by the aging of the population, but these trends persist even after age-adjustment. The likely explanation for this pattern, which is unique among cardiovascular diagnoses, is the improved survival of patients with other chronic cardiovascular conditions, particularly coronary heart disease, hypertension, and diabetes. There has been a significant shift in the etiologic factors for heart failure, from hypertension and valvular heart disease to coronary heart disease and diabetes, over the past several decades. However, survival after symptoms of CHF develop remains poor despite significant advances in therapy.

This litany of worsening statistics raises the question of how to approach CHF as a growing public health problem. As with any epidemic, the focus needs to be extended from the treatment of already affected individuals, whose prognosis is limited, to prevention and early intervention. Efficacy has been demonstrated for a growing number of treatments to prevent cardiac dysfunction or its subsequent progression to clinical CHF. Now the challenge is to implement these approaches in populations at risk.

References

1. Centers for Disease Control (CDC). Trends in ischemic heart disease mortality-United States, 1980–1988. *MMWR* 1992;41:548–549,555–556.
2. Centers for Disease Control (CDC). Cerebrovascular disease mortality and Medicare hospitalization-United States, 1980–1990. *MMWR* 1992;41:477–480.
3. Gillum RF. Trends in acute myocardial infarction and coronary heart disease death in the United States. *J Am Coll Cardiol* 1994;23:1273–1277.
4. Yusuf S, Thom T, Abbott RD. Changes in hypertension treatment and in congestive heart failure mortality in the United States. *Hypertension* 1989;13 (suppl 5):174–179.
5. Ghali JK, Cooper R, Ford E. Trends in hospitalization rates for heart failure in the United States. 1973–1986: Evidence for increasing population prevalence. *Arch Intern Med* 1990;150:769–773.
6. Sytkowski PA, Kannel WB, D'Agostino RB. Changes in risk factors and the decline in mortality from cardiovascular disease: The Framingham Heart Study. *N Engl J Med* 1990;322:1635–1641.
7. McGovern PG, Pankow JS, Shahar E, et al. Recent trends in acute coronary heart disease: Mortality, morbidity, medical care, risk factors. *N Engl J Med* 1996;334:884–890.
8. American Heart Association. Heart and stroke facts: 1996 statistical supplement. Page 15.

9. American College of Cardiology/American Heart Association Committee on Evaluation and Management of Heart Failure. Guidelines for the evaluation and management of heart failure. *J Am Coll Cardiol* 1995;26:1376–1398.

10. Eriksson H. Heart failure: A growing public health problem. *J Intern Med* 1995;237:135–141.

11. Yamani M, Massie BM. Congestive heart failure: Insights from epidemiology, implications for treatment. *Mayo Clin Proc* 1993;68:1214–1218.

12. Rodeheffer RJ, Jacobsen SJ, Gersh BJ, et al. The incidence and prevalence of congestive heart failure in Rochester, Minnesota. *Mayo Clin Proc* 1993;68: 1143–1150.

13. McKee PA, Castelli WP, McNamara PM, Kannel WB. The natural history of congestive heart failure: The Framingham Study. *N Engl J Med* 1971;285: 1441–1446.

14. Ho KKL, Anderson KM, Kannel WB, et al. Survival after the onset of congestive heart failure in Framingham Heart Study subjects. *Circulation* 1993;88: 107–115.

15. Eriksson H, Svardsudd K, Larsson B, et al. Risk factors for heart failure in the general population: The study of men born in 1913. *Eur Heart J* 1989; 10:647–656.

16. Remes J, Reunanen A, Aromaa A, Pyorala K. Incidence of heart failure in eastern Finland: A population-based surveilance study. *Eur Heart J* 1992;20: 301–306.

17. Schocken DD, Arrieta MI, Leaverton PE. Prevalence and mortality rate of congestive heart failure in the United States. *J Am Coll Cardiol* 1992;20: 301–306.

18. Parameshwar J, Shackell MM, Richardson A, et al. Prevalence of heart failure in three general practices in north west London. *Br J Gen Pract* 1992;42: 287–289.

19. Kannel WB, Ho K, Thom T. Changing epidemiological features of cardiac failure. *Am Heart J* 1994;72(suppl):S3–9.

20. Vasan RS, Benjamin EJ, Levy D. Prevalence, clinical features and prognosis of diastolic heart failure and epidemiologic perspective. *J Am Coll Cardiol* 1995;26:1565–1574.

21. CDC. Mortality from Congestive Heart Failure—United States, 1980–1990. *MMWR* 1994;5:77–81.

22. Gillum RF. Heart failure in the United States 1970–1985. *Am Heart J* 1987; 113:1043–1045.

23. Graham D. Utilization of short-stay hospitals. Vital and Health Statistics. Series 13: Data from the National Health Survey, 1985 March (83):1–58.

24. Graves EJ. National Hospital Discharge Survey: Annual summary, 1988. Vital and Health Statistics. Series 13: Data from National Health Survey. 1991 Sep (106):1–55.

25. Graves EJ. National Hospital Discharge Survey: Annual summary, 1993. Vital and Health Statistics. Series 13: Data from National Health Survey. 1995 Aug (121):1–63.

26. The CONSENSUS Trial study group. Effects of enalapril on mortality in severe congestive heart failure: Results of the Cooperative North Scandinavian Enalapril Survival Study (CONSENSUS). *N Engl J Med* 1987;316: 1429–1435.

27. Cohn JN, Archibald DG, Ziesche S, et al. Effect of vasodilator therapy on mortality in chronic congestive heart failure: Results of a Veterans Administration Cooperative Study. *N Engl J Med* 1986;314:1547–1552.

28. The SOLVD Investigators. Effect of enalapril on survival in patients with

reduced left ventricular ejection fractions and congestive heart failure. *N Engl J Med* 1991;325:293–302.

29. Packer M, Carver JR, Rodeheffer RJ, et al. Effect of oral milrinone on mortality in severe chronic heart failure. *N Engl J Med* 1991;325:1468–1475.
30. Cohn JN, Johnson G, Ziesche S, et al. A comparison of enalapril with hydralazine-isosorbide dinitrate in the treatment of chronic congestive heart failure. *N Engl J Med* 1991;325:303–310.
31. CIBIS Investigators and Committees. A randomized trial of beta-blockade in heart failure: The Cardiac Insufficiency Bisoprolol Study (CIBIS). *Circulation* 1994;90:1765–1773.
32. O'Connor CM, Belkin RN, Carson PE, et al. Effect of amlodipine on mode of death in severe chronic heart failure: The PRAISE trial. *Circulation* 1995;92 (suppl I):I-143.
33. Singh SN, Fletcher RD, Fisher SG, et al. Amiodarone in patients with congestive heart failure and asymptomatic ventricular arrhythmia. *N Engl J Med* 1995;333:77–82.
34. Veterans Administration Cooperative Study Group on Antihypertensive Agents: Effects of treatment on morbidity in hypertension. II. Results in patients with diastolic blood pressure averaging 90–115 mm Hg. *J Am Med Assoc* 1970;213:1143–1152.
35. SHEP Cooperative Research Group. Prevention of stroke by antihypertensive treatment in older persons with isolated systolic hypertension: Final results of the Systolic Hypertension in the Elderly Program (SHEP). *J Am Med Assoc* 1991;265:3255–3264.
36. Dahlöf B, Lindholm LH, Hannson L, et al. Morbidity and mortality in the Swedish Trial in Old Patients with Hypertension (STOP Hypertension). *Lancet* 1991;338:1281–1285.
37. Kjekshus J, Pedersen T. Lowering of cholesterol with simvastatin may prevent development of heart failure in patients with coronary heart disease (abstract). *J Am Coll Cardiol* 1995;25:282A.
38. The SOLVD Investigators. Effect of enalapril on mortality and the development of heart failure in asymptomatic patients with reduced left ventricular ejection fractions. *N Engl J Med* 1992;327:685–691.
39. Pfeffer MA, Braunwald E, Moyé LA, et al. Effect of captoprial on mortality and morbidity in patients with left ventricular dysfunction after myocardial infarction: Results of the Survival and Ventricular Enlargement Trial. *N Engl J Med* 1992;327:669–677.
40. Waagstein F, Bristow MW, Swedberg K, et al. Beneficial effects of metoprolol in idiopathic dilated cardiomyopathy. *Lancet* 1993;343:1441–1446.
41. Colucci WS, Packer M, Bristow MR, et al. Carvedilol inhibits clinical progression in patients with mild heart failure. *Circulation* 1995;92(suppl I)I-395.
42. Fowler MB, Gilbert EM, Cohn JN, et al. Effects of carvedilol on cardiovascular hospitalizations in patients with chronic heart failure. *J Am Coll Cardiol* 1996;27:169A.
43. Digitalis Investigation Group (DIG) Trial. Rationale, implementation and baseline characteristics of patients in the DIG Trial: A large, simple trial to evaluate the effect of digitalis on mortality in heart failure. *Clin Trials* (in press).
44. Rich MW, Beckham V, Wittenberg C, et al. A multidisciplinary intervention to prevent the readmission of elderly patients with congestive heart failure. *N Engl J Med* 1995;333:1190–1195.
45. Kornowski R, Zeeli D, Averbuch M, et al. Intensive home-care surveillance prevents hospitalization and improves morbidity rates among elderly patients with severe congestive heart failure. *Am Heart J* 1995;129:762–766.

Chapter 2

Economics of Heart Failure

Marvin A. Konstam, MD and
Carey D. Kimmelstiel, MD

Epidemiology and Overall Cost

Heart failure, a disabling and frequently fatal illness, represents a substantial public health problem in the United States because of its high and increasing prevalence and the substantial financial cost required for its management.

The epidemiology of heart failure has been difficult to describe accurately because there are no diagnostic criteria that have received universal agreement and the vast majority of information that we have relates to patients who have undergone hospitalization, at least once, with the diagnosis of heart failure. Thus, the overall prevalence may be underestimated due to an undercounting of patients who have not yet been hospitalized with this diagnosis, and because epidemiological information that we have may be skewed toward a sicker population. On the other hand, many patients, particularly elderly patients with edema or dyspnea of noncardiac origin, may be counted incorrectly.

Nevertheless, over 2 million Americans have been diagnosed with heart failure, with at least 400,000 new patients diagnosed annually.[1] The prevalence of heart failure has been found to increase in recent years, with this increase spanning both genders and various ethnic groups.[2,3] Heart failure represents the single most frequent hospitalization-related diagnosis among patients over the age of 65 years.[4] Since the early days of the Framingham Study, there has been a substantial shift in the distribution of patients according to etiology.[5] In the 1950s, hypertension represented the predominant risk factor for this condition, by far. With substantial advancement in treatment of hypertension in the United States, hypertension alone has declined as the pre-

From: Balady GJ, Piña IL (eds). *Exercise and Heart Failure*. Armonk, NY: Futura Publishing Company, Inc.; ©1997.

dominant etiologic factor.[5] Likewise, with the virtual eradication of rheumatic heart disease and with effective surgical treatment, valvular disease has declined as an etiologic factor. Today, ischemic heart disease represents the predominant etiology of heart failure in the United States. The increase in prevalence of heart failure, with coronary disease as the predominant factor, despite a decline in overall mortality from ischemic heart disease is, at least in part, due to an increased rate of survival following myocardial infarction, particularly among patients with evidence of hemodynamic compromise. The major factor influencing the increase in the number of heart failure patients is the aging of our population. Although heart failure may affect patients of all ages, its prevalence increases substantially with age (Figure 1),[6] approaching 10% among Americans over the age of 80 years.

The cost of managing patients with heart failure is said to exceed $10 billion annually,[1] with approximately 75% of this cost spent on hospitalized patients (Figure 2). The rising prevalence of this condition, coupled with mounting constraints on overall health care expenditure has created a collision course and a growing interest in developing strategies that will reduce cost.

With an eye on the predominant contribution to the cost of care in heart failure, most cost-cutting strategies are directed toward reducing the number of days spent in the hospital, particularly by reducing the number of hospitalizations. In addition to being the major contributor to

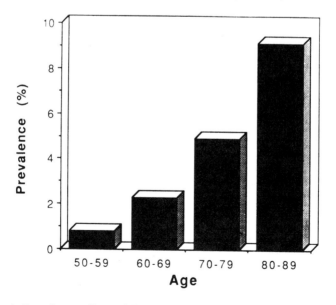

Figure 1: Prevalence of heart failure by age in the Framingham Study. Adapted from Reference 6.

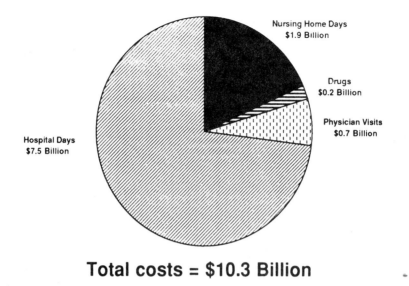

Total costs = $10.3 Billion

Figure 2: Estimated total direct costs of heart failure in the United States. Adapted from Reference 1.

cost, hospitalization frequency has become widely accepted as an important outcome indicator for patients with heart failure. Thus, strategies that reduce hospitalization frequency are presumed to have a favorable impact on both sides of the health care equation: outcome and cost.

Evaluating Treatment Modalities

In the late 1980s and early 1990s, for the first time, medical intervention with angiotensin-converting enzyme (ACE) inhibitors was documented to reduce mortality, reduce the progression to overt heart failure, and reduce hospitalization rates among patients with this disorder.[7-11] An analysis from the Studies of Left Ventricular Dysfunction (SOLVD)[8] indicates that for every 1000 patients with reduced left ventricular systolic function and symptoms of heart failure, treatment with an ACE inhibitor for 3 years will result in 50 fewer deaths and 200 fewer hospitalizations for heart failure. Treatment of 1000 patients with asymptomatic left ventricular systolic dysfunction[9] will result in 90 fewer patients progressing to overt heart failure and 65 fewer hospitalizations for this diagnosis. Recent and ongoing clinical trials hold substantial promise for newer modes of therapy to accomplish even more with regard to these goals.

The potential and actual economic impact of medical therapies for heart failure has been difficult to accurately gauge. To the extent that a therapy reduces hospitalization frequency, overall costs are likely to be substantially reduced. Furthermore, since hospitalization is driven by both disease severity and inability to function at home, an intervention that reduces the rate of hospitalization may be viewed as one that improves clinical outcomes in addition to reducing the major source of cost.

A model[12] based on analysis of hospital costs and the results of the SOLVD,[8] V-HeFTI[13] and V-HeFT II[11] trials revealed that the combination of hydralazine and isosorbide dinitrate produced an average life prolongation of 8 days for a marginal cost of $5600 per year of life gained, compared to digoxin and diuretics alone (Table 1). Use of an ACE inhibitor produced an additional increment in average longevity of 3 months, for a marginal cost of $9700 per year of life prolongation, compared to hydralazine and isosorbide dinitrate. Reduced hospitalization rates by the ACE inhibitor produced a cost reduction within the model, although this reduction was offset by medication costs and prolonged duration of treatment. However, the minimal marginal cost per unit duration of life gained indicates that this treatment modality is extremely cost-effective.

Utilization of Treatment Modalities

Therapies indicated by clinical trials do not always translate themselves into universal clinical practice. In the case of ACE inhibitors, a re-

Table 1
Effectiveness and Costs of Heart Failure Therapy

Therapy	Cost ($)	Effectiveness, Years of Life Saved	Incremental Cost ($)	Incremental Effectiveness, Years of Life Saved	Incremental Cost-effectiveness Ratio, $/Year of Life Saved
Standard	5429	4.364	—	—	—
Standard plus hydralazine-isosorbide dinitrate	5548	4.386	119	0.021 (8 days)	5600
Standard plus enalapril	8117	4.650	2569	0.265 (3 months)	9700

Adapted from Reference 12.

cent analysis[14] has indicated that among patients discharged following myocardial infarction with evidence of clinical heart failure or reduced systolic function—criteria that have been proven to indicate improved outcome with chronic ACE inhibition—only 59% of ideal candidates are prescribed an ACE inhibitor at time of discharge. According to a recent survey,[15] cardiologists (80%) are more likely to prescribe ACE inhibitors for patients with mild to moderate heart failure than are internists (71%) or family medicine practitioners (59%). A similar treatment pattern was noted in the therapy of patients with severe heart failure.

Considerable effort is warranted to identify and implement strategies for educating clinicians and improving utilization of treatment modalities that have documented benefit toward improving outcomes or reducing costs. One such strategy is production and dissemination of clinical practice guidelines, such as the ones for diagnosis and treatment of patients with heart failure recently produced by the Federal Agency for Health Care and Policy Research (AHCPR)[1] and by the American Heart Association and American College of Cardiology.[16,17]

Hospitalization Costs and Strategies to Reduce Hospitalization Frequency

Overall, approximately 75% of the cost expended for care of patients with heart failure is related to hospitalization.[1] A modest estimate of annual costs in heart failure is $10 billion, with approximately $7.5 billion expended for in-patient care.[1] The average cost for a typical hospitalization for heart failure in 1991 (1992 dollars) was estimated at $6429 (Table 2).[12] On the average, a patient with heart failure is hospitalized 1.6 times per year.[18] Analysis of nationwide costs and reimbursements associated with Medicare hospitalizations (by far the most frequent payer for the diagnosis of heart failure), based on data from the Health Care Financing Administration (HCFA), and from estimated actual direct costs for heart failure hospitalizations[12] in 1992 (Table 2) reveals that, on the average, hospitals *lost* approximately $1700 for each heart failure hospitalization; the nationwide annual loss is approximately $1 billion.

Thus, major cost reduction can be expected through interventions designed to reduce hospitalization frequency and length of stay, even if such interventions carry substantial percent increases in ambulatory care expenditures.

It is necessary to identify population characteristics that predict repeat hospitalizations in order to cost-effectively select patients for implementation of such interventions. Conventional means of grading heart failure severity, such as New York Heart Association class, are

Table 2

Hospitalizations and Costs for Heart Failure in the Medicare Population

Total hospitalizations	603,000
Initial hospitalizations	386,000
Rate per 1000 population	11.1
Hospitalizations per patient	1.6
Average length of stay	7.4 days
Readmission rate	36%
Average charge	$8528
Average payment	$4688
Average cost	$6429
Net loss per hospitalization	$1741
Total cost	$3.9 billion
Net annual loss	$1 billion

Adapted from References 12 and 18.

probably not the most effective ways of stratifying populations for re-hospitalization risks. In a pilot study, Rich et al[19] identifies four factors that predict a greater likelihood of repeat hospitalization: prior known history of heart failure; prior history of recent repeated hospitalization: prior known history of heart failure, prior history of recent repeated hospitalizations, for any cause; hospitalization for heart failure associated with acute myocardial infarction; and hospitalization for heart failure associated with uncontrolled hypertension. Using these criteria, these investigators prospectively entered elderly patients ($\geq$70 years) into a 90-day study,[20] and identified four additional risk factors for re-hospitalization (Table 3): elevated blood urea nitrogen; reduced systolic blood pressure; reduced serum sodium; and presence of diabetes mellitus. Application of these criteria to other populations requires caution, with awareness of the special characteristics of the population studied: median age 79 years; 54% African Americans; 63% women; 76% hypertensive; mean ejection fraction 43%. Thus, further investiga-

Table 3

Risk Factors for Readmission for Heart Failure

Blood urea nitrogen
Systolic blood pressure
Serum sodium
Diabetes mellitus

Adapted from Reference 20.

tion is warranted to more clearly define risk factors for repeated hospitalizations across the entire spectrum of heart failure populations.

In addition to the prescription of ACE inhibitors, strategies most likely to result in reduced hospitalization frequency are those that influence improved patient compliance to medication and dietary prescription. Noncompliance has been found to be a major factor contributing to readmission,[2] and educational strategies directed at improving compliance appear to reduce rehospitalization rates.[21]

Rich et al.[20] randomly and prospectively applied an intervention consisting of 1) intensive interdisciplinary education in-hospital, 2) a focused effort to simplify the medical regimen, and 3) an ambulatory case-management strategy, to their population of 282 elderly high-risk patients. They observe an absolute reduction in 90-day readmission rate of 13.2% (42.1% to 28.9%) in the treatment group, compared to the control group. If this treatment effect were sustained, it would be expected to reduce the annual hospitalization frequency within this population by approximately 0.5 per patient, although the cost-efficacy of such an intervention is likely to be maximal during the initial several months following the index hospitalization. In this study, the total excess cost associated with the 90-day combined strategy was estimated at $598 per patient, although spouse or other care giver time contributed $336 to this total, so that the added 90-day cost to the health-care system was $262. This cost was offset by an estimated savings of $1058, resulting from reduction in the number of hospital days, for a total net 90-day savings of $460 per patient ($796 savings to the health care system). The potential cost savings of continuing such an intervention beyond 90 days is unknown, and the exact contribution of each component of the intervention to the savings cannot be determined, although improved compliance to the prescribed medical regimen is likely to have played a substantial role.

Who should implement such interventions? A number of entrepreneurial efforts have emerged nationwide, marketing products designed to assist parties at risk (managed care plans or capitated providers) in reducing costs within their heart failure populations. These have included educational programs, consulting efforts, and case management operations. It remains to be seen whether the marginal savings per patient and the size of the high-risk population support the profitability of broad out-sourced efforts.

Diagnosis and Revascularization in Coronary Artery Disease

No randomized data support a survival benefit from coronary revascularization in patients with heart failure in the absence of limiting angina. However, on the basis of cohort analyses, it is likely that benefit is achieved from revascularization in selected patient groups,[22] particularly those in whom a substantial amount of viable myocardium with reversible ischemia can be identified.[1,23–25] For this reason the AHCPR heart failure guideline[1] advocates consideration of noninvasive testing for reversible ischemia in all patients with heart failure, and proceeding to catheterization only if indicated by results of such testing.

For patients with heart failure but without any further evidence of coronary artery disease, the AHCPR guideline panel calculated the marginal cost per year of life prolongation for the alternative strategy of catheterizing all patients. Assuming a 20% probability of occult coronary artery disease within a particular population and an anticipated 50% reduction in mortality by coronary artery bypass surgery in patients with viable but ischemic myocardium, we estimated the marginal cost per year of life prolongation for performing coronary angiography on all patients, as opposed to noninvasive screening, at $7.2 million. Even if off by an order of magnitude, this analysis argues strongly against the strategy of routine cardiac catheterization in *all* patients with heart failure. However, the potential importance of noninvasive testing must be stressed, and the analysis is likely to change substantially, favoring more liberal use of catheterization in the presence of any clinical evidence supporting the likelihood of coronary artery disease.

Conclusions

Cost-effective strategies for improving the diagnosis and treatment of patients with heart failure are being developed and are likely to have a significant impact on the rising costs of the care of this growing patient population. Efforts are being directed at reducing hospitalization frequency, which represents the dominant source of cost, as well as a major indication of adverse outcome. These efforts will focus both on effective pharmacological therapy and on implementation of systems designed to maximize patient compliance and to respond rapidly to subtle changes in patient condition.

References

1. Konstam MA, Dracup K, Baker D, et al. Heart Failure: Evaluation and Care of Patients With Left Ventricular Systolic Dysfunction. Clinical Practice Guideline No. 11. *AHCPR Publication NO. 94–0612.* Agency for Health Care Policy and Research, Public Health Service, U.S. Dept. of Health and Human Services, Rockville, MD. 1994.

2. Ghali JK, Kadakia S, Cooper R. Precipitating factors leading to decompensation of heart failure: Traits among urban Blacks. *Arch Int Med* 1988;148: 2013–2016.
3. Kimmelstiel CD, Konstam MA. Heart failure in women. *Cardiology* 1995;86: 304–309.
4. Graves EJ. National Center for Health Statistics, Summary: National hospital discharge survey. Advance data from vital and health statistics. No. 199. Hyattsville, MD: Public Health Service : *(DHHS publication no. (PHS) 91–1250.).* 1989;1–12.
5. Ho KKL, Anderson KM, Kannel WB, et al. Survival after the onset of congestive heart failure in Framingham Heart Study subjects. *Circulation* 1993; 88:107–115.
6. Kannel WB, Belanger AJ. Epidemiology of heart failure. *Am Heart J* 1991; 121:951–957.
7. Group CTS. Effects of enalapril on mortality in severe congestive heart failure: Results of the Cooperative North Scandinavian Enalapril Survival Study. *N Engl J Med* 1987;316:1429–1435.
8. Investigators TS. Effect of angiotensin converting enzyme inhibition with enalapril on survival in patients with reduced left ventricular ejection fraction and congestive heart failure: Results of the Treatment Trial of the Studies of Left Ventricular Dysfunction (SOLVD); a randomized double blind trial. *N Engl J Med* 1991;325:293–302.
9. Investigators TS. Effect of enalapril on mortality and the development of heart failure in asymptomatic patients with reduced left ventricular ejection fractions. *N Engl J Med* 1992;327:685–691.
10. Pfeffer MA, Braunwald E, Moye LA, et al. Effect of captopril on mortality and morbidity in patients with left ventricular dysfunction after myocardial infarction. *N Engl J Med* 1992;327:669–677.
11. Cohn JN, Johnson G, Ziesche S, et al. A comparison of enalapril with hydralazine-isosorbide dinitrate in the treatment of chronic congestive heart failure. *N Engl J Med* 1991;325:303–310.
12. Paul SD, Kuntz KM, Eagle KA, et al. Costs and effectiveness of angiotensin converting enzyme inhibition in patients with congestive heart failure. *Arch Int Med* 1994;154:1143–1149.
13. Cohn JN, Archibald DG, Ziesche S, et al. Effect of vasodilator therapy on mortality in chronic congestive heart failure: Results of a Veterans Administration Cooperative Study. *N Engl J Med* 1986;314:1547–1552.
14. Ellerbeck EF, Jencks SF, Radford MJ, et al. Quality of care for medicare patients with acute myocardial infarction: A four-state pilot study from the cooperative cardiovascular project. *JAMA* 1995;273:1509–1514.
15. Edep ME, Shah NB, Tateo I, et al. Differences in practice patterns in managing of heart failure between cardiologists, family practitioners, and internists. *J Am Coll Cardiol* 1996;27:367A.
16. American College of Cardiology/American Heart Association Task Force on Practice Guidelines (Committee on Evaluation and Management of Heart Failure). Guidelines for the evaluation and management of heart failure. *Circulation* 1995;92:2764–2784.
17. American College of Cardiology/American Heart Association Task Force on Practice Guidelines (Committee on Evaluation and Management of Heart Failure). Guidelines for the evaluation and management of heart failure. *J Am Coll Cardiol* 1995;26:1367–1398.
18. HCFA. Medicare CHF Stats. 1992.

19. Rich MW, Vinson JM, Sperry JC, et al. Prevention of readmission in elderly patients with congestive heart failure: Results of a prospective, randomized pilot study. *J Gen Intern Med* 1993;8:585–590.
20. Rich MW, Becham V, Wittenberg C, et al. A multidisciplinary intervention to prevent the readmission of elderly patients with congestive heart failure. *N Engl J Med* 1995;333:1190–1195.
21. Rosenberg S. Patient education leads to better care for heart patients. *HSMHA Health Rep* 1971;86:793–802.
22. Bounous EP, Mark DB, Pollock BG, et al. Surgical survival benefits for coronary disease patients with left ventricular dysfunction. *Circulation* 1988;78 (3Pt2):I-151–I-157.
23. Eitzman D, al-Aouar Z, Kanter HL, et al. Clinical outcome of patients with advanced coronary artery disease after viability studies with positron emission tomography. *J Am Coll Cardiol* 1992;20:559–565.
24. Di Carli MF, Davidson M, Little R, et al. Value of metabolic imaging with positron emission tomography for evaluating prognosis in patients with coronary artery disease and left ventricular dysfunction. *Am J Cardiol* 1994;73:527–533.
25. Di Carli MF, Asgarzadie F, Schelbert HR, et al. Quantitative relation between myocardial viability and improvement in heart failure symptoms after revascularization in patients with ischemic cardiomyopathy. *Circulation* 1995;92:3436–3444.

Heart Failure and Exercise Tolerance

Chapter 3

Systolic Failure

Michael B. Higginbotham, MB, BS

Introduction

Exercise intolerance is frequent in patients with systolic left ventricular dysfunction (SLVD),[1,2] and can be detected by objective testing, even in patients without overt symptoms of heart failure.[3] To develop effective interventions to improve exercise tolerance in these patients, it is important to understand the mechanisms involved in their limitation.

Patients with SLVD complain of fatigue, dyspnea, or both during exercise. The primary limiting symptom varies from one patient to another,[1,2,4-9] and even within individual patients, depending on the type and level of exercise they are performing.[10]

In an effort to explain the pathophysiological basis of exertional symptoms in patients with SLVD, investigators have focused on various "systems" that contribute to the exercise response: the central circulation, the peripheral vasculature and skeletal muscles, and the ventilatory system. Although a wide range of abnormalities has been described in these systems, the contribution of each to specific symptoms remains far from clear.[4-6,11,12] Even less well defined are the factors that determine submaximal as opposed to maximal exercise tolerance.

Changes in Central Circulation in Systolic Failure and Their Influence on Exercise Tolerance

Systolic failure is characterized by abnormal left ventricular (LV) systolic shortening, an increase in end-systolic volume, and an obligatory increase in end-diastolic volume.[7] Ejection fraction is low, generally less than 40%. As increased left ventricular filling pressure gives

From: Balady GJ, Piña IL (eds). *Exercise and Heart Failure.* Armonk, NY: Futura Publishing Company, Inc.; ©1997.

rise to pulmonary venous hypertension and pulmonary arterial hypertension, right ventricular dysfunction may be seen.[7,13] This, in turn, may compromise left ventricular filling because of inadequate right ventricular pressure generation and diastolic encroachment of the left ventricle within a limited pericardial space.[7] Mitral regurgitation may further complicate left ventricular performance due to left ventricular dilatation or papillary muscle dysfunction.[7] Abnormalities in diastolic relaxation[14] and exertional ischemia in patients with coronary artery disease can produce additional compromise.[15]

Because of these many factors determining cardiac pump function in systolic failure no single variable, such as ejection fraction, correlates strongly with maximal oxygen consumption.[13,16,17] However, descriptors of overall cardiac pump function, such as cardiac output and stroke volume, correlate very well with maximal oxygen uptake ($\dot{V}O_{2max}$),[1,18] and translate directly into decrease in limb blood flow.[4,18] Of the two components of the Fick equation, cardiac output and arteriovenous O_2 difference, only the former differs among subjects with varying values of $\dot{V}O_{2max}$.[1,18]

The above observations indicate that central factors appear to be the primary determinants of peak cardiovascular performance or cardiovascular reserve. Interventional studies have also supported the importance of oxygen delivery rather than peripheral uptake in determining exercise tolerance. Mancini et al. demonstrate a close relationship between increases in skeletal muscle blood flow and improved exercise tolerance following ACE inhibitor therapy;[19] changes in pacemaker function, a purely central intervention, have been demonstrated to produce acute changes in maximal oxygen uptake.[20,21] Finally, the strong association between $\dot{V}O_{2max}$ and prognosis in patients with SLVD strongly suggests a link between exercise tolerance and cardiac function.[22,23]

While increases in pulmonary capillary wedge pressure appear to have some important limitation of exercise tolerance in extreme situations such as mitral stenosis,[24] filling pressures are often normal in treated heart failure patients, and correlate poorly with exercise tolerance.[1,9,25]

The influence of central factors on submaximal exercise tolerance is less clear. Low oxygen uptake during submaximal exercise[18,26] and a low anaerobic threshold[1,27] suggest the possibility that oxygen delivery is, in fact, important in heart failure, even during submaximal exercise. Although tissue hypoxia has not been demonstrated at these levels of exercise, a critical capillary PO_2 may be essential to proper oxygen transport.[28,29] A recent study by Cohen-Solal et al.[30] demonstrates an acute decrease in oxygen consumption during submaximal exercise when patients developed complete heart block, supporting the role of oxygen delivery in maintaining $\dot{V}O_{2max}$ during this phase of exercise.

While these observations suggest a link between oxygen delivery and uptake, a correlation between these factors and submaximal exercise endurance has not been established. Indeed, the observation that decreases in $\dot{V}O_{2max}$ and anaerobic threshold in heart failure patients appear to be dissociated suggests that they are influenced at least in part by different mechanisms.

Peripheral Changes in Systolic Failure and Their Influence on Exercise Tolerance

A wide range of peripheral changes has been observed in patients with SLVD. Alterations in vascular tone and compliance[31] give rise to increases in systemic vascular resistance, both at rest and during exercise,[31] and some mediators of vasoconstriction such as plasma norepinephrine[6,32] and endothelin[33] are elevated. Abnormalities in the skeletal muscles themselves have also been uniformly observed in heart failure, ranging from altered metabolism and changes in fiber type to atrophy and fibrosis.[5,34-36]

Despite these widespread and marked peripheral abnormalities and their correlation with maximal exercise capacity in heart failure patients,[6,36] it remains to be demonstrated that they actually contribute to exercise tolerance rather than being secondary adaptations to a low cardiac output. This distinction is vital to the concept of peripheral abnormalities being targeted for therapy with the hope of improving exercise tolerance.

In fact, studies of blood flow distribution and oxygen extraction do not favor a primary role for peripheral factors in limiting exercise tolerance in patients with SLVD. In such patients systemic arteriovenous difference is normal[1,18] and does not vary among patients with widely differing exercise capacities (such patients are instead characterized by differences in cardiac output reserve). Also, femoral vein oxygen content is lower in heart failure patients than in normal subjects,[18] ruling out inadequate peripheral oxygen extraction as a contributing factor to exercise intolerance. Finally, decreases in limb blood flow during exercise in heart failure patients are dictated by low cardiac output reserve,[18] given the need for minimal and constant amount of nonlimb blood flow.

Thus, peripheral abnormalities do not appear to determine $\dot{V}O_{2max}$, and the relationship between peripheral abnormalities and $\dot{V}O_{2max}$ reflects a secondary adaptive response. It may be more appropriate to view vascular and muscular changes in heart failure as peripheral abnormalities accompanying exercise tolerance rather than peripheral abnormalities responsible for exercise intolerance. Exceptions to this general principle may be seen in two situations: (1) when patients with heart failure are subjected to unnecessary restriction of activity and become severely deconditioned, and (2) when cardiac output improves as a result of drug therapy[37] or cardiac transplantation.[38,39] In these two situations, pre-existing and irreversible peripheral abnormalities, which initially parallel decreases in cardiac output, may become limiting.

The role of peripheral factors in determining submaximal exercise tolerance is unclear. The anaerobic threshold, which determines the level of work below which exercise is sustainable for long periods,[40] is low in heart failure[1,27,41,42] and may depend more on peripheral factors than on central oxygen delivery. This is supported by the dissociation between abnormalities in anaerobic threshold and VO_{2max} in heart failure patients.[1,27] Correspondingly, local muscle training may improve submaximal exercise tolerance without challenging the constraint imposed by the central circulation, and it represents a promising therapeutic intervention.

Ventilatory Changes in Systolic Failure and Their Influence on Exercise Tolerance

Many abnormalities in ventilation have been documented in patients with SLVD, and have been the topic of excellent recent reviews.[8] These abnormalities include changes in structure due to persistent pulmonary venous hypertension, and giving rise to obstructive and restrictive abnormalities; alveolar-capillary membrane function;[43] hyperventilation[9] resulting from increased physiological dead space due to VQ mismatch and from early onset of anaerobic metabolism; and ventilatory muscle fatigue and weakness.[44]

The link between the above-mentioned pathophysiological abnormalities and the complex integrated symptom of dyspnea has, however, been very elusive. For example, even in patients limited by dyspnea, ventilatory reserve appears normal.[45] In addition, no descriptor of ventilation f including ventilation itself, or the ratio of ventilation to CO_2 production f has correlated with quantitative indices of dyspnea.[46] Nor have these measures differed in patients limited by dyspnea, compared with those who are fatigue-limited.[9,46]

This baffling lack of relationship between hyperventilation and dyspnea has led many to conclude that dyspnea and fatigue may be merely different central interpretations of the same peripheral signal,[46] or that respiratory muscle fatigue or ischemia may be responsible for dyspnea, independent of the amount of ventilation.[8]

Despite the frequency of dyspnea accompanying exercise, it is unlikely that pulmonary factors commonly limit maximal exercise performance in heart failure. Ventilatory reserve is generally high even at maximal exercise;[45] PO_2 and PCO_2 remain normal;[9] the anaerobic threshold occurs early in exercise;[1,2,27] systemic and regional venous desaturation are maximal;[18] and $\dot{V}O_{2max}$ often plateaus at maximal exercise.[1,2] This all suggests that circulatory rather than pulmonary factors limit exercise tolerance in most patients with LVSD.

Although the symptoms that arise from ventilatory limitation would be expected to express themselves more during extended exercise, such a relationship should also be present for peripheral muscle fatigue. Therefore, there appears to be little or no theoretical basis for believing that pulmonary symptoms should be especially limiting during sustained submaximal exercise. In addition, it has been demonstrated that rapid exercise rather than sustained exercise is more likely to result in shortness of breath.[10]

Summary

Despite many potential limitations to exercise tolerance in patients with LVSD, peak exercise capacity appears to be determined primarily by cardiac output reserve, which in turn depends on complex interactions within the left ventricle and between the left ventricle and the right ventricle. Secondary peripheral abnormalities do not appear to be primary limitations to maximal exercise, except perhaps in patients with unnecessary immobilization and those with partially corrected central hemodynamics, such as which may be seen after inotropic therapy or cardiac transplantation. In contrast, secondary peripheral abnormalities may well be primary determinants of submaximal exercise tolerance; they would be expected to be related to the primary cardiac abnormality, but may be amenable to low level or regional skeletal muscle training, which should not challenge this central circulation.

Abnormalities in pulmonary structure and function are seen in patients with LVSD and are likely to contribute to dyspnea. However, even in patients limited primarily by the symptom of shortness of breath, the central circulation appears to be the predominant mechanism of exercise limitation.

Challenges for Future Research

Definition of the factors that limit exercise tolerance in patients with LVSD remains a difficult but important challenge for biomedical research. Three major challenges must be overcome. First, current measures of exercise tolerance, either maximal or submaximal, suffer from technical limitations of reproducibility and theoretical limitations of relevance to heart failure patients, whose perceived exertional symptoms may not reflect their actual exercise capacity.[47] In addition, interventions in heart failure do not produce consistent benefits, necessitating the use of large studies to produce significant changes. In such studies, mechanisms are very difficult to address. Finally, even if these first two limitations could be overcome, it is very likely that individual variations in the mechanisms of exercise limitation will prevent the development of a standardized concept of exercise limitation, and consequently the broad application of any intervention to improve exercise tolerance in this group will remain difficult.

References

1. Weber KT, Kinasewitz GT, Janicki JS, et al. Oxygen utilization during exercise in patients with chronic cardiac failure. *Circulation* 1982;65(suppl 6): 1213–1223.
2. Weber KT, Wilson JR, Janicki JS, et al. Exercise testing in the evaluation of patients with chronic cardiac failure. *Am Rev Respir Dis* 1984;129:S60-S62.
3. LeJemtel TH, Liang CS, Stewart DK, et al. (for the SOLVD Investigators). Reduced peak aerobic capacity in asymptomatic left ventricular systolic dysfunction. *Circulation* 1994;90:2757–2760.
4. Wilson JR, Martin JL, Schwartz D, et al. Exercise intolerance in patients with chronic heart failure: Role of impaired nutritive flow to skeletal muscle. *Circulation* 1984;69(suppl 6):1079–1087.
5. Mancini DM, Walter G, Reicheck N, et al. Contribution of skeletal muscle atrophy to exercise intolerance and altered muscle metabolism in heart failure. *Circulation* 1992;85:1364–1373.
6. Kraemer MD, Kubo SH, Rector TS, et al. Pulmonary and peripheral vascular factors are important determinants of peak exercise oxygen uptake in patients with heart failure. *J Am Coll Cardiol* 1993;21:641–648.
7. Weber KT, Janicki JS: Cardiopulmonary Exercise Testing: Physiologic Principles and Clinical Applications. Philadelphia, WB Saunders, 1986.
8. Mancini DM. Pulmonary factors limiting exercise capacity in patients with heart failure. *Prog Cardiovasc Dis* 1995;37(56):347–370.
9. Sullivan MJ, Higginbotham MB, Cobb FR. Increased exercise ventilation in patients with chronic heart failure: Intact ventilatory control despite hemodynamic and pulmonary abnormalities. *Circulation* 1988;77(suppl 3): 552–559.
10. Lipkin DB, Canepa-Anson R, Stephens MR, et al. Factors determining symptoms in heart failure: Comparison of fast and slow exercise tests. *Br Heart J* 1986;55:439–445.
11. Poole-Wilson PA, Buller NP. Causes of symptoms in chronic congestive heart failure and implications for treatment. *Am J Cardiol* 1988;62:31A-34A.
12. Mancini DM, Walker G, Reicheck N, et al. Contribution of skeletal muscle atrophy to exercise intolerance and altered muscle metabolism in heart failure. *Circulation* 1992;85:1364–1373.
13. Baker B, Wilen M, Boyd C, et al. Relation of right ventricular ejection frac-

tion to exercise capacity in chronic left ventricular failure. *Am J Cardiol* 1984;54:596–599.

14. Rihal CS, Nishimura RA, Hatle LK, et al. Systolic and diastolic dysfunction in patients with clinical diagnosis of dilated cardiomyopathy. Relation to symptoms and prognosis. *Circulation* 1994;90:2772–2779.

15. Fragasso G, Benti R, Sciammarella M, et al. Symptom-limited exercise testing causes sustained diastolic dysfunction in patients with coronary disease and low effort tolerance. *J Am Coll Cardiol* 1991;17:1251–1255.

16. Franciosa JA, Park M, Levine TB. Lack of correlation between exercise capacity and indexes of resting left ventricular performance in heart failure. *Am J Cardiol* 1981;47:33–38.

17. Higginbotham MB, Morris KG, Conn EH, et al. Determinants of variable exercise performance among patients with severe left ventricular dysfunction. *Am J Cardiol* 1983;51:52–60.

18. Sullivan MJ, Knight D, Higginbotham MB, et al. Relation between central and peripheral hemodynamics during exercise in patients with severe heart failure. *Circulation* 1989;80(suppl 4):769–781.

19. Mancini DM, Davis L, Wexler JP, et al. Dependence of enhanced maximal exercise performance on increased peak skeletal muscle perfusion during long-term captopril therapy in heart failure. *J Am Coll Cardiol* 1987;10:845–850.

20. Norlander R, Hedmon A, Pehrsson SK. Rate-variable pacing and exercise capacity, a comment. *PACE* 1989;12:749–751.

21. Treese N, Coutinho M, Stegmeier A, et al. Influence of rate-responsive pacing on aerobic capacity in patients with chronotropic incompetence. In Winter U, Wasserman K, Treese N, Höpp H eds: *Computerized Cardiopulmonary Exercise Testing*. Darmstadt, Germany: Steinkopff Verlag; 1991:139–144.

22. Mancini DM, Eisen H, Kussmaul W, et al. Value of peak exercise oxygen consumption for optimal timing of cardiac transplantation in ambulatory patients with heart failure. *Circulation* 1991;83:778–786.

23. Stevenson L, Steimle A, Chelimsky-Fallick C, et al. Outcomes predicted by oxygen consumption during evaluation of 333 patients with advanced heart failure. *Circulation* 1993;88:94A.

24. Reed JW, Ablett M, Cotes JE. Ventilatory responses to exercise and to carbon dioxide in mitral stenosis before and after valvulotomy; causes of tachypnoea. *Clin Sci Molecular Med* 1987;54:9–16.

25. Fink LI, Wilson JR, Ferraro N. Exercise ventilation and pulmonary artery wedge pressure in chronic stable congestive heart failure. *Am J Cardiol* 1986;57:249–253.

26. Cohen-Solal A, Chabernaud JM, Gourgon R. Comparison of oxygen uptake during bicycle exercise in patients with chronic heart failure and in normal subjects. *J Am Coll Cardiol* 1990;16:80–85.

27. Simonton CA, Higginbotham MB, Cobb FR. The ventilatory threshold: Quantitative analysis of reproducibility and relation to arterial lactate concentration in normal subjects and in patients with chronic congestive heart failure. *Am J Cardiol* 1988;62:100–107.

28. Wasserman K, Stringer WW. Critical capillary PO_2, net lactate production, and oxyhemoglobin dissociation. In Wasserman K, ed: *Exercise Gas Exchange in Heart Disease*. New York: Futura Publishing Co., Inc.; 1996:157–181.

29. Wittenberg BA, Wittenberg JB. Transplant of oxygen in muscle. *Ann Rev Physiol* 1989;51:857–878.

30. Cohen-Solal A, Aufertit JF, Page E, et al. (for the VO_2 French Group). Tran-

sient fall in oxygen consumption during exercise in heart failure: Evidence for oxygen consumption dependence upon oxygen transport. *Chest* 1996; In Press.

31. Mason DT, Zelis, Longhurst P, Lee G. Cardiocirculatory responses to muscular exercise in congestive heart failure. *Prog Cardiovasc Dis* 1977;19:475–489.
32. Francis GS, Goldsmith SR, Cohn J. Relationship of exercise capacity to resting left ventricular performance and basal plasma norepinephrine levels in patients with congestive heart failure. *Am Heart J* 1982;104:725–731.
33. Krum H, Goldsmith R, Wilshire-Clement M, et al. Role of endothelin in the exercise intolerance of chronic heart failure. *Am J Cardiol* 1995;75:1282–1283.
34. Massie BM, Conway M, Rapagopalen B, et al. Skeletal muscle metabolism during exercise under ischemic conditions in congestive heart failure. *Circulation* 1988;78:320–326.
35. Sullivan M, Green H, Cobb F. Skeletal muscle biochemistry and histology in ambulatory patients with long term heart failure. *Circulation* 1990;81:518–527.
36. Volterrani M, Clark AL, Ludman PF, et al. Predictors of exercise capacity in chronic heart failure. *Eur Heart J* 1994;15:801–809.
37. Maskin CS, Forman R, Sonnenblick EH, et al. Failure of dobutamine to increase exercise capacity despite hemodynamic improvement in severe chronic heart failure. *Am J Cardiol* 1983;51:177–182.
38. Kao AC, Van Trigt P, Shaeffer-McCall GS, et al. Central and peripheral limitations to upright exercise in untrained cardiac transplant recipients. *Circulation* 1994;89(suppl 6):2605–2615.
39. Stratton JR, Kemp GJ, Daly RC, et al. Effects of cardiac transplantation on bioenergetic abnormalities of skeletal muscle in congestive heart failure. *Circulation* 1994;89:1624–1631.
40. Wasserman K. The anaerobic threshold measurement in exercise testing. *Clin Chest Med* 1984;5:77–88.
41. Weber KT, Janicki JS. Lactate production during maximal and submaximal exercise in patients with chronic heart failure. *J Am Coll Cardiol* 1985;6:717–724.
42. Sullivan MJ, Higginbotham MB, Cobb FR. Exercise training in patients with chronic heart failure delays ventilatory anaerobic threshold and improves submaximal exercise performance. *Circulation* 1989;79(suppl 2):324–329.
43. Puri S, Baker L, Dutka DP, et al. Reduced alveolar capillary membrane diffusing capacity in chronic heart failure. *Circulation* 1995;91:2769–2774.
44. Mancini DM, Henson D, LaManca J, et al. Respiratory muscle function and dyspnea in patients with chronic congestive heart failure. *Circulation* 1992;86: 909–918.
45. Wassermann K. Dyspnea on exertion: Is it the heart or the lungs? *J Am Med Assoc* 1982;248:2039–2043.
46. Clark AL, Sparrow JL, Coats AJS. Muscle fatigue and dyspnea in chronic heart failure: Two sides of the same coin? *Eur Heart J* 1955;16:49–52.
47. Wilson JR, Rayos E, Yeoh TK, et al. Dissociation between exertional symptoms and circulatory function in patients with heart failure. *Circulation* 1995;92:47–53.

Chapter 4

Exercise, Diastolic Function, and Dysfunction

Carl S. Apstein, MD, Joseph R. Libonati, PhD, Niraj Varma, MD, and Franz R. Eberli, MD

Introduction

Several important interactions connect exercise and diastole. During exercise diastolic function must be enhanced so that left ventricular (LV) input remains precisely matched to LV output, despite the shortened duration of diastole resulting from the tachycardia of exercise, and without increasing left atrial pressure and compromising pulmonary function. Several elegant mechanisms combine to promote LV diastolic filling during exercise. These mechanisms are lost in patients with pressure overload hypertrophy (pathological hypertrophy) and/or ischemia; consequently, such patients have dyspnea with exertion as the most common manifestation of their diastolic dysfunction. Long-term exercise training produces physiological cardiac hypertrophy with enhanced diastolic function, and such exercise conditioning has the potential to reverse the diastolic dysfunction of pathological hypertrophy. The physiological and subcellular mechanisms responsible for these interactions between exercise and diastole, and the diagnosis and management of diastolic dysfunction will be reviewed. Appropriate management can improve the exercise tolerance of patients with diastolic dysfunction and potentially allow them to gain more from exercise training programs.

Cardiac failure is the result of either systolic or diastolic dysfunction or both. Systolic dysfunction can be defined as a decreased ejection from one or both ventricles. Diastolic dysfunction can be defined as an impaired filling of one or both ventricles. Systolic dysfunction is easily

From: Balady GJ, Piña IL (eds). *Exercise and Heart Failure*. Armonk, NY: Futura Publishing Company, Inc.; ©1997.

assessed by measuring ejection fraction and regional wall motion abnormalities. Clinical manifestations of pure LV systolic dysfunction include a decreased cardiac output, increased heart rate, and peripheral vasoconstriction. However, patients hospitalized for congestive heart failure almost always present with the additional symptom of shortness of breath, at rest or with exertion due to pulmonary congestion as a result of LV diastolic dysfunction (Table 1).[1,2] In fact, approximately one third of all cases of congestive heart failure are due primarily to diastolic dysfunction. Classic examples of isolated diastolic dysfunction are hypertrophic cardiomyopathy, the hypertensive hypertrophic cardiomyopathy of the elderly, and aortic stenosis with a normal ejection fraction.[3-5] Such patients have normal systolic function despite clinical signs and symptoms of left-sided heart failure, ie dyspnea on exertion or pulmonary congestion. The fraction of patients with congestive heart failure due primarily to diastolic dysfunction is higher in elderly patients than in the general population.[6]

Understanding the pathophysiology of diastolic dysfunction is important because it affects therapy and prognosis. Diastolic properties are determined by a complex interplay of functional and structural components. The major components contributing to diastolic dysfunction are: (1) slowed and incomplete myocardial relaxation; (2) impaired left ventricular filling; and (3) altered passive elastic properties of the ventricle resulting in increased passive stiffness. Table 2 lists the most common etiologies leading to these forms of diastolic dysfunction and some of the parameters used to measure diastolic dysfunction. Measurements of diastolic properties are more complicated than those of systolic function. Usually high-fidelity pressure measurements and/or simultaneous LV pressure-volume measurements are required. Changes in the isovolumic relaxation are most often assessed by changes in the time constant of the isovolumic LV pressure decay (tau), filling abnormalities by changes in the filling rate and the time-to-peak filling, and changes in passive elastic properties by changes in the diastolic pressure-volume relationship. In a given patient, impairment of one or more of these parameters will result in decreased LV chamber distensibility as manifested by an increase in diastolic pressure at any given LV volume (see below).

Table 1

Clinical Manifestations of Diastolic Dysfunction

1. Exertional dyspnea
2. Congestive heart failure
3. Acute ischemic pulmonary edema
4. Respiratory symptoms of angina pectoris
5. Postcardiac surgery dysfunction

Table 2

Diastolic Dysfunction: Parameters and Etiology

Physiological Abnormality	Alteration in Parameter of Assessment	Common Etiology
Delayed or incomplete relaxation	↑ Tau ↑ IVRT ↓ E/A ratio	LV hypertrophy Myocardial ischemia LV asynchrony Abnormal loading
Early diastolic filling abnormalities	↓ Peak filling rate ↑ Time to peak filling ↓ E/A ratio	Delayed relaxation LV asynchrony
Late diastolic filling abnormalities	↑ Diastolic P/V relationship Normal or ↑ E/A ratio	LV chamber dilation Restrictive/constrictive filling pattern
Increased LV passive chamber stiffness	↑ Diastolic P/V relationship ↑ Stiffness constant	↑ Collagen and fibrosis Myocardial infiltration (e.g. amyloid) ↑ Vascular turgor Concentric LVH Post-MI hypertrophy and fibrosis LV chamber dilation

LV = left ventricular; LVH = left ventricular hypertrophy; Tau = time constant of isovolumic pressure decay; IVRT = isovolumic relaxation time; E/A ratio = ratio of early and late left ventricular inflow as detected by Doppler echocardiography; peak filling rate = dV/dt max; time to peak filling = time to dV/dt max; ↑ diastolic P/V relationship = upward shift and/or increased slope of LV diastolic pressure/volume relationship; stiffness constant = Kp = constant of chamber stiffness calculated from simple exponential of pressure-volume relationship (lnP = Kp.V + ln c).

Myocardial Abnormalities: Hypertrophy and Ischemia

Widespread use of noninvasive methods of cardiac imaging has lead to the recognition that LV diastolic dysfunction commonly occurs as a result of myocardial hypertrophy and/or ischemia. Myocardial resistance to diastolic filling is usually the result of common structural abnormalities such as hypertrophy and interstitial fibrosis and/or impaired myocyte relaxation as a result of ischemia. The increased mass of the hypertrophied myocardium and the increased collagen content that frequently accompanies hypertrophy both represent structural abnormalities that reduce diastolic distensibility. Ischemia also causes a functional impairment of myocyte relaxation. Important interactions connect hypertrophy and ischemia. The left ventricle with concentric hypertrophy is more susceptible to ischemia, especially subendocardial ischemia, and such myocardium generally exhibits exaggerated ischemic diastolic dysfunction[1,6,7] For a given degree of ischemia, the functional impairment of relaxation is more severe in the hypertrophied heart than occurs in the absence of hypertrophy.[7,8] Thus, patients with concentric left ventricular hypertroohy (LVH) secondary to chronic hypertension or aortic stenosis are particularly susceptible to ischemic diastolic dysfunction.

Ischemic diastolic dysfunction is a reversible impairment of myocyte relaxation caused by ischemia. The slowing or failure of myocyte relaxation means that a fraction of actin-myosin cross-bridges persist and continue to generate tension throughout diastole, especially in early diastole, creating a state of "partial persistent systole." As a result, LV pressure decay, as assessed by tau, is impaired and the LV is functionally stiffer than normal during diastole. Such ischemic diastolic dysfunction can continue during and after reperfusion, resulting in a phase of post-ischemic diastolic "stunning", analogous to post-ischemic "stunning" of contractile function. For example, diastolic dysfunction is usually present early after cardiac surgery, after the myocardium has been exposed to cardioplegic arrest, ie to ischemia and reperfusion.[9,10]

This chapter will consider the clinical syndromes listed in Table 1 by reviewing the physiology of ischemic diastolic dysfunction, the subcellular mechanisms responsible for it, and current therapy.

Normal LV Diastolic Function: Matching Input to Output

Cardiac function, especially during exercise, is critically dependent on diastolic physiological mechanisms to increase LV filling (cardiac input) in parallel with LV ejection (cardiac output). Furthermore, adequate pulmonary function is also dependent on LV diastolic function because LV diastolic pressure directly affects pulmonary capillary pressure. Figure 1 presents this relationship by illustrating the heart and lungs during diastole (the mitral valve is open). During diastole the left ventricle, left atrium, and pulmonary veins form a "common chamber," which is continuous with the pulmonary capillary bed. Therefore, an increase in LV diastolic pressure will increase pulmonary capillary pressure, and if high enough, will cause pulmonary congestion and edema.

LV diastolic pressure is determined by the volume of blood in the left ventricle during diastole and by LV diastolic distensibility or compliance. At the onset of diastole, relaxation of the contracted myocardium occurs. This is a dynamic process that takes place during isovolumic relaxation (between aortic valve closure and mitral valve opening) and during early rapid filling of the ventricle. The rapid pressure decay and the concomitant "untwisting" and elastic recoil of the left ventricle produce a ventricular suction that augments the left atrial-ventricular pres-

LV Diastolic Pressure and Pulmonary Congestion

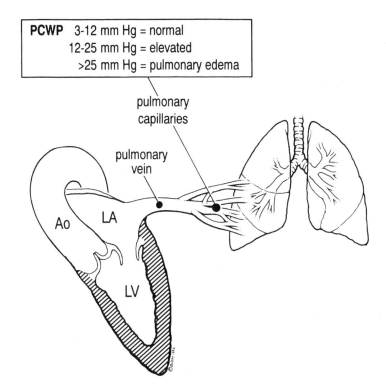

PCWP 3-12 mm Hg = normal
12-25 mm Hg = elevated
>25 mm Hg = pulmonary edema

pulmonary
capillaries

pulmonary
vein

Ao   LA

LV

Figure 1: Left ventricular diastolic pressure and pulmonary congestion. The heart is drawn in diastole with the mitral valve open to illustrate that during diastole the left ventricle, the left atrium, and pulmonary veins form a common chamber, continuous with the pulmonary capillary bed. Thus, left ventricular diastolic pressure determines pulmonary capillary pressure and the presence or absence of pulmonary congestion or edema.

sure gradient, and thus enhances diastolic filling. During the later phases of diastole the normal LV is composed of completely relaxed myocytes and is very compliant and easily distensible, offering minimal resistance to LV filling over a normal volume range. Therefore, LV filling can normally be accomplished by very low filling pressures in the left atrium and pulmonary veins, preserving a low pulmonary capillary pressure (normal pulmonary capillary pressure is <12 mm Hg), and a high degree of lung distensibility. A loss of normal LV diastolic relaxation and distensibility due to either structural or functional causes, impairs LV filling, resulting in increases in LV diastolic, left atrial, and pulmonary venous pressures, which directly increase pulmonary capillary pressure.

Measurement of LV Diastolic Distensibility

LV diastolic distensibility is quantified by the position and slope of the LV filling curve, or diastolic pressure-volume (P-V) curve, which plots LV diastolic pressure as a function of LV diastolic volume throughout diastole. A relatively stiff, nondistensible ventricle will require higher pressures to achieve filling of a given volume. Therefore an increase in LV diastolic chamber stiffness (or decrease in distensibility or compliance) shifts the LV diastolic P-V curve upwards, and often also increases its slope. Definition of LV filling curves in humans requires the simultaneous measurement of LV diastolic pressure and volume. Such LV volume measurements have been achieved by angiography, echocardiography, or radionuclide imaging techniques simultaneous with measurements of LV diastolic pressure. Figure 2 illustrates LV filling curves in a patient at rest and during myocardial ischemia caused by exercise. During exercise the diastolic P-V curve is shifted upwards, indicating decreased LV diastolic distensibility.

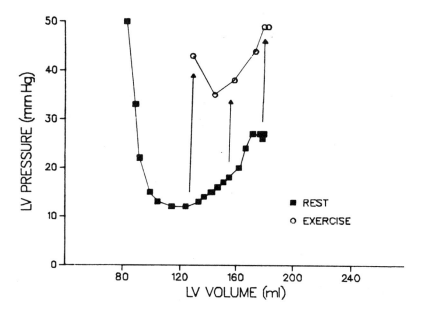

Figure 2: The classic LV diastolic pressure-volume shift of ischemia is illustrated by this patient. At all diastolic volumes pressure is clearly elevated compared to the resting coordinates. Adapted from Carroll JD, Carroll EP: *Herz* 1991;16:1.

LV Filling Dynamics

The normal left ventricle has a characteristic pattern of inflow velocities, which are altered with the development of diastolic dysfunction. Because inflow velocities are readily measured by Doppler echocardiography, a characteristic abnormal inflow pattern provides diagnostic evidence for the presence of diastolic dysfunction. The altered inflow pattern also has important physiological consequences.

Figure 3 depicts an idealized change of LV volume versus time during systole and diastole. Normally, LV inflow velocity and the volume rate of LV filling is greatest early in diastole, immediately after mitral valve opening, and is responsible for the normally tall E wave of the Doppler echocardiogram. Relatively little LV filling occurs in late diastole because most atrial-to-ventricular transfer of blood has occurred in early and mid-diastole. The amount of blood transported by atrial contraction is relatively small, the velocity imparted by the atrial contraction (the A wave of the Doppler echocardiogram) is relatively low, and the normal E/A wave ratio is greater than 1 and approaches a value of 2 in younger individuals.[11–13]

With the diastolic dysfunction that accompanies ischemia and/or hypertrophy, myocardial relaxation is characteristically impaired and the rate and amount of early diastolic LV filling are reduced, with a resultant shift of LV filling to the later part of diastole. The Doppler E wave is decreased, the hemodynamic load on the atrium is increased, and atrial contraction makes a more important contribution to ventricular filling than in normals. This is reflected by an increase in the Doppler A wave, and decrease in the E/A ratio. A typical example of changes in the mitral flow velocities during short periods of ischemia (ie balloon angioplasty) is given in Figure 4. The chronic atrial overload often eventually results in atrial fibrillation, and the loss of atrial contraction can dramatically reduce LV filling, left atrial emptying, and LV stroke-volume. The redistribution of filling from early to late diastole also means that LV filling and left atrial emptying are compromised more in patients with diastolic dysfunction than in normals by the occurrence of tachycardia; an increased heart rate shortens the duration of diastole and truncates the important late phase of diastolic filling.

Doppler-echocardiographic assessment of LV filling has its limitations since diastolic filling parameters are a function of multiple determinants. The typical, but nonspecific, mitral filling patterns, such as the pattern of increased isovolumic relaxation time and the decreased E/A ratio can be altered, ie pseudonormalized, by changes in atrial pressure. When severe LV systolic dysfunction and a restrictive pattern exists, the isovolumic relaxation time might even be decreased and the E/A

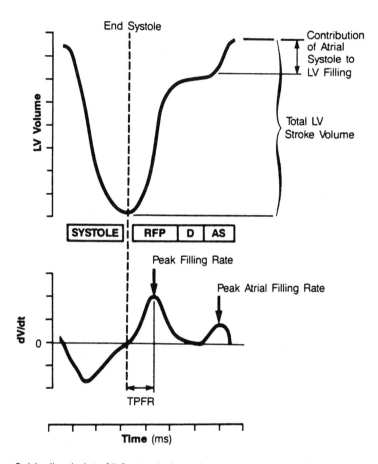

Figure 3: Idealized plot of left ventricular volume versus time (top) and the rate of change of volume (dV/dt) versus time (bottom) as might be obtained from contrast or radionuclide ventriculography. The representative cardiac cycle begins at end diastole. Subsequent events as depicted by the bars in the center of the figure are: (1) systole, during which LV volume decreases to a minimum and (2) diastole, the beginning of which is signaled by the opening of the mitral valve and the onset of left ventricular filling. Diastole has three distinct phases in normal individuals: (1) the rapid filling phase (RFP) during which left ventricle fills rapidly, dV/dt reaches its maximum, and the peak filling rate occurs; (2) diastasis (D) during which relatively little LV volume change occurs; and (3) atrial systole (AS) in which active atrial contraction fills the left ventricle to its end-diastolic volume. The diastolic parameters that have been derived from such analysis are the peak filling rate, the time to peak filling rate (TPFR), the percent contribution of atrial systole, and the first third filling fraction. Adapted from Reference 13.

ratio increased.[12] A detailed discussion of Doppler echocardiography is beyond the scope of this chapter and the interested reader is referred to recent reviews of Doppler echocardiographic assessment of diastolic dysfunction.[11,12]

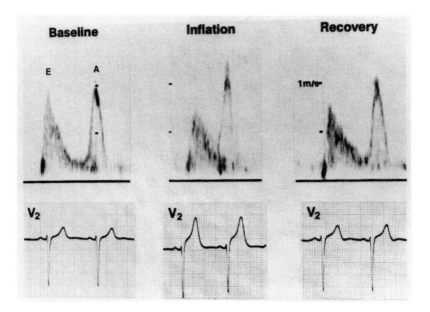

Figure 4: Pulsed Doppler ultrasound recording of LV inflow velocities with accompanying electrocardiographic lead V_2 during left anterior descending coronary artery occlusion (inflation of angioplasty balloon). Note the marked reversal of early (E) and atrial (A) peak velocities and ST segment elevation with coronary occlusion. With permission from Labovitz AJ et al.: J Am Coll Cardiol 1987;10:748.

Importance of LV Diastolic Function During Exercise

During exercise the cardiac output can increase several-fold. The increase in LV output must be matched by an increase in LV input. The increase in LV output during exercise is accomplished by an increase in heart rate, a modest increase in stroke volume, a decrease in peripheral vascular resistance, and an increase in contractile force, which increases LV systolic pressure and the force of ejection. However, the LV cannot accomplish an increase in input by those mechanisms that increase output during exercise. Tachycardia shortens the duration of diastole ie,the time in which LV filling must occur, thereby mandating that the diastolic filling rate during exercise be increased out of proportion to cardiac output. Nor can an increase in left atrial pressure be used as a mechanism to increase LV filling without the sacrifice of a low pulmonary capillary pressure.

How can this requirement for a marked increase in LV input (diastolic filling rate) during exercise be accomplished? An increase in flow rate across the mitral valve requires that the transmitral diastolic pressure gra-

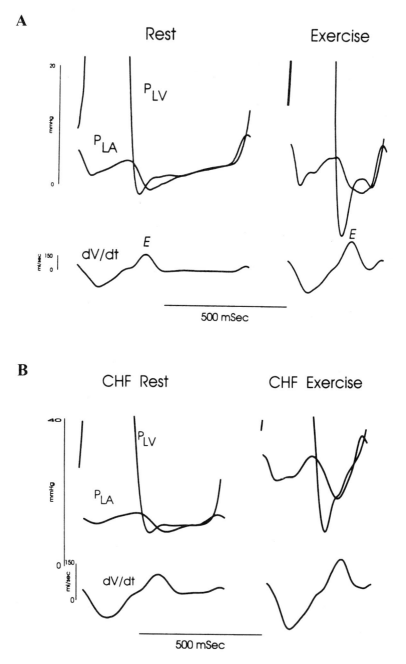

Figure 5: Effects of exercise with and without heart failure on LV filling dynamics. *A. Upper panel:* Recording of left ventricular pressure (P_{LV}) and left atrial pressure (P_{LA}) and the rate of change of left ventricular volume (dV/dt) at rest and during exercise. During exercise, minimal P_{LV} decreases without any increase in P_{LA}. This leads to an increase in the peak mitral valve gradient and produces a larger peak filling rate (E). *B. Lower panel:* Effect of heart failure. In a format similar to upper panel A, data are shown at rest and after

dient increase. However, this increase in transmitral gradient can not be achieved by increasing the pressure in the left atrium, for that would increase pulmonary capillary pressure, cause pulmonary congestion, and precipitate dyspnea and respiratory compromise during exercise. Rather, the normal LV accomplishes a remarkable increase in diastolic filling rate during exercise by rapidly and markedly decreasing intra-LV pressure during early diastole. This early diastolic LV pressure decrease creates a relative LV "suction" effect, which increases the transmitral pressure gradient without increasing left atrial pressure (Figure 5).[14–17] In other words, during exercise the LV increases its force of ejection during systole to "push" the LV output more forcefully, but it also "pulls" blood in during diastole more forcefully to increase input in parallel with output. This LV diastolic "suction" occurs as a result of several mechanisms. During exercise, the increased force of contraction during systole (observed clinically as an increase in systolic LV and arterial pressure) increases early diastolic myocardial elastic recoil due to the greater systolic shortening forces and extent of systolic fiber shortening, manifested as a smaller end-systolic volume, which occurs during exercise.[16] Also, an acceleration of myocyte relaxation occurs during exercise, due to an increased rate of calcium uptake by the sarcoplasmic reticulum (SR). Increased cyclic adenosine monophosphate (AMP), generated by the β-adrenergic response to exercise, phosphorylates the regulatory SR membrane protein, phospholamban, to increase the rate of calcium uptake by the SR during diastole.[18]

Thus, during exercise the normal heart has an elegant balance and symmetry of physiological mechanisms to ensure that cardiac input keeps pace with cardiac output, with preservation of a low pulmonary capillary pressure. The β-adrenergic system increases cyclic AMP levels to increase systolic calcium entry and SR calcium release, with a consequent increase in contractility and systolic fiber shortening. The rate of diastolic SR calcium reuptake is also accelerated by the cyclic AMP increase, and the greater extent of systolic fiber shortening results in the early diastolic recoil mechanism. This decreases intra-LV pressure in early diastole to pull blood into the LV and facilitate LV filling. These mechanisms result in an increase in measured LV distensibility during exercise in normal patients, as manifested by a downward shift of the LV diastolic P-V curve, especially during early diastole (Figure 6, left panel).[19,20]

(Figure 5 *Continued.*) exercise in a dog following the development of congestive heart failure (CHF). CHF was induced by several weeks of rapid pacing. During exercise after CHF, peak LV filling rate (E wave) increases due to an increase in the early transmitral valve pressure gradient. However, the gradient is produced by an increase in left atrial pressure, instead of a decrease in LV pressure as occurred during exercise prior to CHF, as shown in upper panel A. Adapted from References 14–16.

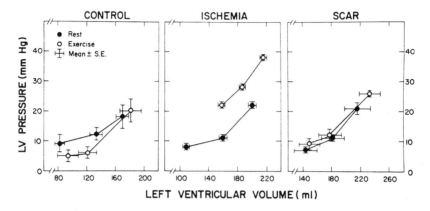

Figure 6: The LV diastolic pressure-volume relation in controls, patients with exercise-induced ischemia, and in patients with scar from prior infarction, but no exercise-induced ischemia. The coordinates of pressure and volume are averages at three diastolic points: the early diastolic pressure nadir, mid-diastole, and end-diastole. For details see text. Adapted from Reference 19.

Effects of Heart Failure

When congestive heart failure (CHF) develops, the left ventricle loses the ability to augment diastolic filling in response to exercise by the normal mechanism of accentuated elastic recoil and early diastolic suction. Early diastolic filling is increased during exercise in CHF, but the responsible mechanism is an increase in left atrial pressure to create the requisite transmitral gradient, rather than an exercise-induced decrease in early diastolic LV as occurs in normals. Consequently, the increase in left atrial pressure results in pulmonary congestion with exercise, a hallmark of CHF (Figure 5).

Effects of Ischemia

If ischemia occurs during exercise, not only is the normal increase in LV distensibility lost, but even worse, a rapid and marked increase in LV diastolic chamber stiffness occurs and LV diastolic pressures quickly increase, resulting in acute pulmonary congestion (Figure 2). The responses of LV diastolic distensibility during exercise in normal patients, in patients with coronary artery disease and exercise-induced ischemia, and in patients with healed myocardial infarction but without ischemia during exercise, are illustrated in Figure 6.

Figure 6 illustrates LV diastolic P-V curves in the three patient groups at rest and during exercise.[20] The simultaneous measures of LV diastolic pressure and volume define LV distensibility or compliance. In normal patients (control), during the rest state, LV pressure was approximately 9 mm Hg in early diastole, and increased to about 15 mm Hg at end-diastole. Exercise caused a marked downward shift of the LV diastolic P-V curve in early diastole, and a lesser decrease of mean LV diastolic pressure relative to the rest state. During exercise, these control patients increased their cardiac output between three-fold and four-fold. Because of this physiological increase in LV diastolic distensibility, the increase in cardiac output was accomplished without an increase of LV diastolic pressure and pulmonary capillary pressure.

In contrast, the middle panel shows the LV diastolic P-V curves in patients with coronary artery disease who developed angina and ischemia with exercise. The P-V curve at rest was similar to that of the control patients, but with exercise a marked upward shift occurred, such that LV end-diastolic pressure was 40 mm Hg, and LV mean diastolic pressure was approximately 30 mm Hg. As discussed above (Figure 1), such an increase in LV diastolic pressure would cause significant pulmonary congestion.

This upward shift of the LV diastolic P-V curve and the consequent pulmonary congestion during exercise-induced ischemia explains why many patients with coronary disease have respiratory symptoms with their anginal pain, and often complain of wheezing, chest tightness, inability to take a deep breath, or shortness of breath. Such respiratory symptoms may occur in the absence of anginal pain and are often referred to as "anginal equivalents." Often these "anginal" symptoms are quite similar to symptoms of heart failure, which is not surprising since in both cases the responsible mechanism is an increase of pulmonary capillary pressure. The acute decrease in LV distensibility during angina and its consequences on pulmonary mechanics are documented by Pepine.[21] He showed that airway resistance and lung compliance decrease during an anginal episode concomitant with the increase in LV diastolic chamber stiffness and LV diastolic pressure.[21] Thus, during angina acute left-sided diastolic heart failure often occurs as the result of an acute increase in LV diastolic chamber stiffness, as illustrated in Figure 2 and the middle panel of Figure 6. This upward shift of the LV diastolic P-V curve is completely reversible with recovery after exercise.

The right panel of Figure 6 illustrates the LV diastolic P-V curves in patients with a healed myocardial infarction but without exercise-induced ischemia. Such patients lost the early diastolic increase in distensibility during exercise that was seen in the control patients, so that LV diastolic filling was not facilitated by an increase in distensibility. Because exercise-induced ischemia did not occur, there was no upward shift of the LV diastolic P-V curve.

Hypertrophy-Ischemia Interactions and Their Effects on LV Diastolic Dysfunction

The conditions of LVH and ischemia have important interactions. Hearts with concentric LVH (secondary to chronic hypertension or aortic stenosis) are highly susceptible to subendocardial ischemia for several reasons, as outlined in Table 3 (Adapted from Isoyama[22]): (1) There is some evidence that an inadequate coronary growth relative to muscle mass, with a resulting decrease in capillary density and increased capillary to myocyte oxygen diffusion distance, renders the hypertrophied myocyte more susceptible to ischemia.[23] (2) The increase in ventricular wall thickness results in an increased epicardial-endocardial distance. The coronary arterial circulation consists of epicardial vessels which penetrate transmurally, giving rise to mid-myocardial branches which perfuse the thickened LV wall before serving the subendocardium. Thus, coronary perfusion pressure is dissipated in proportion to LV wall thickness, leaving the subendocardium as the region most vulnerable to ischemia.[22] (3) Coronary arterial remodeling accompanies concentric hypertrophy and is manifested by an increase in coronary arterial medial thickness and perivascular fibrosis, which can restrict the extent of coronary arterial vasodilatation. (4) Coronary vasodilator reserve is usually diminished with concentric LVH, because vascular tone at rest is usually abnormally reduced and coronary flow at rest is increased.[23–25] The increased coronary flow is required in the resting state to supply the increased muscle mass. Since maximal achievable coronary flow is similar to that of normal ventricles, coronary flow reserve is decreased. When metabolic demand and the need for oxygen increases, coronary reserve is often inadequate to meet the increased oxygen requirements, and ischemia occurs.[25] Additionally, increased LV diastolic pressures can cause vascular compression, thereby reducing coronary flow and perfusion of the subendocardial layer.[22] Furthermore, a decrease in

---

Table 3

Mechanisms for Increased Susceptibility of LVH to Ischemia

---

1. Inadequate coronary growth relative to muscle mass
2. Increased epi- to endocardial coronary artery perfusion pressure dissipation
3. Coronary artery remodeling
4. Decreased coronary vasodilator reserve
5. Increased LV diastolic pressure
6. Increased coronary atherosclerosis with hypertensive LVH

LV = left ventricle; LVH = left ventricular hypertrophy.

coronary flow reserve is partly due to an endothelial dysfunction in the vasculature of hearts with LV hypertrophy secondary to pressure overload hypertrophy.[26]

Coronary atherosclerosis incidence and severity is increased in the presence of systemic arterial hypertension, which is often the cause of concentric LVH. Thus, patients with concentric LVH on a hypertensive basis often have significant concomitant coronary artery disease.

Taken together, these factors make the heart with concentric LVH exquisitely sensitive to subendocardial ischemia. Such hearts also have a structural basis for diastolic dysfunction because of their increased mass and increased interstitial and subendocardial fibrosis that commonly accompany concentric LVH, particularly when it results from hypertension.[7] The combination of structural abnormality, susceptibility to subendocardial ischemia, and exaggerated impairment of myocyte relaxation in response to ischemia, make the heart with concentric LVH highly vulnerable to frequent and severe ischemic diastolic dysfunction.

The exaggerated ischemic diastolic dysfunction of concentric LVH has been demonstrated in several clinical settings and experimental models.[7] For example, during pacing-induced ischemia, patients with aortic stenosis and concentric LVH developed marked increases in LV end-diastolic pressure and a substantial upward shift of the LV diastolic P-V curve.[3] In experimental studies, rat hearts with concentric LVH due to sodium overload hypertension developed greater diastolic dysfunction during hypoxia[27–29] and ischemia[30] than control rat hearts . Hearts from rabbits with LVH secondary to renal vascular hypertension exhibited exaggerated diastolic dysfunction during demand ischemia.[31] Rat hearts with concentric LVH due to aortic banding had exaggerated ischemic LV diastolic dysfunction when subjected to low-flow ischemia.[8]

A clinical example of exercise-induced pulmonary congestion in patients with LVH and diastolic dysfunction is illustrated in Figure 7. The patients in this study had severe clinical heart failure (New York Heart Association Class III or Class IV), but normal systolic function (normal ejection fractions) and no significant valvular, pericardial or coronary artery disease. Most had concentric LVH secondary to hypertension, but four elderly patients had only chronic hypertension. These patients were compared to age- and gender-matched controls during symptom-limited upright bicycle exercise. The controls had more distensible left ventricles at rest, as manifested by a lower pulmonary capillary wedge pressure (PCWP) at a larger LV end-diastolic volume (LVEDV). During exercise, the control subjects increased their LVEDV, consistent with use of the Frank-Starling mechanism, and the increase in LVEDV was associated with a modest and proportional increase in PCWP, which stayed within the normal range. In contrast, during ex-

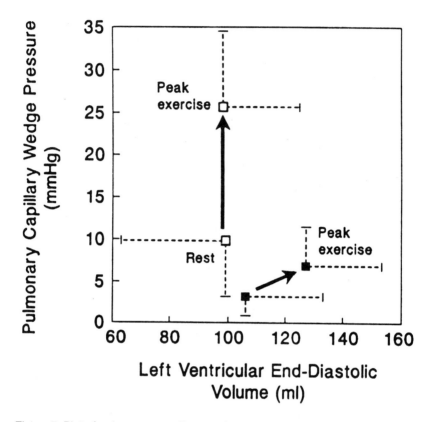

Figure 7: Plot of pulmonary capillary wedge pressure versus LV end-diastolic volume, with arrows indicating the changes from rest to peak exercise in patients and control subjects during symptom-limited upright bicycle exercise. These patients had normal systolic function, but symptomatic severe CHF due to diastolic dysfunction in the setting of hypertension and LVH. See text for discussion. Adapted from Reference 143.

ercise the patients with diastolic dysfunction did not increase their LVEDV; they were unable to use the Frank-Starling mechanism, presumably because their stiff, non-distensible ventricles resisted any increase in EDV. Rather, during exercise in these patients, the PCWP increased markedly, to pulmonary edema levels. This dramatic increase in PCWP, undoubtedly reflecting a comparable increase in LV diastolic pressures, suggests a very stiff ventricle that is unable to accomodate even a small increase in volume. Alternatively, the marked increase in PCWP at a constant LVEDV is also consistent with an exercise-induced increase in LV diastolic stiffness, and suggests the occurrence of subendocardial ischemia and an "exaggerated" impairment of diastolic relaxation of the hypertrophied myocardium, as discussed above.

Subcellular Mechanisms Potentially Responsible for Ischemic Diastolic Dysfunction in Normal and Hypertrophied Hearts

Myocyte relaxation occurs by reversal of those processes which cause contraction. The sodium and calcium movements that comprise excitation-contraction coupling are reversed to effect repolarization-relaxation coupling, the tension generating actin-myosin interaction abates, and myofilament tension is dissipated. Hypertrophy and ischemia can alter myocyte sodium and calcium movements, high energy phosphate metabolism (levels of ATP, ADP, creatine phosphate, and inorganic phosphate ($[P_i]$)), and intracellular pH, all of which can affect the rate and extent of myocyte relaxation. Furthermore, both pH and $[P_i]$ alter myofilament sensitivity to calcium and can thereby influence both systolic and diastolic myofilament tension at any calcium level. (For recent review, see Apstein et al[32]). Diastolic dysfunction at the myofilament level can result from either the persistence of excessive cytosolic calcium or the persistence of actin-myosin rigor complexes throughout diastole (Figure 8).

Role of Calcium

The major calcium movements regulating contraction and relaxation are illustrated in Figure 9. Contraction is initiated during myocyte activation. An inward calcium current occurs during the action potential, when the sarcolemmal voltage-dependent calcium channel opens, and calcium diffuses into the cell, driven by its 10,000-fold transmembrane concentration gradient. This calcium influx triggers a much greater amount of calcium release from the sarcoplasmic reticulum (SR). Cytosolic calcium levels rise rapidly and calcium binds to its myofilament receptor on troponin-C, activating contractile protein tension generation via the actin-myosin cross-bridge cycle, as illustrated in Figure 10. For complete myocyte relaxation to occur, the cytosol must be cleared of calcium so that calcium dissociates from troponin-C, and all tension-generating actin-myosin bonds must be lysed. The diastolic clearance of cytosolic calcium requires ATP to fuel the SR and sarcolemma calcium ATPases, which transport calcium into the sarcoplasmic reticulum or across the sarcolemma, respectively. Calcium removal may also occur via Na^+/Ca^{2+} exchange, and ATP is required to fuel the Na^+ pump that maintains a low intracellular Na^+ level which is favorable to Ca^2 extrusion by this mechanism.

During ischemia and hypoxia, an intracellular accumulation of calcium occurs. This increase in cytosolic calcium could potentially result

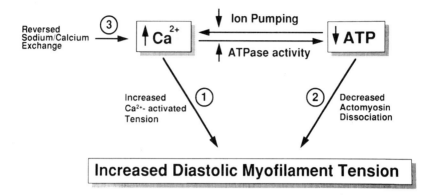

Figure 8: Synergistic interaction between an increase in cytosolic calcium and a decrease in ATP availability to increase diastolic myofilament tension. This Figure illustrates how an increased cytosolic calcium level or a decrease in ATP availability can directly increase diastolic myofilament tension and cause or exacerbate ischemic diastolic dysfunction. (1) An increase in diastolic calcium can directly increase diastolic myofilament tension by binding to Troponin C and/or can accelerate a decrease in ATP levels by activating a number of myocyte calcium ATPases. (2) A decrease in ATP availability can directly increase diastolic tension by decreasing the rate or amount of actomyosin dissociation from the rigor complex state. A decrease in ATP availability can also impair the calcium removal from the cytosol by the sarcolemmal and sarcoplasmic reticular calcium ATPases. (3) A decrease in ATP availability can also decrease the sarcolemmal sodium-potassium ATPase (sodium pump) activity resulting in an increase in intracellular sodium, which increases intracellular calcium by means of sodium-calcium exchange. Thus either cytosolic calcium overload or a decrease in ATP availability can initiate a "vicious cycle" of calcium-ATP interactions, which are synergistic in causing or exacerbating diastolic dysfunction.

from either excessive calcium entry into the cytosol, from a decrease in calcium efflux, or from inadequate calcium reuptake by the sarcoplasmic reticulum during diastole, but it seems not to be due to an excessive calcium influx via slow "L"-type calcium channels.[33] The reversible increase in diastolic chamber stiffness observed in patients with angina,[3,20,34] as well as the similar reversible increase in diastolic chamber stiffness in experimental models of ischemia, have been explained by an increase in intracellular calcium $[Ca^{2+}]_i$ and a consequent increase in calcium activated cross-bridge cycling and tension development.[24,35-41] $[Ca^{2+}]_i$ measurements by [19]-F nuclear magnetic resonance (NMR) spectroscopy, bioluminescent, and fluorescent calcium indicators that showed an increase of $[Ca^{2+}]_i$ both during hypoxia and during zero-flow ischemia in the whole heart, have supported this notion.[37,42-46] More recently, Camacho et al also reported an increase in $[Ca^{2+}]_i$ during low-flow ischemia in the rabbit heart, and they found a correlation between the impaired re-

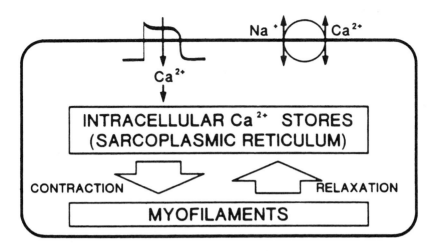

Figure 9: Major steps of excitation-contraction coupling in mammalian working myocardium. Adapted from Morgan J et al. *Am J Cardiol* 1984;3:410.

laxation of the left ventricle as assessed by the constant of the pressure decay, tau, and the intracellular calcium reuptake.[47]

In addition to their potential for persistently activating the actin-myosin cross-bridge interaction, excessive calcium levels can decrease phosphocreatine and ATP levels and increase ADP levels by increasing the activities of Ca^{2+}-activated ATPases such as the SR and SL calcium pumps, as well as other ATPases.[48] Thus, an increase in cell calcium can also impair relaxation indirectly by decreasing phosphocreatine and/or the ATP/ADP ratio, because such changes in the levels of high energy phosphate metabolites affect the actin-myosin cross-bridge cycle (Figure 10).

Much recent research has been devoted to determining the relative roles of disordered calcium regulation and/or abnormalities of high-energy phosphate metabolism as primary mechanisms for diastolic dysfunction during demand and supply ischemia and during post-ischemic reperfusion. For example, in some studies, the increases in diastolic calcium level preceded and did not occur simultaneously with the onset of contracture.[37,43] Conversely other studies have shown increase in intracellular calcium before the onset of increased diastolic force in isolated hearts,[49] or contracture occurring before any increase in intracellular calcium in isolated myocytes.[50,51] Furthermore, in recent studies from our laboratory, interventions which altered intracellular calcium after the onset of ischemic diastolic dysfunction in isolated heart models of both supply and demand ischemia did not affect the degree of ischemic diastolic dysfunction. However, during post-ischemic reperfusion, after both demand and supply ischemia, an exper-

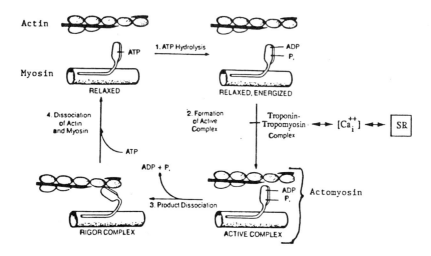

Figure 10: Contraction and relaxation at the molecular level: Role of ATP and calcium in the cross-bridge cycle. This diagram illustrates the cross-bridge cycle, ie, contraction and relaxation at the molecular level. The sequence begins at the upper left, where ATP binding to myosin has dissociated the thick and thin filaments (ie, the myosin and actin filaments), causing the muscle to relax. Hydrolysis of myosin bound ATP (Step 1) transfers the energy of the ATP molecule to the cross-bridge, which remains in a relaxed, unattached, but energized state (upper right). The affinity for ATP of the myosin head is very high, requiring only micromolar concentrations of ATP for this step in the molecular cardiac cycle. Interaction of the energized myosin cross-bridge with actin in the thin filament (Step 2) leads to the formation of the actomyosin active complex (lower right), in which the energy derived from ATP is still associated with the cross-bridge, which has yet to move. This step is regulated by the troponin-tropomyosin regulatory protein complex, whose interaction with actin is regulated by the binding of troponin-C to calcium; such binding is regulated by the cytosolic calcium concentration. When the cytosolic calcium concentration is low, as in normal diastole, troponin-C has minimal or no calcium bound to it, the troponin-tropomyosin complex inhibits the formation of the actomyosin complex, and the myofilaments remain in a relaxed, but energized state. Systolic contraction is initiated by the release of calcium from the sarcoplasmic reticulum. The calcium binds to troponin C, the configuration of the troponin-tropomyosin complex changes such that the inhibition of the actin-myosin interaction is removed, and formation of the active complex of actomyosin at Step 2 occurs. Step 2 is also referred to as the step of "calcium-activated tension" because of the central role of calcium in regulating this reaction by means of the troponin-tropomyosin complex. Failure to lower cytosolic calcium adequately during diastole results in the continuous formation of active actomyosin complexes throughout the cardiac cycle because a persistently elevated calcium level prevents the troponin-tropomyosin complex from completely inhibiting Step 2 as is required for normal diastolic relaxation. At Step 3, dissociation of ADP and $[P_i]$, the products of ATP hydrolysis, leads to formation of a rigor complex in which the chemical energy of the energized cross-bridge has been expended to perform mechanical work, the motion of the cross-bridge. This rigor bond complex represents a low energy state of acto

imentally-imposed calcium load immediately worsened the degree of diastolic dysfunction, suggesting that it was calcium-driven during reperfusion.[52–57]

The Role of Decreased ATP and Increased ADP in Increased Ischemic Diastolic Chamber Stiffness

As previously discussed, ATP and ADP play a critical role in myocyte relaxation. ATP is required to fuel the ion pumps that regulate diastolic levels of cytosolic calcium. ATP and ADP also have a complex number of interactions with the contractile proteins.

It was recognized early that the beginning of ischemic or hypoxic contracture was associated with a fall of ATP below a critical level. Therefore a decrease in tissue ATP levels, which causes actin-myosin crossbridges to "lock" in a noncycling rigor state, was proposed as the mechanism for the initiation of increased diastolic chamber stiffness.[58,59] In support of an ATP-based, rather than calcium-based mechanism of contracture, Koretsune and Marban, using NMR spectroscopy in ferret hearts, showed that $[Ca^{2+}]_i$ began to rise after about 10 minutes of zero-flow ischemia, and peaked in a steady-state level of about two-fold sys-

---

(Figure 10 *Continued.*) myosin. It is the state of the actomyosin complex at "end-systole" of the cross-bridge cycle. For relaxation to occur, the actomyosin rigor complex must be dissociated by ATP (Step 4). At Step 4, a rapid binding of ATP to the high-affinity myosin head of the rigor complex occurs, causing the rigor complex to dissociate to actin and myosin and the muscle to relax. This dissociation is facilitated by millimolar concentrations of ATP. This action of ATP has been called its "plasticizing effect," and is caused by an allosteric action of ATP. The ATP concentrations needed for the "plasticizing effect" are much higher than those needed to saturate the high affinity substrate site of myosin. Thus, if ATP depletion occurs, rigor complexes can still form because of the high affinity of the myosin head for ATP, but the dissociation of actin and myosin caused by the plasticizing effect of ATP is reduced. Increased levels of ADP also inhibit ATP binding to myosin. Thus, the initial net effect of ATP depletion is to cause inadequate relaxation or diastolic dysfunction. This Figure indicates that diastolic dysfunction and impaired relaxation can occur by two distinct mechanisms. An inadequate lowering of cytosolic calcium during diastole can lead to persistent formation of active complexes of actomyosin throughout diastole because of failure of adequate inhibition of Step 2 by the troponin-tropomyosin complex caused by persistent binding of calcium to troponin C. A second mechanism that can cause diastolic dysfunction occurs when ATP levels are diminished such that the "plasticizing effect" of ATP to dissociate actomyosin at Step 4 is reduced. An increase in ADP level may also impair actomyosin dissociation. All of these mechanisms can occur simultaneously and may be synergistic, as illustrated in Figure 8. Adapted from Katz AM: *Physiology of the Heart.* New York, Raven Press, 1992, pp151–177.

tolic concentration after 30 minutes to 35 minutes; in contrast, in this model contracture began only after 40 minutes.[49] This dissociation of $[Ca^{2+}]_i$ and contracture has also been observed in ferret papillary muscle[60] and in isolated myocytes during anoxia or metabolic inhibition.[50,61,62] These studies support the concept that contracture occurs when cytosolic ATP decreases below a critical level. The critical decrease in ATP level in whole-heart preparations for contracture to develop has been found to be from 10% to 50%, depending on metabolic parameters such as glycolytic activity.[49,58,59,63] However, these decreases result in ATP levels that are higher than [ATP] associated with contracture in skinned-muscle fiber preparations or isolated myocytes. In skinned-muscle fibers ATP had to fall below 0.1 mM before rigor developed; alternatively it could be prevented by adding 30 μM ATP.[64,65] In metabolically-inhibited isolated myocytes, contracture occurred when ATP had dropped to about 0.2 mM.[66]

There are several possible hypothetical explanations for this discrepancy, ie, how increased diastolic chamber stiffness could arise at ATP levels in the millimolar range, as measured in whole-heart preparations. First, it is conceivable that the increase in diastolic chamber stiffness observed in a whole heart at ATP levels in the millimolar range simply represents a number of myocytes that have depleted their ATP and have gone in contracture, and a number of myocytes that have preserved ATP and preserved contractile function. This explanation of loss of ATP substrate and classic rigor formation in a subset of myocytes is supported by the observations that after ATP depletion, isolated myocytes go into contracture within a short period of time.[50,61,62,66] Second, during ischemia, increased diastolic chamber stiffness could result from a loss of the plasticizing effect of ATP (Figure 10).[18] The plasticizing effect of ATP describes the role of ATP in the relaxation of myofilaments, as opposed to its role in their contraction. For relaxation to occur, ATP has to bind to the myosin head to initiate acto-myosin dissociation. This plasticizing effect is facilitated by ATP concentrations in the millimolar range, which are much higher concentrations than are needed to saturate the substrate site of myosin, which requires only micromolar concentrations of ATP. A third explanation is a classic product inhibition of the myofibrillar ATPase (ie, on the myosin head), whereby MgADP competes for the binding of MgATP to the actomyosin complex or for an allosteric regulatory site on the actomyosin complex.[67,68] As MgADP increases during ischemia, the decreased binding of MgATP to the rigor complex would decrease dissociation of the rigor complex and result in an increased tension of diastolic chamber stiffness.[67,68] Finally, there could be a compartmentation of ATP within the myocyte (mitochondrial versus cytosolic ATP pool).[69] Localization of glycolytic enzymes and the creatine kinase system have both been proposed to contribute to a compartmentation of ATP pools (see below).[70-73]

In addition to these effects at the level of the actin-myosin cross-bridge cycle, ATP is necessary to fuel the ion pumps that maintain normal intracellular calcium movements, which are the SR Ca-ATPase and the sarcolemmal Ca^{2+} and Na_+ pumps discussed above. Thus, a decrease in [ATP] can result in cytosolic calcium overload and impaired relaxation because of a failure to maintain normal ionic homeostasis.

Demand and Supply Ischemia

The term "ischemic diastolic dysfunction" implies a single pathophysiological process, but recent studies suggest that diastolic function may be affected somewhat differently by supply and demand ischemia. Demand ischemia typically occurs during exercise or pacing-induced angina resulting from an increase in oxygen demand in the setting of limited coronary flow, (due to a coronary stenosis) which reduces or eliminates coronary vasodilator reserve. In contrast, supply ischemia results from a marked reduction of coronary flow, eg, a coronary occlusion, resulting in inadequate coronary perfusion even for the resting state, such that ischemia occurs without any increase in myocardial oxygen demand.

The initial effects of acute ischemia on diastolic compliance differ, depending on whether it is of the supply or demand type. Experimental coronary ligation, resulting in acute supply ischemia, caused an initial downward and rightward shift of the diastolic P-V curve such that end-diastolic volume increased relative to end-diastolic pressure, indicating an increase in diastolic compliance. Conversely, during demand ischemia, diastolic compliance acutely decreased in patients with coronary artery disease during pacing or exercise-induced angina, in dogs with coronary arterial stenoses and pacing tachycardia, and in isolated hearts with low coronary flow and tachycardia.[35,55-57,74]

These opposite initial compliance changes with demand and supply ischemia may be explained by differences in the pressure and volume within the coronary vasculature, by the mechanical effects of the normal nonischemic myocardium, which is adjacent to the ischemic region, and by tissue metabolic factors. An acute coronary occlusion (supply ischemia) increases diastolic compliance initially because (1) the coronary vasculature distal to the occlusion is collapsed, causing a loss of coronary turgor; (2) the marked decrease in ischemic segmental force development permits repetitive systolic stretching, resulting in ischemic segment lengthening; and (3) tissue acidosis and increased inorganic phosphate levels decrease any calcium mediated diastolic fiber tension. In contrast, with demand ischemia there is less acidosis and less of an increase in inorganic phosphate. The coronary vascular space is not collapsed, and the ischemic segment is not stretched by the surrounding nonischemic myocardium. The sum of these processes results in an acute decrease in diastolic compliance during demand ischemia.[35] After more sustained ischemia (30 minutes to 60 minutes or longer) both demand and supply ischemia result in decreased diastolic compliance.

Importance of Glycolysis in Ischemic Diastolic Dysfunction

Additional evidence that altered ATP levels have a critical role in causing ischemic diastolic dysfunction comes from studies of ischemic glycolysis. During conditions of oxygen supply limitation such as ischemia, the glycolytic pathway becomes a relatively more important source of ATP synthesis because of its ability to achieve ATP synthesis anaerobically. In general, the rate of development of ischemic contracture or diastolic dysfunction is inversely related to the activity of the glycolytic pathway. Metabolic interventions that inhibited glycolysis accelerated the development of ischemic contracture, and provision of additional exogenous glycolytic substrate (a high level of glucose with or without insulin) increased levels of ATP, and partially or completely prevented ischemic contracture.[36,75–78] In studies that compared the sources and rates of ATP production during low-flow ischemia, the rate of glycolytic flux from glucose was the metabolic parameter that best correlated with the prevention or delay of ischemic contracture.[79] Glycolysis also plays a very important role in the diastolic function of certain forms of pressure-overload hypertrophy. Inhibition of glycolysis in hypertrophied hearts resulted in a much greater impairment of diastolic relaxation than in controls.[80] Furthermore, the exaggerated ischemic diastolic chamber stiffness in hypertrophied hearts could be attenuated by the provision of an abundance of glycolytic substrate.[27] In dogs with decompensated hypertrophy after chronic aortic stenosis, exaggerated ischemic diastolic dysfunction was associated with a loss of glycolytic flux.[81]

These results are consistent with the hypothesis that the glycolytic pathway may provide a small but critically localized pool of ATP, which may have a high turnover rate relative to its pool size.[73] In support of this hypothesis, it has been shown in skeletal muscle that certain glycolytic enzymes are bound to the contractile apparatus[72] and that membrane fragments consisting of transverse tubules connected to adjacent terminal cisternae of the sarcoplasmic reticulum contain a compartmentalized glycolytic reaction that is not in equilibrium with the bulk cell ATP stores.[71]

However, although these studies demonstrate the importance of an active glycolytic pathway in protecting against ischemic diastolic dysfunction, they do not define the mechanism of protection ordistinguish between an effect on high energy phosphate metabolites at the level of the myofilaments versus an improvement in sodium and/or calcium homeostasis secondary to increased glycolytic energy supply. Evidence that the protective effect of glycolysis during low-flow ischemia is mediated, at least in part, by improving cation homeostasis comes from recent NMR studies.[48] Provision of glucose to rat hearts during low-flow ischemia protected against ischemic diastolic dysfunction, and this protection was associated with a more active sarcolemmal Na^+/K^+ ATPase activity (sodium pump activity), which prevented an increase in intracellular Na^+ during ischemia. Since intracellular Na^+ excess can lead to cell Ca^{2+} uptake via Na^+/Ca^{2+} exchange, the glucose probably also protected against calcium overload.

From this discussion it is clear that calcium homeostasis, high energy phosphate metabolism, and myocardial relaxation are intimately related and interdependent. During ischemia, either or both processes may become primarily or secondarily abnormal with resultant diastolic dysfunction. The relative importance of primary disturbances of calcium regulation in comparison with high-energy phosphate metabolism, under different circumstances of ischemia and hypertrophy, remains an area of active research.

The Effects of Long-Term Exercise Conditioning on Diastolic Function and Dysfunction

Physiological versus Pathological Hypertrophy: The "Athletic Heart"

In contrast to pressure-overload hypertrophy and its associated diastolic dysfunction, discussed in detail above, the cardiac hypertrophy that occurs in response to endurance exercise training is associated with normal or improved diastolic function. These differences in diastolic function with each type of hypertrophy probably result from differences in the type of overload imposed on the heart. In pathological states such as hypertension or aortic stenosis, a constant, chronic, unrelenting pressure-overload is imposed; with exercise training intermittent, repetitve hormonal, heart rate, volume, and pressure overloads occur, resulting in the "physiological" hypertrophy of the "athletic heart syndrome,"[82] which differs geometrically, morphologically, metabolically, and functionally from the heart with pathological pressure-overload hypertrophy.

During exercise, the heart and circulatory system increase their hemodynamic work to provide the active skeletal musculature with sufficient energy. This task is accomplished by increasing cardiac ouput, stroke volume, heart rate, and arteriovenous oxygen extraction above resting levels. The cardiac output is redistributed primarily from the splanchnic and renal circulation toward the metabolically active skeletal muscle . These circulatory shifts result in acute reductions in renal blood flow and glomerular filtration, which activate the renin-angiotensin-aldosterone system.[83] Coupled with the thermal stress of exercise, these hormonal changes lead to a chronic expansion of the blood volume. With training, blood volume increases approximately 7%,[84] and like other volume loads, may increase end-diastolic wall stress and induce myocardial hypertrophy by augmenting sarcomere replication in series.[85] In addition to the observed four-fold increase in cardiac output with exercise, athletes have a 20% increase in mean arterial pressure and a 70% increase in supine LV filling pressure.[86] Thus, the hemodynamic burden of dynamic endurance exercise is one of a repetitive, intermittent combined volume and pressure overload, resulting in exercise-induced myocardial hypertrophy or the "athletic heart syndrome".[82]

Geometric Features of the Athletic Heart: Consequences for Diastole

Exercise training alters LV geometry, and such geometric changes have the potential to affect diastolic function. The type and extent of geometric alteration depends on the specific sport[87] and whether the associated training requires isotonic, dynamic endurance training, such as distance running or cycling, as opposed to "static-type" exercise, eg, weight lifting. In general, dynamic endurance training causes parallel increases in LV end-diastolic radius and wall thickness such that wall stress, as calculated by the Laplace relation, remains normal. In contrast, static exercise training results in an increase in LV wall thickness relative to radius, similar to the geometric changes that occur with pressure-overload hypertrophy (Figure 11).

Echocardiographic studies have documented LV dimension and wall thickness increases in distance runners,[88] cyclists,[88] and professional basketball players.[89] Morganroth et al[87] characterize these geometric changes as "sport specific" because LV end-diastolic volume and mass, but not wall thickness, were increased in swimmers and runners while wall thickness, but not LV end-diastolic volume was increased in wrestlers and shot-putters. Spirito et al compare cardiac dimensions in 947 elite athletes in 27 sports (Figure 11). Isotonic (dynamic) sports such as endurance cycling, rowing, and swimming significantly increased both LV cavity diastolic dimensions and wall thickness, but track sprint-

Sport	Impact on LVIDd (mm)	Sport	Impact on Wall Thickness (mm)
1) Endurance cycling	5.91	Rowing	2.13
2) Cross-country skiing	5.41	Endurance cycling	2.02
3) Swimming	4.90	Swimming	1.71
4) Pentathlon	4.35	Canoeing	1.70
5) Canoeing	4.23	Long-distance track	1.49
6) Sprint cycling	3.97	Water polo	1.38
7) Rowing	3.87	Sprint cycling	1.35
8) Long-distance track	3.47	Weightlifting	1.23
9) Soccer	3.11	Wrestling/judo	1.21
10) Team handball	2.87	Tennis	1.00
11) Tennis	2.69	Pentathlon	0.98
12) Roller hockey	2.41	Cross-country skiing	0.98
13) Boxing	2.25	Boxing	0.94
14) Alpine skiing	2.13	Roller skating	0.88
15) Fencing	2.09	Soccer	0.76
16) Taekwondo	2.07	Roller hockey	0.69
17) Water polo	2.02	Fencing	0.63
18) Diving	1.70	Sprint track	0.54
19) Roller skating	1.68	Volleyball	0.39
20) Volleyball	1.43	Diving	0.38
21) Bobsledding	1.35	Alpine skiing	0.29
22) Weightlifting	1.32	Field weight events	0.25
23) Wrestling/judo	1.25	Taekwondo	0.23
24) Equestrian	0.43	Team handball	0.19
25) Field weight events	0.18	Equestrian	0.13
26) Yachting	0.10	Bobsledding	0.07
27) Sprint track	0.00	Yachting	0.00

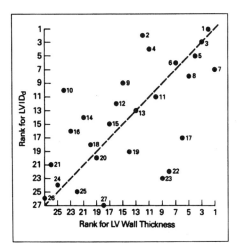

Figure 11. Sport-specific changes in LV geometry after exercise training in 947 elite athletes. In the upper panel 27 sports are ranked on the basis of the impact of training on LV internal diastolic cavity dimension (LVIDd) and LV wall thickness. In the lower panel LVIDd is plotted against LV wall thickness. Most points are near the 45° line of identity, indicating that these sports have a similar impact on LVIDd and wall thickness. Points to the right of the line have a relatively greater increase in wall thickness than in cavity diameter. The 27 sports and their corresponding numbers are listed in the left column of the upper panel. Adapted from Reference 90.

ing, field weights and diving had minimal effects. Sports involving static exertion and valsalva manuevers, such as weightlifting and wrestling, increased wall thickness out of proportion to cavity dimension.[90] Longhurst et al[91] also report that both isotonic and static exercise training increased LV mass; isotonic training increased LV mass out of proportion to lean body mass, whereas, static training increased LV mass proportionally to lean muscle mass.[91]

Diastolic Function Following Exercise Training

The cardiovascular changes which result from endurance exercise training are functionally beneficial in several ways. The increase in end-diastolic volume and stroke-volume improves oxygen uptake ($\dot{V}O_2$), functional capacity, and aerobic capacity.[92,93] Training also induces a relative sinus bradycardia, secondary to increased vagal tone[94] or volume-induced baroreceptor activation, which prolongs the time for diastolic filling.

The physiological hypertrophy associated with dynamic exercise training does not result in impaired diastolic function[92,93,95–102,104] in contrast to the pathological hypertrophy that accompanies chronic hypertension, aortic stenosis, and hypertrophic cardiomyopathy. Although rate-dependent isovolumic relaxation time has been shown to be longer in endurance runners than in control subjects,[103] most studies report that dynamic indices of diastolic filling are either unchanged[97,99,104] or enhanced[92,93,95,96,98,100–102,105,106] following training. When averaged, radionuclide estimates of LV filling were found to be unaltered in long distance runners.[97] However, resting indices of early diastolic filling, ie, transmitral flow velocities, have been found to be slightly increased in endurance runners,[98,101] cyclists,[99] and ultra-endurance athletes.[96] Also, during dynamic exercise in athletes with LV hypertrophy, the echocardiographic peak filling rate, Doppler derived peak filling, and the E/A ratio were greater than age-matched controls, despite a lack of training-induced changes in LV diastolic filling at rest.[102] Other studies have reported that resting and exercise LV diastolic function is improved in trained individuals.[93,101] Matsuda et al[101] report that early diastolic filling is greater in runners at rest and during low level exercise, and Levy et al[93] find that six months of endurance training increases the resting peak early filling rate and peak exercise peak filling rate by approximately 14%.

The Aging Heart: Exercise and Diastole

Exercise training may alter the natural progression of diastolic dysfunction that occurs with age.[93,100,106] As discussed above, aging is associated with an increase in LV mass, LV stiffness, and diastolic dysfunction. A hallmark of age is impaired diastolic filling ie, prolonged time constant of relaxation,[107] decreased peak early filling rate,[108] an increased peak atrial filling rate,[100,109] and a decreased E/A ratio.[100,109] These age-associated alterations in diastolic filling may contribute to the 40% of individuals with CHF and normal systolic function.[110] A comparison of sedentary and distance running 60-year-olds showed that late diastolic filling (Doppler A wave) was reduced by approximately 25% in the runners, however there was no difference in early diastolic filling (Doppler E wave) between groups. Because of the A wave difference, the E/A ratio was greater in the runners.[106] Levy et al[93] observe an improvement in absolute early diastolic filling rates at rest and at all exercise heart rates in the elderly after exercise training. Because maximal oxygen consumption is highly correlated with both resting and exercise measurements of diastolic filling,[93] and both diastolic filling and functional capacity deteriorate with age,[93,106,108] exercise training may have some potential to counteract the functional aerobic impaiment frequently observed in the elderly.

Mechanisms of Improved Diastolic Function by Exercise Training

The mechanistic basis for the improved diastolic function after exercise training is not completely defined, but may be related to exercise-induced changes in myocardial collagen, calcium regulation and/or contractile protein changes. Relatively few studies have examined the effects of exercise on the collagen concentration of the heart. Tomanek[111] shows that exercise training only slightly attenuated the increase in myocardial collagen content that occurs with aging in the rat; nor did training appear to reduce collagen content in young rats[111] or mice.[112] Likewise, swimming did not affect LV type III collagen content,[113] although treadmill running resulted in a small reduction in left and right ventricular collagen content.[114] In dogs, endurance training increased prolyl 4-hydroxylase activity[115] and collagen cross-linking was reduced in rats following training.[116]

Comparison of exercise-trained rats with hypertensive rats showed a marked increase in LV collagen and a reduced rate of LV pressure decay $(-dP/dt)$ with hypertension, but not with exercise training.[117] After exercise training the LV relaxation response to an isoproterenol challenge was improved without alteration of collagen concentration or collagen type.[117]

Changes in excitation-contraction coupling and myocyte metabolism may also contribute to enhanced relaxation in trained hearts. In rats, exercise training improved the rate of LV pressure decay $(-dP/dt)$[118] and the time constant of relaxation,[118] while increasing calcium reuptake by the sarcoplasmic reticulum[119] and Ca^{2+} stimulated myosin ATPase activity.[120] Exercise training also increased LV cytochrome c concentrations and rate of fatty acid oxidation.[121]

Reversal of Pathological Hypertrophy by Exercise Training

Exercise conditioning of rats (8 week to 10 week swimming program) reversed several abnormalities associated with pathological, pressure-overload hypertrophy due to renovascular hypertension, such as the LVH associated decrease in myocardial actomyosin, Ca^{2+} myosin, and actin-activated Mg^{++-} myosin ATPase activities and the increase in myosin isoform V_3 content.[122] The swimming program also partially or completely reversed the LVH-associated abnormalities of cardiac function, coronary flow and oxygen consumption.[123] A similar improvement in cardiac function was observed when swim conditioning was superimposed on the concentric LVH caused by aortic stenosis.[124]

Long-Term Exercise Training and Protection Against Hypoxic and Ischemic Injury

As discussed above, pressure overload hypertrophy has generally been associated with a decreased cardiac tolerance to hypoxia or ischemia and reperfusion. By contrast, exercise training and physiological hypertrophy may increase the heart's tolerance to both hypoxia and ischemia/reperfusion (For review see Starnes, et al [125]). Both swimming[126] and treadmill running[127,128] protected the rat heart from the contractile dysfunction associated with hypoxia and reoxygenation. Swim-trained rat hearts generated greater cardiac outputs and performed more work than untrained controls during hypoxia. Oxygen delivery and energy production were similar between trained and untrained animals, suggesting that training resulted in more efficient myocardial energy utilization.[126] Similarly, treadmill running conditioning of rats reduced the extent of hypoxia-induced contractile dysfunction without differences in myocardial oxygen utilization or energy availability consistent with more efficient myocardial energy utilization with training.[127] Thus, despite one report to the contrary[129] there is strong evidence that both treadmill running and swimming reduce hypoxia-induced contractile dysfunction in the rat.[126-128,130]

Similarly, exercise training appears to reduce the contractile dysfunction caused by ischemia and reperfusion, and the degree of anti-ischemic protection is related to the intensity of the exercise training regimen.[131,132] Although low-intensity running conferred some protection from post-ischemic systolic contractile dysfunction, greater protection was observed with more intense training, ie, interval running. Interval running was also associated with greater post-ischemic phosphocreatine and ATP concentrations, which correlated closely with the level of post-ischemic hemodynamic recovery.[131] Libonati et al report that only treadmill running at high exercise intensities conferred protection from ischemia/reperfusion-induced systolic and diastolic dysfunction.[132] Both isolated hearts and single cardiomyocytes from high intensity trained animals exhibited enhanced post-ischemic contractile function without a change in calcium transient magnitude from the untrained animals. These studies suggest that post-ischemic myofilament calcium senstivity was better maintained in trained hearts, possibly by attenuating calcium overload upon reperfusion.[132] Bowles and Starnes also recently show that moderate-intensity endurance training increased hemodynamic recovery and high energy phosphate content, and was associated with reduced $^{45}Ca^{2+}$ uptake and an increased inotropic response to extracellular calcium during post-ischemic reperfusion.[133] Studies using less intense training programs have not consistently observed protection from ischemia/reperfusion contractile dysfunction.[127,132,134,135]

Anti-oxidant effects may contribute to the mechanisms by which exercise training protects against hypoxic/ischemic/reperfusion injury. Oxygen-derived free radicals are thought to play a potentially important role in acute ischemic-reperfusion injury. Swim training protected the rat heart from oxidative stress.[130] Following 45 minutes of hypoxia, trained rat hearts had less lipid peroxidation and creatine phosphokinase release, concomitant with increased levels of reduced glutathione.[130] Some studies report an increase in antioxidant enzyme levels with training,[130,136,137]while others have found no change[136,138,139] or a decreased antioxidant capacity.[140] The intensity and duration of training appears to affect the anti-oxidant level. Eight weeks of swim training in the mouse heart did not affect antioxidant status, while 21 weeks of swimming increased superoxide dismutase, catalase, and glutathione peroxidase.[136] Only high-intensity training, or moderate-intensity training over long durations, induced increases in LV superoxide dismutase.[132,137] Generally studies utilizing less intense training regimens have found no change[136,138,139] or a decreased antioxidant capacity,[139] suggesting that the level of work performed during training is crucial in determining the antioxidant levels of the heart.[139]

Clinical Considerations: The Diagnosis and Management of Ischemic Diastolic Dysfunction

In 1923, Henderson[141] observed, "If an old man's heart relaxes slowly, his capacity for physical exertion is thus limited, . . . even though the systolic contractions were still like those of youth," and thus recognized that dyspnea with exertion (also occuring at rest in severe cases) is the most characteristic symptom of LV diastolic dysfunction. The shortness of breath results from pulmonary congestion due to elevated pressures in the pulmonary capillaries, pulmonary veins, left atrium and ventricle because of the impairment of LV diastolic filling as illustrated in Figure 1 and Figure 2. Clinical management requires recognition of this condition and therapeutic measures which improve the diastolic physiology and relieve the pulmonary congestion. A general approach to the treatment of diastolic dysfunction is outlined in Table 4 and is adapted from the recommendations of Levine and Gaasch.[142]

Table 4

A General Approach to the Treatment of Diastolic Dysfunction

Treatment Goals	Treatment Methods
1. Reduce central vascular volume to decrease pulmonary capillary pressure	Venodilators (nitrates, ACEI) Diuretics Morphine Tourniquets Salt restriction
2. Maintain atrial contraction	Cardioversion of atrial fibrillation Atrial antiarrhythmics Avoid atrial distension
3. Enhance ventricular systolic emptying	Antihypertensive therapy
4. Regression of hypertrophy	Antihypertensive therapy
5. Control heart rate	Exercise limitation Beta adrenergic blocker Cardioversion of atrial fibrillation Rate control of atrial fibrillation
6. Prevent/treat ischemia	Antihypertensive therapy Control heart rate Lipid-lowering therapy Beta-adrenergic blockers Calcium channel blockers Nitrates Revascularization
7. Improve myocardial relaxation	Calcium channel blockers (?) ACE inhibitors (?)

Adapted from Reference 142.

Diagnosis

The patient with symptomatic LV diastolic dysfunction usually presents with dyspnea on exertion, or in severe cases, at rest. The signs and symptoms are those of left-sided CHF with pulmonary congestion ranging from mild to severe, and are typically worse with exertion. The diagnosis of diastolic dysfunction is made when further evaluation, usually by echocardiography, reveals normal systolic function, ie, a normal ejection fraction, and the absence of valvular disease. In most cases, LV hypertrophy is present on the echocardiogram and/or electrocardiogram, but occasionally it is not. Doppler echocardiography of mitral valve inflow may demonstrate diminished early diastolic filling velocities (an abnormally low E wave) and increased late diastolic filling, as manifest by an increased A wave, if the patient is in normal sinus rhythm. Evidence of ischemia is often present in the form of typical electrocardiographic abnormalities (ST segment and T wave changes), by myocardial perfusion scan defects, and by symptoms of angina pectoris. In patients with marked LVH, subendocardial ischemia is often a contributing or precipitating factor.

Long-Term Management of Patients with Exertional Dyspnea Due to LV Diastolic Dysfunction

During exercise, the aging or hypertensive heart characteristically has preserved systolic function (ejection fraction, cardiac output), but diastolic function is usually impaired.[143,144] Therefore it is not surprising that patients presenting with exertional dyspnea and a normal ejection fraction are more often elderly and/or have LV hypertrophy. Characteristically, these patients show no signs of pulmonary congestion at rest. They may, however, show cardiomegaly by chest x-ray, falsely suggesting LV systolic pump failure. Direct objective assessment of systolic function is very important, since treatment of dyspnea on exertion secondary to pure diastolic dysfunction differs from treatment of dyspnea due to systolic pump failure.

The most important principle is the prevention of recurrent episodes of pulmonary congestion by decreasing or reversing those factors which predispose to diastolic dysfunction. The goals of long-term management of the patient with LV diastolic dysfunction are outlined in Table 4.

In patients with hypertensive LVH, antihypertensive therapy is the mainstay of treatment. The choice of a specific antihypertensive agent must be individualized, as each has specific characteristics relevant to the management of diastolic dysfunction. Regression of LVH is an important therapeutic goal and can be accomplished by effective antihypertensive treatment with diuretics, calcium channel blockers, β-adrenergic blockers, or angiontensin converting enzyme (ACE) inhibitors.[145]

ACE inhibitors possess some features which make them particularly attractive for treating patients with diastolic dysfunction due to hypertensive LVH. Some experimental evidence suggests that ACE inhibitors may reduce the myocardial fibrosis that accompanies hypertensive LVH;[146] this action, if verified clinically, could be a theoretical advantage. Recently, ACE inhibitors have been shown to improve LV diastolic dysfunction in patients with ischemic heart disease,[147] in patients with LVH due to aortic stenosis,[148] and during experimental low-flow ischemia in hypertrophied hearts with ischemic diastolic dysfunction.[8] Furthermore, unlike β-adrenergic and calcium channel blockers, the use of ACE inhibitors is not proscribed by the presence of concomitant systolic dysfunction.

Ischemia often precipitates and/or contributes to diastolic dysfunction. Ischemia can result from the presence of coronary atherosclerosis, LVH with subendocardial ischemia (Table 3), or both. Therefore, drugs with anti-ischemic effects such as the β-adrenergic blockers, calcium antagonists, and nitrates are useful agents.

In addition to their anti-hypertensive action, β-adrenergic blockers provide salutary bradycardic and negative inotropic actions, which reduce myocardial oxygen demand by these mechanisms. Slowing of the heart rate is particularly important in the treatment of pulmonary congestion due to ischemic diastolic dysfunction. In addition to decreasing myocardial oxygen demand, a relative bradycardia increases the duration of diastole, thereby increasing the time available for both coronary flow and LV filling, both of which are usually compromised, especially in patients with LVH and ischemic diastolic dysfunction. Furthermore, the amount of myocyte calcium and sodium entry is directly proportional to the frequency of depolarization or heart rate, and tachycardia can contribute to cellular calcium overload by this mechanism. Thus β-blockers and calcium channel blockers with strong bradycardic actions are particularly useful.

Calcium channel blockers, especially verapamil, have been reported to be useful in the treatment of pure diastolic dysfunction. In a randomized placebo-controlled prospective, cross-over trial in patients with primary diastolic dysfunction, verapamil significantly reduced the signs and symptoms of heart failure and increased LV diastolic filling rate and treadmill exercise time, providing objective evidence of this drug's efficacy in this syndrome.[149] In hypertrophic cardiomyopathy verapamil improved acutely LV diastolic function and prolonged long-term survival.[150] Calcium antagonists have been purported to have a direct "lusitropic" (relaxation enhancing) effect, but it is difficult to distinguish between such an action and benefit that is secondary to reduction or prevention of ischemia.

Both short- and long-acting nitrates may be useful in the management of ischemic diastolic dysfunction because of multiple effects. Their venodilating action reduces central blood volume and pulmonary capillary pressure concomitant with relief of ischemia. Relief of ischemia results from both a decrease in myocardial oxygen demand and improved myocardial perfusion. Oxygen demand is decreasd because the venodilating effect reduces LV volume and wall stress. Myocardial perfusion can be increased by virtue of coronary arterial dilation, relief of coronary vasospasm, and improved collateral flow. The nitrate-induced reduction of LV diastolic pressure also relieves subendocardial vascular compression and improves subendocardial perfusion by this mechanism.

Relief of ischemia by means of coronary artery bypass graft surgery or angioplasty may be required for management of severe drug-resistant ischemic diastolic dysfunction.

An important caveat is that the patient with LV diastolic dysfunction with a small, stiff LV chamber is particularly susceptible to excessive preload reduction with resultant underfilling of the left ventricle, a consequent decrease in stroke-volume and cardiac output, and subsequent hypotension. In patients with severe LV hypertrophy, excessive pre-load reduction can also create a subaortic outflow obstruction. Thus treatment with diuretics or venodilators such as the nitrates, calcium antagonists, and ACE inhibitors must be done cautiously, with careful attention to symptoms of ventricular underfilling such as weakness, dizziness, near-syncope, and syncope.

In patients with chronic atrial fibrillation, where sinus rhythm cannot be restored and maintained, heart rate control is particularly important because the loss of atrial contraction is cumulative with the myocardial resistance to LV filling in contributing to diastolic dysfunction. Digitalis, β-adrenergic blockers, and verapamil are useful in blocking A-V nodal conduction and controlling ventricular rate. It is important to measure heart rate during moderate exercise and to not assume that heart rate control is adequate based on the resting state. Often a combination of these drugs is required to achieve adequate heart rate control.

Management of Patients with Acute Pulmonary Edema

Despite the best management strategy, patients with LV diastolic dysfunction often present with severe pulmonary congestion or pulmonary edema requiring emergent treatment. The treatment goal of acute pulmonary edema for such patients is identical to that for all forms of cardiogenic pulmonary edema: reduction of pulmonary capillary pressure by means of diuretics and vasodilators. Commonly such patients have chronic, inadequately controlled hypertension with secondary LVH. The acute episode of pulmonary edema frequently occurs with concomitant exacerbation of hypertension, and aggresive antihypertensive therapy may be required as part of the treatment of pulmonary edema.

However, as discussed above, the patient with a small, stiff LV chamber is particularly susceptible to excessive preload reduction with resultant underfilling of the left ventricle. Such patients should have frequent monitoring of arterial blood pressure; if hypotension occurs, it can usually be promptly reversed by decreasing the dosage of preload reducing agents and by intravenous volume replacement with saline. Often such patients are hemodynamically unstable and small changes in intravascular volume can have profound effects on the arterial blood pressure and/or on the pulmonary capillary pressure. In such cases, continuous monitoring of the pulmonary capillary pressure and intra-arterial pressure is useful in guiding the administration of vasodilators and intravenous volume replacement.

When a patient presents with acute pulmonary edema, it is often unclear as to whether systolic or diastolic dysfunction (or both) is primarily responsible, and the presence and significance of any concomitant myocardial ischemia may also be uncertain. The relative roles of systolic versus diastolic dysfunction can be rapidly clarified by echocardiography. Until such clarification, treatment with diuretics and vasodilators should proceed to relieve the pulmonary congestion. Intravenous nitroglycerin is particularly useful because it also treats any concomitant ischemia, and its vasodilatory effects can be rapidly and readily titrated in response to hemodynamic changes. The use of ACE inhibitors is not proscribed by the presence of concomitant systolic dysfunction; thus, these agents are theoretically attractive, but their efficacy in the setting of acute pulmonary edema due to diastolic dysfunction has not been definitively established. Similarly, calcium channel blockers without negative inotropic effects (eg, felodipine and amlodipine) have been shown to reduce experimental ischemic diastolic dysfunction without worsening residual ischemic contractile function;[151] such agents are also theoretically attractive, but need to be tested in this specific clinical setting. Both ACE inhibitors and these calcium channel blockers may be useful when anti-hypertensive therapy is required.

Other drugs useful in the treatment of acute pulmonary edema due to diastolic dysfunction are those discussed above under long-term management. In the absence of significant systolic dysfunction, β-adrenergic blockers and calcium channel blockers with negative inotropic effects such as diltiazem and verapamil are potentially useful. These drugs are anti-hypertensive, anti-ischemic, and anti-tachycardic, thus they reverse the triad of factors often responsible for decompensation in pateints with diastolic dysfunction.

The occurrence of atrial fibrillation can precipitate acute pulmonary edema in patients with LVH and diastolic dysfunction as a result of the associated tachycardia, and also because of the loss of atrial contraction. Atrial contraction is particularly important for atrial emptying in such patients because early LV filling is impaired; a disproportionate amount of LV filling and left atrial emptying occurs in late diastole and is dependent on atrial contraction. A decrease in atrial emptying due to atrial fibrillation can result in both increased pulmonary capillary pressure and relative LV underfilling, with a resultant sympathetic drive to increased heart rate. Therefore, rapid restoration of normal sinus rhythm is an important treatment goal.

From this discussion it should be apparent that no simple or single therapeutic plan exists for the management of this condition. Because the major symptom of chronic diastolic dysfunction is dyspnea with exertion, a practical clinical approach is to use the patient's exercise tolerance as a guide to the efficacy of drug therapy, adjusting dosage and adding "combination therapy" accordingly.

Is exercise training potential therapy for CHF due to diastolic dysfunction? The answer is not known, but some observations would support such an approach. As discussed above, a number of clinical studies have reported enhanced dynamic indices of diastolic filling with endurance training.[92,93,95,96,98,100–102,105,106] Furthermore, the elegant experimental work of Scheuer et al[122–124] demonstrates that exercise conditioning can reverse several biochemical and functional features of the pathological hypertrophy that is associated with diastolic dysfunction. Any exercise training program for the potential treatment of diastolic dysfunction should be based on dynamic isotonic exercise, not static exercise, since the latter causes changes in cardiac geometry similar to those of hypertensive LVH (Figure 11).[90] Definitive information regarding the value of exercise training for diastolic dysfunction will require further clinical investigation. Such research would appear to be warranted in light of the importance and prevalance of this clinical syndrome.

References

1. Grossman W. Diastolic dysfunction in congestive heart failure. *New Engl J Med* 1991;325:1557–1564.
2. Packer M. Abnormalities in diastolic function as a potential cause of exercise intolerance in chronic heart failure. *Circulation* 1990;81(suppl III): III-78–III-86.
3. Fifer MA, Bourdillon PD, Lorell BH. Altered left ventricular diastolic properties during pacing-induced angina in patients with aortic stenosis. *Circulation* 1986;74:675–683.
4. Hess OM, Murakami T, Krayenbuehl HP. Does verapamil improve left ventricular relaxation in patients with myocardial hypertrophy? *Circulation* 1986;74:530–543.
5. Topol EJ, Traill TA, Fortuin NJ. Hypertensive hypertrophic cardiomyopathy of the elderly. *N Engl J Med* 1985;312:277–282.
6. Gaasch WH. Diagnosis and treatment of heart failure based on left ventricular systolic or diastolic function. *JAMA* 1994;271:1276–1280.
7. Lorell BH. Left ventricular hypertrophy: The consequences for diastole. In Gaasch WH, LeWinter MM (eds): Left Ventricular Diastolic Dysfunction and Heart Failure. Philadelphia, Lea and Febiger, pp 345–353, 1994.
8. Eberli FR, Apstein CS, Ngoy S, Lorell BH. Exacerbation of left ventricular ischemic diastolic dysfunction by pressure-overload hypertrophy: Modification by specific inhibition of cardiac angiotensin converting enzyme. *Circ Res* 1992;70:931–943.
9. McKenney P, Apstein CS, Mendes LA, et al. Increased left ventricular diastolic chamber stiffness immediately after coronary artery bypass surgery. *J Am Coll Cardiol* 1994;24:1189–1194.

10. McKenney P, Apstein CS, Mendes LA, et al. Marked diastolic dysfunction immediately after aortic valve replacement for aortic stenosis. *J Am Coll Cardiol* 1994(suppl I):278A.

11. Cohen GI, Pietrolungo JF, Thomas JD, Klein AL. A practical guide to assessment of ventricular diastolic function using Doppler echocardiography. *J Am Coll Cardiol* 1996;27: 1753–1760.

12. Hatle L. Doppler echocardiographic evaluation of diastolic function in hypertensive cardiomyopathies. *Eur Heart J* 1993;14(suppl J):88–94.

13. Labovitz AJ, Pearson AC. Evaluation of left ventricular diastolic function: Clinical relevance and recent Doppler echocardiographic insights. *Am Heart J* 1987;114:836–851.

14. Cheng CP, Igarashi Y, Little WC. Mechanism of augmented rate of left ventricle filling during exercise. *Circ Res* 1992;70:9–19.

15. Cheng CP, Noda T, Nozawa T, Little WC. Effect of heart failure on the mechanism of exercise induced augmentation of mitral valve flow. *Circ Res* 1993;72:795–806.

16. Little WC, Cheng CP. Modulation of diastolic dysfunction in the intact heart. In Lorell BH, Grossman W (eds): Diastolic Relaxation of the Heart (Second Edition). Boston, Kluwer Academic Publishers, pp 167–176, 1994.

17. Yellin EL, Nikolic, SD. Diastolic suction and the dynamics of left ventricular filling. In Gaasch WH, LeWinter MM (eds): Left Ventricular Diastolic Dysfunction and Heart Failure. Philadelphia, Lea and Febiger, pp 89–102, 1994.

18. Katz, AM. *Physiology of the Heart*. New York: Raven Press; 1992: pp 178–195.

19. Carroll JD, Hess OM, Hirzel HO, Krayenbuehl HP. Dynamics of left ventricular filling at rest and during exercise. *Circulation* 1983;68:59–67.

20. Carroll JD, Hess OM, Hirzel HO, Krayenbuehl HP. Exercise-induced ischemia: The influence of altered relaxation on early diastolic pressures. *Circulation* 1983;67:521–528.

21. Pepine C, Wiener L. Relationship of anginal symptoms to lung mechanics during myocardial ischemia. *Circulation* 1972;46:863–869.

22. Isoyama S. Interplay of hypertrophy and myocardial ischemia. In Lorell BH, Grossman, W (eds): *Diastolic Relaxation of the Heart (Second Edition)*. Boston, Kluwer Academic Publishers, 1992: 203–211.

23. Tomanek RJ, Wessel TJ, Harrison DG. Capilary growth and geometry during long-term hypertension and myocardial hypertrophy in dogs. *Am J Physiol* 1991;261:H1011–H1018.

24. Eberli FR, Ritter M, Schwitter J, et al. Coronary reserve in patients with aortic valve disease before and after successful aortic valve replacement. *Eur Heart J* 1991;12:127–138.

25. Marcus ML, Koyanagi S, Harrison DG, et al. Abnormalities in the coronary circulation that occur as a consequence of cardiac hypertrophy. *Am J Med* 1983;75:62–66.

26. Ishihara K, Zile MR, Nagatsu M, et al. Coronary blood flow after the regression of pressure-overload left ventricular hypertrophy. *Circ Res* 1992; 71:1472–1481.

27. Cunningham MJ, Apstein CS, Weinberg EO, et al. Influence of glucose and insulin on exaggerated diastolic and systolic dysfunction of hypertrophied rat hearts during hypoxia. *Circ Res* 1990;66:406–415.

28. Lorell BH, Wexler LF, Momomura S, et al. The influence of pressure overload left ventricular hypertrophy on diastolic properties during hypoxia in isovolumically contracting rat hearts. *Circ Res* 1986;58:653–663.

29. Wexler LF, Lorell BH, Momomura S, et al. Enhanced sensitivity to hypoxia-induced diastolic dysfunction in pressure overload hypertrophy in the rat: Role of high energy phosphate depletion. *Circ Res* 1988;62:766–775.
30. Libonati JR, Apstein CS, Ngoy S, et al. No effect of angiotensin II on ischemic diastolic dysfunction in hypertrophied and infarcted rat hearts. *J Am Coll Cardiol* 1996;27:733–3140A.
31. Lorell BH, Grice WN, Apstein CS. Influence of hypertension with minimal hypertrophy during demand ischemia. *Hypertension* 1989;13:361–370.
32. Apstein CS, Morgan JP. Cellular mechanisms underlying left ventricular diastolic dysfunction. In Gaasch WH, LeWinter, MM (eds): *Left Ventricular Diastolic Dysfunction and Heart Failure.* Philadelphia: Lea and Febiger; 1994: 3–24.
33. Applegate RJ, Walsh RA, O'Rourke RA. Effects of nifedipine on diastolic function during brief periods of flow-limiting ischemia in the conscious dog. *Circulation* 1987;76:1409–1421.
34. Bronzwaer JGF, de Bruyne B, Ascoop CAPL, Paulus WJ. Comparative effects of pacing-induced and balloon coronary occlusion ischemia on left ventricular diastolic function in man. *Circulation* 1991;84:211–222.
35. Apstein CS, Grossman W. Opposite initial effects of supply and demand ischemia on left ventricular diastolic compliance: The ischemia-diastolic paradox. *J Mol Cell Cardiol* 1987;19:119–128.
36. Eberli FR, Weinberg EO, Grice WN, et al. Protective effect of increased glycolytic substrate against systolic and diastolic dysfunction and increased coronary resistance from prolonged global underperfusion and reperfusion in isolated rabbit hearts perfused with erythrocyte suspensions. *Circ Res* 1991;68:466–481
37. Kihara Y, Grossman W, Morgan JP. Direct measurement of changes in $[Ca^{2+}]_i$ during hypoxia, ischemia, and reperfusion of the intact mammalian heart. *Circ Res* 1989; 65:1029–1044.
38. Mochizuki T, Eberli FR, Apstein CS, Lorell BH. Exacerbation of ischemic dysfunction by angiotensin II in red cell-perfused rabbit hearts: Effects of coronary flow, contractility, and high-energy phosphate metabolism. *J Clin Invest* 1992;89:490–498.
39. Paulus, WJ, Takashi S, Grossman W. Altered left ventricular diastolic properties during pacing-induced ischemia in dogs with coronary stenoses: Potentiation by caffeine. *Circ Res* 1982;50:218–227.
40. Serizawa T, Vogel WM, Apstein CS, Grossman W. Comparison of acute alterations in left ventricular diastolic chamber stiffness induced by hypoxia and ischemia. *J Clin Invest* 1981;68:91–102.
41. Wexler LF, Weinberg EO, Ingwall JS, Apstein CS. Acute alterations in diastolic left ventricular chamber distensibility: Mechanistic differences between hypoxemia and ischemia in isolated perfused rabbit and rat hearts. *Circ Res* 1986;59:515–528.
42. Camacho SA, Figueredo VM, Brandes R, Weiner MW. Ca^{2+}-dependent fluorescence transients and phosphate metabolism during low-flow ischemia in rat hearts. *Am J Physiol* 1993;265:H114–H122.
43. Lee HC, Mohabir R, Smith N, et al. Effect of ischemia on calcium-dependent fluorescence transients in rabbit hearts containing Indo-1. *Circulation* 1988;78:1047–1059.
44. Marban E, Kitakaze M, Kusuoka H, et al. Intracellular free calcium concentration mesured with ^{19}F NMR spectroscopy in intact ferret heart. *Proc Natl Acad Sci USA* 1987;84:6005–6009.

45. Mohabir R, Lee HC, Kurz RW, Clusin WT. Effects of ischemia and hyperbaric acidosis on myocyte calcium transients, contraction, and pH_i in perfused rabbit hearts. *Circ Res* 1991;69:1525–1537.
46. Steenbergen C, Murphy E, Levy L, London RE. Elevation in cytosolic free calcium concentration early in myocardial ischemia in perfused rat heart. *Circ Res* 1987;60:700–707.
47. Camacho SA, Brandes R, Figueredo VM, Weiner MW. Ca^{2+} transient decline and myocardial relaxation are slowed during low flow ischemia in rat hearts. *J. Clin. Invest.* 1994;93:951–957.
48. Cross HR, Radda GK, Clarke K. The role of Na^+/K^+ ATPase activity during low flow ischemia in preventing myocardial injury: A ^{31}P, ^{23}Na and ^{87}Rb NMR spectroscopic study. *Magnetic Resonance in Medicine* 1995;34:673–685.
49. Koretsune Y, Marban E. Mechanism of ischemic contracture in ferret hearts: Relative roles of $[Ca^{2+}]_i$ elevation and ATP depletion. *Am J Physiol* 1990;258:H9–H16.
50. Allshire A, Piper HM, Cuthbertson KSR, Cobbold PH. Cytosolic free Ca^{2+} in single rat heart cells during anoxia and reoxygenation. *Biochem J* 1987; 244:381–385.
51. Miyata H, Lakatta EG, Stern MD, Silverman HS. Relation of mitochondrial and cytosolic free calcium to cardiac myocyte recovery after exposure to anoxia. *Circ Res* 1992;71:605–613.
52. Eberli FR, Ferrell MA, Apstein CS. Role of calcium in diastolic dysfunction. *Circulation* 1990;82(suppl III):III-605.
53. Eberli FR, Ferrell MA, Ngoy S, Apstein CS. Role of calcium and calcium-sodium exchange on diastolic dysfunction. *Circulation* 1991;84(suppl II):II-211.
54. Eberli FR, Ngoy S, Bernstein E, Apstein CS. More evidence against calcium overload as direct cause of ischemic diastolic dysfunction. *Circulation* 1992; 86:(suppl I):I-480.
55. Varma N, Eberli FR, Apstein CS. Calcium sensitivity of diastolic dysfunction is dissociated in demand ischemia compared to reperfusion, suggesting differing roles for increased myocyte calcium. *Circulation* 1994;90(suppl I):I-432.
56. Varma N, Eberli FR, Apstein CS. Diastolic dysfunction during demand ischemia is due to a reversible rigor force and is not a calcium activated tension. *J Am Coll Cardiol* 1995; Special Issue, 27A.
57. Varma N, Eberli FR, Ngoy S, Apstein CS. Subcellular mechanisms of ischemic diastolic dysfunction: Further evidence for rigor force in pathogenesis and not for Ca^{2+} activated diastolic tension. *Circulation* 1995;92(suppl I):I-657.
58. Hearse DJ, Garlick PB, Humphrey SM. Ischemic contracture of the myocardium: Mechanisms and prevention. *Am J Cardiol* 1977;39:986–993.
59. Lowe JE, Jennings RB, Reimer KA. Cardiac rigor mortis in dogs. *J Mol Cell Cardiol* 1979;11:1017–1031.
60. Allen DG, Orchard CH. Intracellular calcium concentration during hypoxia and metabolic inhibition in mammalian ventricular muscle. *J Physiol (Lond)* 1983;339:107–122.
61. Cobbold PH, Bourne PK. Aequorin measurements of free calcium in single heart cells. *Nature* 1984;312:444–446.
62. Haigney MCP, Miyata H, Lakatta EG, et al Dependence of hypoxic cellular calcium loading on Na^+-Ca^{2+} exchange. *Circ Res* 1992;71:547–557.
63. Kingsley PB, Sako EY, Yang MQ, et al Ischemic contracture begins when anaerobic glycolysis stops: A ^{31}P-NMR study of isolated rat hearts. *Am J Physiol* 1991;261:H469-H478.

64. Allen DG, Orchard CH. Myocardial contractile function during ischemia and hypoxia. *Circ Res* 1987;60:153–168.
65. Ventura-Clapier R, Mekhfi H, Vassort G. Role of creatine kinase in chemically skinned rat cardiac muscle. *J Gen Physiol* 1987;89:815–837.
66. Bowers KC, Allshire AP, Cobbold PH. Bioluminescent measurement in single cardiomyocytes of sudden cytosolic ATP depletion coincident with rigor. *J Mol Cell Cardiol* 1991;24:213–218.
67. Ventura-Clapier R, Veksler V. Myocardial ischemic contracture metabolites affect rigor tension development and stiffness. *Circ Res* 1994;74: 920–929.
68. Yamashita H, Sata M, Sugiura S, et al. ADP inhibits the sliding velocity of fluorescent actin filaments on cardiac and skeletal myosins. *Circ Res* 1994;74: 1027–1033.
69. Illingworth JA, Ford WCB, Kobayashi K, Williamson JR. Regulation of myocardial energy metabolism. *Recent Adv Stud Card Struct Metab* 1975;8: 271–290.
70. Bessman SP, Yang WCT, Geiger PJ, Erickson-Viitanen S. Intimate coupling of creatine phosphokinase and myofibrillar adenosintriphophatase. *Biochem Biophysic Res Comm* 1980;96:1414–1420.
71. Han JW, Thielczek R, Varsanyi M, Herlmeyer LMG. Compartmentalized ATP synthesis in skeletal muscle triads. *Biochemistry* 1992;31:377–384.
72. Kurganov BI, Sugrobova NP, Mil'man LS. Supramolecular organization of glycolytic enzymes. *J Theor Biol* 1985;116:509–526.
73. Weiss J, Hiltbrand B. Functional compartmentation of glycolytic versus oxidative metabolism in isolated rabbit heart. *J Clin Invest* 1985;75:436–447.
74. Isoyama S, Apstein CS, Wexler LF, et al. Acute decrease in left ventricular diastolic chamber distensibility during simulated angina in isolated hearts. *Circ Res* 1987;61:925–933.
75. Apstein CS, Deckelbaum L, Hagopian L, Hood WB Jr. Acute cardiac ischemia and reperfusion. Contractility, relaxation and glycolysis. *Am J Physiol* 1978;235 *(Heart Circ Physiol 6):*H637–H648.
76. Apstein CS, Gravino FN, Haudenschild CC. Determinants of protective effect of glucose and insulin on the ischemic myocardium: Effects on contractile function, diastolic compliance, metabolism and ultrastructure during ischemia and reperfusion. *Circ Res* 1983;52:515–526.
77. Schaefer S, Prussel E, Carr LJ. Requirement of glycolytic substrate for metabolic recovery during moderate low flow ischemia. *J Mol Cell Cardiol* 1995; 27:2167–2176.
78. Vanoverschelde J-L J, Janier MF, Bakke JE, et al. Rate of glycolysis during ischemia determines extent of ischemic injury and functional recovery after reperfusion. *Am J Physiol* 1994;267*(Heart Circ Physiol 36):*H1785–H1794.
79. Owen P, Dennis S, Opie LH. Glucose flux regulates onset of ischemic contracture in globally underperfused rat hearts. *Circ Res* 1990;66:406–415.
80. Kagaya Y, Weinberg EO, Ito N, et al. Glycolytic inhibition: Effects on diastolic relaxation and intracellular calcium handling in hypertrophied rat ventricular myocytes. *J Clin Invest* 1995 95:2766–2776.
81. Gaasch WH, Zile MR, Hoshino PK, et al. Tolerance of the hypertrophic heart to ischemia. *Circulation* 1990;81:1644–1653.
82. Maron BJ. Structural features of the athlete heart as defined by echocardiography. *J Am Coll Cardiol* 1986,7:190–203.
83. McArdle WD, Katch FI, Katch VL. *Essentials of Exercise Physiology.* Philadelphia: Lea and Febiger; 1994.

84. Convertino VA. Blood volume: Its adaptation to endurance training. *Med Sci Sports Exerc* 1991:23:1338–1348.
85. Grossman W, Jones D, McLaurin LP. Wall Stress and patterns of hypertrophy in the human left ventricle. *J Clin Invest* 1975,56:56–64.
86. Bevegard S, Holmgren A, Jonsson B. Circulatory studies in well trained athletes at rest and during heavy exercise, with special reference to stroke volume and the influence of body position. *Acta Physiol Scand* 1963;57: 26–50.
87. Morganroth J, Maron BJ, Henry WL, Epstein SE. Comparative left ventricular dimensions in trained athletes. *Ann Intern Med* 1975:82;521–524.
88. Snoeckx LHEH, Abeling HFM, Lambregts JAC, et al. Echocardiographic dimensions in athletes in relation to their training programs. *Med Sci Sports Exer* 1982;14:428–434.
89. Roeske WR, O'Rourke RA, Klein A, et al. Noninvasive evaluation of ventricular hypertrophy in professional athletes. *Circulation* 1976;53:286–292.
90. Spirito P, Pelliccia A, Proschan MA, et al. Morphology of the "athlete's heart" assessed by echocardiography in 947 elite athletes representing 27 sports. *Am J Cardiol* 1994;74:802–806.
91. Longhurst JC, Kelly AR, Gonyea WJ, Mitchell JH. Chronic training with static and dynamic exercise: Cardiovascular adaptation and response to exercise. *Circ Res* 1981;48 (suppl I):I171–178.
92. Di Bello V, Santoro G, Talarico L, et al. Left ventricular function during exercise in athletes and in sedentary men. *Med Sci Sports Exerc* 1996;28: 190–196.
93. Levy WC, Cerqueira MD, Abrass IB, et al. Endurance exercise training augments diastolic filling at rest and during exercise in healthy young and older men. *Circulation* 1993;88:116–126.
94. Smith ML, Hudson DL, Graitzer HM, Raven PB. Exercise training bradycardia: The role of autonomic balance. *Med Sci Sports Exer* 1989;21:40–44.
95. Colan SD, Sanders SP, MacPherson D, Borow KM. Left ventricular diastolic function in elite athletes with physiologic cardiac hypertrophy. *J Am Coll Cardiol* 1985;6:545–549.
96. Douglas PA, O'Toole ML, Hiller DB, Reichek N. Left ventricular stucture and function by echocardiography in ultraendurance athletes. *Am J Cardiol* 1986;58:805–809.
97. Granger CB, Karimeddini MK, Smith VE, et al. Rapid ventricular filling in left ventricular hypertrophy: I. Physiologic hypertrophy. *J Am Coll Cardiol* 1985;5:862–868.
98. Finkelhor RS, Hanack LJ, Bahler RC. Left ventricular filling in endurance-trained subjects. *J Am Coll Cardiol* 1986;8289–8293.
99. Fagard R, Broeke CVD, Bielen E, et al. Assessment of stiffness of the hypertrophied left ventricle of bicyclists using left ventricular inflow doppler velocimetry. *J Am Coll Cardiol* 1987;9:1250–1254.
100. Foreman DE, Manning WJ, Hauser R, et al. Enhanced left ventricular diastolic filling associated with long-term endurance training. *J Gerntol* 1992;47:M56–M58.
101. Matsuda M, Sugishita Y, Koseki S, et al. Effect of exercise on left ventricular diastolic filling in athletes and nonathletes. *J Appl Physiol (Respirat Environ Exercise Physiol* 1983;55:323–328.
102. Nixon JV, Wright AR, Porter TR, et al. Effects of exercise on left ventricular diastolic performance in trained athletes. *Am J Cardiol* 1991:68;945–949.
103. Underwood RH Schwade JL. Noninvasive analysis of cardiac function in

elite distance runners-echocardiography, vectorcardiography, and cardiac intervals. *Ann NY Acad Sci* 1977;301:297–309.

104. Shapiro LM, Smith RG. Effect of training on left ventricular structure and function: An echocardiographic study. *Br Heart J* 1983;50:534–539.
105. Senior DG, Waters KL, Cassidy M, et al. Effect of aerobic training on left ventricular diastolic filling. *Conn Med* 1989;53:67–70.
106. Takemoto KA, Berstein L, Lopez JF, et al. Abnormalities of diastolic filling of the left ventricle associated with aging are less pronounced in exercise trained individuals. *Am Heart J* 1992;124:143–148.
107. Hirota Y. A clinical study of left ventricular relaxation. *Circulation* 1980;62: 756–763.
108. Arora RR, Machac J, Goldman ME, et al. Atrial kinetics and left ventricular diastolic filling in the healthy elderly. *J Am Coll Cardiol* 1987;9:1255–1260.
109. Iskandrian AS, Hakki AH. Age-related changes in left ventricular diastolic performance. *Am Heart J* 1986;112:75–78.
110. Dougherty AH, Naccerelli GV, Gray EL, et al. Congestive heart failure with normal systolic function. Am J Cardiol 1984:54:778–782.
111. Tomanek RJ, Taunton CA, Liskop KS. Relationship between age, chronic exercise, and connective tssue of the heart. *J Gerontol* 1972;27:33–38.
112. Kiiskinen A, Heikkinen E. Physical Training and connective tissues in young mice heart. *Eur J Appl Physiol* 1976;35:167–171.
113. Medugorac I, Jacob R. Characterization of left ventricular collagen in the rat. *Cardiovasc Res* 1983;17:15–21.
114. Masumura S, Furui T, Hara K, et al. Collagen content in the hearts of exercised rats. *Int Res Commun Syst Med Sci* 1983:11:995–996.
115. Takala TES, Ramo P, Kiviluoma K, et al. Effects of training and anabolic steriods on collagen synthesis in dog heart. *Eur J Appl Physiol* 1991;62:1–6.
116. Thomas DP, McCormick RJ, Zimmerman SD, et al. Aging-and training-induced alterations in collagen characteristics of the rat left ventricle and papillary muscle. *Am J Physiol* 1992:263:H778–H783.
117. Burgess ML, Buggy J, Price RL, et al. Exercise-and hypertension-induced collagen changes are related to left ventricular function in rat hearts. *Am J Physiol* 1996; 270:H151–H159.
118. Bersohn MM, Scheuer J. Effects of physical training on end-diastolic volume and myocardial performance of isolated rat hearts. *Circ Res* 1977;40: 510–516.
119. Penpargkul S, Repke DI, Katz AM, Scheuer J. Effect of physical training on calcium transport by rat cardiac sarcoplasmic reticulum. *Circ Res* 1977;40: 134–138.
120. Pagani ED, Solaro RJ. Swimming exercise, thyroid state and the distribution of myosin isoenzymes in rat heart. *Am J. Physiol* 1983;245:H713–H720.
121. Starnes JW, Beyer RE, Edington DW. Myocardial adaptations to endurance exercise in aged rats. Am J. Physiol 1983;245:H560–H566.
122. Scheuer J, Malhotra A, Hirsch G, et al. Physiologic cardiac hypertrophy corrects contractile protein abnormalities associated with pathologic hypertrophy in rats. *J Clin Invest* 1982;70:1300–1306.
123. Schaible TF, Ciabbrone GJ, Capasso JM, Scheuer J. Cardiac conditioning ameliorates cardiac dysfucntion associated with renal hypertension in rats. *J Clin Invest* 73:1086–1094.
124. Buttrick PM, Malhotra A Scheuer J. Effects of systolic overload and swim training on cardiac mechanics and biochemistry in rats. *J Appl Physiol* 64:1466–1471.

125. Starnes JW, Bowles DK. Role of Exercise in the Cause and Prevention of Cardiac Dysfunction. In JP Holloszy ed: *Exercise and Sport Sciences Reviews,V23.* Baltimore: Williams and Wilkens, Baltimore; 349–373.
126. Scheuer JA,.Stezoski S. Effect of physical training on the mechanical and metabolic response of the rat heart to hypoxia. *Circ Res* 1972;30:418–429.
127. Carey RA, Tipton CM, Lund DR. Influence of training on myocardial responses of rats subjected to conditions of ischemia and hypoxia. *Cardiovasc Res* 1976;10:359–367.
128. Cutiletta AF, Edmistion K, Dowell RT. Effect of a mild exercise program on myocardial function and the development of hypertrophy. *J Appl Physiol* 1979;46:354–360.
129. Fuller EO, Nutter DO. Endurance training in the rat II: Performance of isolated and intact heart. *J Appl Physiol* 1981;51:941–947.
130. Kihlstrom M. Protection effect of endurance training against reoxygenation-induced injuries in rat heart. *J Appl Physiol* 1990;68:1672–1678.
131. Bowles DK, Farrar RP, Fordyce DE, Starnes JW. Exercise training improves cardiac function after ischemia in the isolated, working rat heart. *Am J Physiol* 1992;263:804–809.
132. Libonati JR, Gaughan JP, Hefner CA, et al. Reduced ischemia and reperfusion injury following exercise training. *Med Sci Sports Exer* 1996;in press.
133. Bowles DK, Starnes JW. Exercise training improves metabolic response after ischemia in isolated, working rat heart. *J Appl Physiol* 1994:76(4):1608–1614.
134. Korge P, Mannick G. The effect of regular physical exercise on the sensitivity to ischemia in the rat's heart. *Eur J Appl Physiol* 1990;61:42–47.
135. Paulson DJ, Kopp SJ, Peace CG, Tow JP. Improved postischemic recovery of cardiac pump function in exercise trained diabetic rats. *J Appl Physiol* 1988;65:187–193.
136. Kanter MM, Hamlin RL, Unverferth DV et al. Effect of exercise training on antioxidant enzymes and cardiotoxicity of doxorubicin. *J Appl Physiol* 1985;59:1298–1303.
137. Powers SK, Criswell D, Lawler J, et al. Rigorous exercise training increases superoxide dismutase activity in ventricular myocardium. *Am J Physiol* 1993;265:H2094–H2098.
138. Higuchi M,Cartier LJ, Chen M, Holloszy JO. Superoxide dismutase and catalase in skeletal muscle: Adaptive response to exercise. *J Gerontol* 1985;40:281–286.
139. Ji, LL. Exercise and oxidative stress: Role of the cellular antioxidant systems. *Exerc Sport Sci Rev* 1995;23:135–166
140. Ji LL, Fu RG, Mitchell E,et al. Cardiac hypertrophy alters myocardial response to ischemia and reperfusion in vivo. *Acta Physiol Scand* 1994;151:279–290.
141. Henderson Y. Volume changes of the heart. *Physiol Rev* 1923;3:165–208.
142. Levine HJ and Gaasch WH. Clinical recognition and treatment of diastolic dysfunction and heart failure. In Gaasch WH, LeWinter MM eds: *Left Ventricular Diastolic Dysfunction and Heart Failure.* Philadelphia: Lea and Febiger; 1994;439–454.
143. Kitzman DW, Higginbotham MB, Cobb FR, et al. Exercise intolerance in patients with heart failure and preserved left ventricular systolic function: Failure of the Frank-Starling mechanism. *J Am Coll Cardiol* 1991;17:1065–1072.
144. Nixon JV, Burns CA. Cardiac effects of aging and diastolic dysfunction in

the elderly. In Gaasch WH, LeWinter MM eds: *Left Ventricular Diastolic Dysfunction and Heart Failure*. Philadelphia: Lea and Febiger;1994:427–435.

145. Dahloef B, Pennert K, Hansson L. Reversal of left ventricular hypertrophy in hypertensive patients. A metaanalysis of 109 treatment studies. *Am Heart J* 1992;5:95–110.

146. Weber KT, Brilla CG. Pathological hypertrophy and cardiac interstitium. *Circulation* 1991;83:1849–1865.

147. Rousseau MF, Gurne O, van Eyll C, et al. Effects of Benazeprilat on left ventricular systolic and diastolic function and neurohumoral status in patients with ischemic heart diesease. *Circulation* 1990;81(suppl III):III-123–129.

148. Friedrich SP, Lorell BH, Rousseau MF, et al. Intracardiac angiotensin-converting enzyme inhibition improves diastolic function in patients with left ventricular hypertrophy due to aortic stenosis. *Circulation* 1994;90: 2761–2771.

149. Setaro JF, Zaret BL, Schulman DS et al.Usefulness of verapamil for congestive heart failure associated with abnormal left ventricular diastolic filling and normal left ventricular systolic performance. *Am J Cardiol* 1990;66:981–986.

150. Hess OM, Krayenbuehl HP. Beta-adrenergic receptor blockers and calcium channel blockers in left ventricular hypertrophy. In Gaasch WH, LeWinter MM eds: *Left Ventricular Diastolic Dysfunction and Heart Failure*. Philadelphia: Lea and Febiger; 1994:455–464.

151. Bernstein EA, Eberli FR, Silverman AM, et al.The calcium channel blocker felodipine protects against ischemia-reperfusion injury by a mechanism other than reducing O_2 demand. *Cardiovasc Drugs Ther* 1996; in press.

Chapter 5

Neurohormonal Responses to Exercise in Heart Failure

Gary S. Francis, MD

Introduction

Patients with congestive heart failure are well known to have breathlessness and fatigue at rest or with minimal exercise. Over the years there has been extraordinary effort on the part of many investigators to better understand the mechanism of exertional dyspnea in heart failure. It now seems clear that, except for the case of pulmonary edema, this is not simply due to excessive pulmonary capillary wedge pressure or inadequate cardiac output. Multiple mechanisms are likely to account for exercise intolerance in the syndrome of heart failure. These include abnormalities of the central circulation; skeletal muscles; physical deconditioning; increased ventilatory dead space; exaggerated ventilatory response; diminished performance of respiratory muscles; increased interstitial fluid in the lungs; and perhaps abnormal reflex control mechanisms involving J-receptors in the lungs.

It has long been known that systemic neuroendocrine activation occurs in patients with heart failure. It therefore seems logical that the measurement of neurohormones at rest and during exercise may lead to further enlightenment regarding the possible role of neuroendocrine activation as a mechanism contributing to exercise intolerance in the syndrome of heart failure.

Plasma Norepinephrine

Plasma norepinephrine concentration and many other neurohormones and cytokines are known to be increased in patients with chronic

From: Balady GJ, Piña IL (eds). *Exercise and Heart Failure*. Armonk, NY: Futura Publishing Company, Inc.; ©1997.

heart failure who are in the resting state (Table 1). Changes in plasma norepinephrine occurring with progression of the syndrome may be due to either reduced clearance or increased production of the neurotransmitter.[1] It now seems clear that increases in certain neurohormones, particularly norepinephrine, may have important implications regarding the pathophysiology of heart failure.[2] More is known about the role of plasma norepinephrine in heart failure than other neurohormones.[3-9]

The response of neurohormones to exercise in patients with heart failure has been less well-studied. It was reported by Rowell[10] in 1974 that patients with heart failure have greater intensity of splanchnic vasoconstriction than normal subjects during exercise, suggesting heightened sympathetic drive to certain vascular regions during exercise. One decade earlier, Chidsey and colleagues[11] reported an augmented generalized sympathetic response to exercise in patients with heart failure as measured by increased plasma norepinephrine. These authors consider an excessive sympathetic response to have a "supportive" role during exercise.[11] Since then, numerous authors have demonstrated increased plasma norepinephrine in the syndrome of heart failure at rest and during exercise. The increase in plasma norepinephrine during exercise is thought largely to be due to enhanced release rather than reduced clearance.[12] The actual mechanism and the clinical importance of this observation have, however, remained unclear.

In 1982 Francis and colleagues[13] confirm the earlier work of Chidsey et al,[11] and extend the results to indicate that patients with heart failure have higher basal levels of plasma norepinephrine which abruptly increase with even limited exercise. It was observed, however, that maximal plasma norepinephrine levels during exercise in patients with heart failure failed to achieve the much higher peak values observed in strenuously exercised normal subjects.[13] In the study by Francis et al, patients

Table 1

Neuroendocrine Factors Known to be Increased in Patients with Heart Failure

Norepinephrine	Endothelin
Epinephrine	β-endorphins
Renin activity	Calcitonin gene-related peptide
Angiotensin II	Growth hormone
Aldosterone	Cortisol
Arginine vasopressin	Tumor necrosis factor-alpha (TNF-α)
Neuropeptide Y	Neurokinin A
Vasoactive intestinal peptide	Substance P
Prostaglandins	Adrenomedullin
Atrial natriuretic factor	TNF-α soluble receptors/receptor antagonists

with heart failure increased their basal plasma norepinephrine levels from 650 ± 95 ($\pm$SEM) to 1721 ± 198 pg/mL at an average maximum oxygen consumption ($\dot{V}O_{2max}$) of 10.3 mL/kg/min, whereas normal subjects increased their plasma norepinephrine from 318 ± 36 to 3230 ± 418 pg/mL while achieving an average $\dot{V}O_{2max}$ of 35.0 mL/kg/min (Figure 1). Of course, the patients with heart failure were unable to exercise to the same maximal extent as normals, which may have limited the rate of rise of their plasma norepinephrine concentration.

Although it seems clear that patients with heart failure have an augmented sympathetic response to exercise as measured by the observed abrupt rise in plasma norepinephrine, such patients exercise far less maximally than normal subjects. Therefore, it was considered useful to compare normal subjects to patients with heart failure when they were

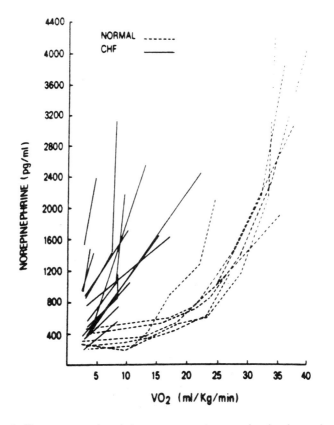

Figure 1: Plasma norepinephrine response to exercise is shown in dashed lines for normal subjects and in solid lines for patients with congestive heart failure (CHF). $\dot{V}O_2$ = total body oxygen consumption. From Reference 13, with permission.

exercising in the same physiologic framework, ie, at an equivalent level of work. To perform this comparison, Francis et al[14] incrementally exercised both patients with heart failure and normal subjects, and express the plasma norepinephrine data for both groups as percent peak $\dot{V}O_{2max}$, rather than as a function of absolute oxygen consumption. When the plasma norepinephrine (NE) data were expressed as a function of percent peak $\dot{V}O_{2max}$, patients with heart failure demonstrated a slower rate of rise of plasma norepinephrine, as manifested by a flatter slope than normal (p = 0.002) in response to exercise (Figure 2).[14] One interpretation of these data is that patients with heart failure may actually have a relative attenuation of sympathetic nervous system activity during exercise for any given amount of work. However, others have demonstrated that the overall sympathetic response during steady-state exercise in patients with heart failure results in more release and higher plasma norepinephrine concentrations when using the norepinephrine spillover technique,[12] thus implying that differing methodologies may produce varying results. This controversy has remained unresolved.

A.   **B.**

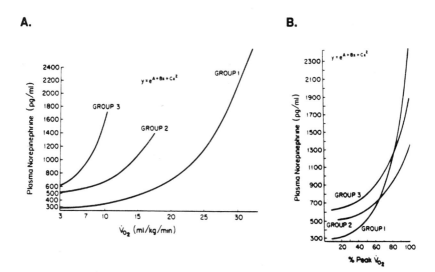

Figure 2: Three groups of patients are studied: group 1 is 10 healthy normal subjects; group 2 is 11 patients with mild heart failure (able to exercise at least 100 watts); group 3 is 20 patients with severe heart failure (failure to exercise to 75 watts). In A, there is a clear separation of the curves (p = 0.004), with the patients having severe heart failure demonstrating a much lower $\dot{V}O_{2max}$ and an abrupt increase in plasma norepinephrine. In B, the same patients are plotted as a function of relative work intensity, expressed as % $\dot{V}O_{2max}$ (all are in a comparable physiological framework as % $\dot{V}O_{2max}$). Now the patients with heart failure have a flatter slope (p = 0.002) than normal subjects, suggesting an attenuated sympathetic response to exercise. From Reference 14, with permission.

One matter of concern is that group mean plasma norepinephrine levels may be reproducible from one week to another, but individual plasma norepinephrine levels are not.[15] Moreover, the onset of dynamic exercise does not produce mass uniform sympathetic discharge in humans, but muscle chemoreflexes and central command appear to produce differential effects on sympathetic and parasympathetic responses.[16] During the initiation of dynamic exercise in humans there is a concomitant delay in the onset of sympathetic activation to nonexercising skeletal muscle and to the heart.[16] Age[17] and gender [18] may also influence the response of catecholamines to exercise. Therefore, measuring simple plasma norepinephrine values at rest and at peak exercise may not represent the overall picture.

There have been very few studies investigating the relationship between treatment and exercise-induced catecholamines in patients with heart failure. One study demonstrated no significant reduction in plasma norepinephrine in response to exercise following the use of single-dose captopril.[19] Creager and colleagues[19] studied 12 patients with heart failure during supine bicycle exercise before and after administration of 25 mg of captopril. The angiotensin-converting enzyme (ACE) inhibitor failed to change plasma norepinephrine either at rest or following exercise.[19] On the contrary, McGrath and Arnolda demonstrate that enalapril, also an ACE inhibitor, reduces the catecholamine response to exercise in patients with heart failure.[20] The chronic pharmacologically-induced reduction in plasma norepinephrine at rest in patients with heart failure is now known to be small, and it may be very difficult to further demonstrate a meaningful reduction in plasma norepinephrine with drugs during maximal exercise.

The Renin-Angiotensin-Aldosterone System and Arginine Vasopressin

While the plasma renin-angiotensin system is well known to be activated in patients with advanced heart failure at rest,[21] there is little information regarding its measurement during exercise in such patients. The same is true for arginine vasopressin (AVP). Their measurement is confounded by the fact that maximal exercise may alter plasma osmolality and blood volume, which in turn can influence AVP and renin activity. Kirlin and associates[22] were the first to measure plasma osmolality, plasma AVP, and plasma renin activity in patients with heart failure at rest and during strenuous exercise. Of interest, there were no significant differences in plasma osmolality at rest or during exercise between normal subjects and 14 patients with New York Heart Association Class II and III heart failure (Figure 3). Similar to the findings of

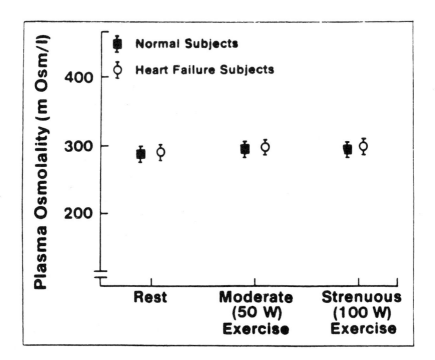

Figure 3: Plasma osmolality at rest and during exercise in normal subjects (■) and patients with heart failure (O). No significant differences were seen either at rest or during exercise. Data are mean ± SEM. From Reference 22, with permission.

others,[23-25] these investigators found baseline plasma AVP to be increased in patients with heart failure at rest. During moderate exercise (50 watts), the difference between normal subjects and patients with heart failure persisted, but during strenuous exercise, normal subjects increased their plasma AVP levels, whereas patients with heart failure had unchanged plasma AVP levels (Figure 4).

Plasma renin activity, as expected, was elevated at rest in the patients with heart failure. Moderate exercise did not change plasma renin activity in either normal subjects or patients with heart failure (Figure 5), but strenuous exercise (100 watts) substantially increased the plasma renin activity in patients with heart failure. The two-fold rise in plasma renin activity during exercise in patients with heart failure suggests activation of renin secretion. Although the clinical implications of this finding are not clear, the observations are consistent with the concept that markedly diminished renal blood flow occurs during exercise in animal models of heart failure.[26] Bayliss and co-workers[27] note that plasma aldosterone concentrations also rise during exercise in

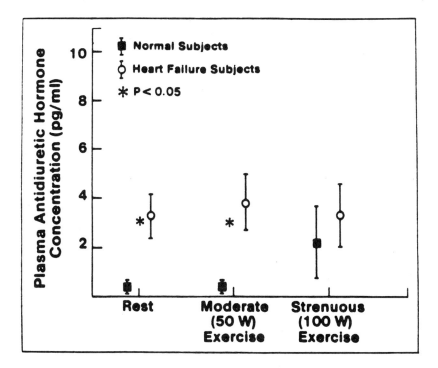

Figure 4: Plasma AVP concentration at rest and during exercise. Patients with heart failure had significantly higher concentrations at rest and during moderate (50 watts) exercise. However, during strenuous (100 watts) exercise, there was an increase in normal subjects, whereas patients with heart failure demonstrated no change. Data are mean ± SEM. From Reference 22, with permission.

patients with heart failure, which suggests that the circulating peptide angiotensin II remains biologically active during exercise. However, it is questionable whether angiotensin II plays a role in interfering with blood flow to working skeletal muscle during exercise in patients with heart failure.[28]

Interpretation of the Data

Measuring neurohormones during exercise in patients with heart failure is relatively straightforward, but interpreting the data can be difficult. Exercise intolerance is a hallmark of heart failure, and it has become common to measure exercise time or $\dot{V}O_{2max}$ in clinical drug trials. Patients with chronic heart failure are frequently limited during maximal exercise even when they are only minimally symptomatic at rest. The mechanism of exercise intolerance in patients with heart fail-

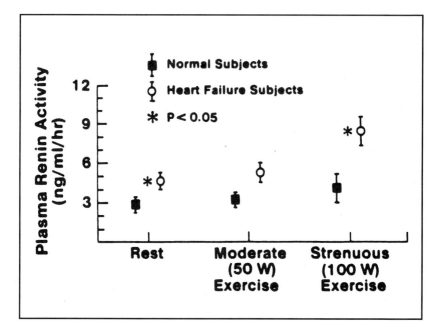

Figure 5: Plasma renin activity at rest and during exercise. Patients with heart failure have significantly elevated levels at rest, with a substantial increase during strenuous exercise (100 watts). Normal subjects have only a slight increase during exercise. Data are mean ± SEM. From Reference 22, with permission.

ure has been very difficult to define.[28] The severity of exercise intolerance and fatigue correlate poorly with indexes of resting cardiac function. There may be reduced flow to exercising muscle,[29] but there are also important primary abnormalities of skeletal muscle.[30] Many investigators have measured diminished skeletal muscle blood flow in heart failure, but description of the actual mechanism for the impairment in flow has been elusive. Skeletal muscle vasodilator capacity does not seem to be intrinsically impaired in patients with nonedematous chronic heart failure.[31] Acute increments in blood flow induced by dopamine or dobutamine do not improve exercise tolerance in patients with heart failure.

Reduced blood flow to peripheral tissues occurs both at rest and during exercise in patients with heart failure. Reduced flow leads to recruitment of compensatory vasoconstrictor mechanisms which may "protect" central blood pressure and redirect flow to most vital organs. These so-called "compensatory" mechanisms include activation of the sympathetic nervous system and the renin-angiotensin system. It is therefore natural that investigators would be interested in measuring plasma norepinephrine and plasma renin activity at rest and during the stress of exercise. These neurohormone measurements, in my opinion, have, however, failed to provide much enlightenment regarding the mechanism of how exercise intolerance occurs. The role of the renin-angiotensin system during exercise is questionable, since angiotensin II does not seemingly interfere with blood flow to working skeletal muscle.[28] The "augmented" rise in plasma norepinephrine observed during exercise in patients with heart failure may serve to benefit the patient by sustaining arterial blood pressure.[32] At the very least, the increased sympathetic drive during exercise does not seem to adversely affect blood flow to working skeletal muscles. It is therefore tempting to conclude that the excessive neuroendocrine activation during exercise is not directly related to exercise intolerance that is typically manifested in the syndrome of heart failure. Rather, heightened neuroendocrine activity during exercise may simply be a marker of severity of disease. This concept gains support from the observation that carvedilol, a drug which provides nearly complete adrenergic blockade, is generally not accompanied by any substantial short- or long-term improvement in maximal exercise tolerance.[33]

Conclusions

Patients with heart failure have increased resting plasma levels of many neurohormones, including norepinephrine, renin activity, and AVP. It now seems clear that plasma norepinephrine and plasma renin activity are increased during strenuous dynamic exercise in patients with heart failure. The real question is whether or not these increased levels are playing a pathophysiological role in the well-known reduced exercise tolerance of heart failure. This question remains unanswered to date, in part because we lack the methodology to study regional circulatory changes in detail, and also because we have no pharmacological means to consistently inhibit their augmentation during exercise without further altering peripheral flow mechanisms.

References

1. Hasking GJ, Esler MD, Jennings GL, et al. Norepinephrine spillover to plasma in patients with congestive heart failure: Evidence of increased overall and cardiorenal sympathetic nervous activity. *Circulation* 1986;4: 615–621.
2. Packer M. The neurohormonal hypothesis: A theory to explain the mechanism of disease progression in heart failure. *J Am Coll Cardiol* 1992;20: 248–254.
3. Francis GS. Neurohormones in congestive heart failure. *Cardiol Rev* 1993;1:5: 278–289.

4. Thomas JA, Marks BH. Plasma norepinephrine in congestive heart failure. *Am J Cardiol* 1978;41:233–243.
5. Levine TB, Francis GS, Goldsmith SR, et al. Activity of the sympathetic nervous system and renin-angiotensin system assessed by plasma hormone levels and their relation to hemodynamic abnormalities in congestive heart failure. *Am J Cardiol* 1982;49:1659–1666.
6. Meredith IT, Eisenhofer G, Lambert GW, et al. Cardiac sympathetic nervous activity in congestive heart failure. *Circulation* 1993;88:136–145.
7. Leimbach WN, Wallin BG, Victor RG, et al. Direct evidence from intraneural recordings for increased central sympathetic outflow in patients with heart failure. *Circulation* 1986;73:5:913–919.
8. Ferguson DW, Berg WJ, Sanders JS. Clinical and hemodynamic correlates of sympathetic nerve activity in normal humans and patients with heart failure: Evidence from direct microneurographic recordings. *J Am Coll Cardiol* 1990;16:1125–1134.
9. Kaye DM, Lefkovits J, Jennings GL, et al. Adverse consequences of high sympathetic nervous activity in the failing human heart. *J Am Coll Cardiol* 1995;26:1257–1263.
10. Rowell LB. Human cardiovascular adjustments to exercise and thermal stress. *Physiol Rev* 1974;54:75–1959.
11. Chidsey CA, Harrison DC, Braunwald E. Augmentation of the plasma norepinephrine response to exercise in patients with congestive heart failure. *N Engl J Med* 1962;267:650–654.
12. Hasking GJ, Esler MD, Jennings GL, et al. Norepinephrine spillover to plasma during steady-state supine bicycle exercise. *Circulation* 1988;78: 516–521.
13. Francis GS, Goldsmith SR, Ziesche SM, Cohn JN. Response of plasma norepinephrine and epinephrine to dynamic exercise in patients with congestive heart failure. *Am J Cardiol* 1982;49:1152–1156.
14. Francis GS, Goldsmith SR, Ziesche S, et al. Relative attenuation of sympathetic drive during exercise in patients with congestive heart failure. *J Am Coll Cardiol* 1985;5:832–839.
15. Peronnet F, Blier P, Brisson G, et al. Reproducibility of plasma catecholamine concentrations at rest and during exercise in man. *Eur J Appli Physiol* 1986;54:555–558.
16. Victor RG, Seals DR, Mark AL. Differential control of heart rate and sympathetic nerve activity during dynamic exercise. *J Clin Invest* 1987;79:508–516.
17. Lehmann M, Keul J, Korste-Reck U. The influence of graduated treadmill exercise on plasma catecholamines, aerobic and anaerobic capacity in boys and adults. *Eur J Appl Physiol* 1981;47:301–311.
18. Lehmann M, Keul J, Berg A, et al. Plasma catecholamines and aerobic-anaerobic capacity in women during graduated treadmill exercise. *Eur J Appl Physiol* 1981;46:305–315.
19. Creager MA, Faxon DP, Weiner DA, et al. Haemodynamic and neurohumoral response to exercise in patients with congestive heart failure treated with captopril. *Br Heart J* 1985;53:431–435.
20. McGrath BP, Arnolda LF. Enalapril reduces the catecholamine response to exercise in patients with heart failure. *Eur J Clin Pharmacol* 1986;30:485–487.
21. Dzau VJ, Colluci WS, Hollenberg NK, et al. Relation of the renin-angiotensin-aldosterone system to clinical state in congestive heart failure. *Circulation* 1981;63:645–651.

22. Kirlin PC, Grekin R, Das S, et al. Neurohumoral activation during exercise in congestive heart failure. *Am J Med* 1986;81:623–629.
23. Szatalowica VL, Arnold PE, Chaimovita C, et al. Radioimmunoassay of plasma arginine vasopressin in hyponatremic patients with congestive heart failure. *N Engl J Med* 1981;305:263–266.
24. Riegger GAJ, Liebau G, Kochsiek K. Antidiuretic hormone in congestive heart failure. *Am J Med* 1982;72:49–52.
25. Goldsmith SR, Francis GS, Cowley AW, et al. Increased plasma arginine vasopressin levels in patients with congestive heart failure. *J Am Coll Cardiol* 1983;1:1385–1390.
26. Higgins CB, Vatner SF, Franklin D, Braunwald E. Effects of experimentally produced heart failure on the peripheral vascular response to severe exercise in conscious dogs. *Circulation* 1972;31:186–194.
27. Bayliss J, Norell M, Canepa-Anson R, et al. Neuroendocrine and hemodynamic interactions at rest and during exercise in chronic heart failure: Double-blind comparison of captopril and prazosin (abstr). *Circulation* 1984;70 (suppl II):II-1673.
28. Zelis R, Sinoway LI, Musch TI. Why do patients with congestive heart failure stop exercising? *J Am Coll Cardiol* 1988;12:359–361.
28. Wilson JR, Ferraro N. Effect of the renin-angiotensin system on limb circulation and metabolism during exercise in patients with heart failure. *J Am Coll Cardiol* 1985;6:556–563.
29. Wilson JR, Martin JL, Schwartz D, et al. Exercise intolerance in patients with chronic heart failure: Role of impaired nutritive flow to skeletal muscle. *Circulation* 1984;69:1079–1087.
30. Massie BM, Simonini A, Sahgal P, et al. Relation of systemic and local muscle exercise capacity to skeletal muscle characteristics in men with congestive heart failure. *J Am Coll Cardiol* 1996;27:140–145.
31. Wilson JR, Wiener DH, Fink LI, et al. Vasodilatory behavior or skeletal muscle arterioles in patients with nonedematous chronic heart failure. *Circulation* 1986;74:775–779.
32. Wilson JR, Ferraro N, Wiener DH. Effect of the sympathetic nervous system on limb circulation and metabolism during exercise in patients with heart failure. *Circulation* 1985;1:72–81.
33. Olsen SL, Gilbert EM, Renlund DG, et al. Carvedilol improves left ventricular function and symptoms in chronic heart failure: A double-blind randomized study. *J Am Coll Cardiol* 1995;25:1225–1231.

Chapter 6

The Transplanted Heart

Jon A. Kobashigawa, MD

Introduction

Cardiac transplantation is the therapy of choice for end-stage heart disease. Despite major advances in organ preservation and immuno-suppression, the function of the cardiac allograft is not normal. The donor heart is denervated and has altered physiology,[1] which has significant effects on exercise tolerance. The physiological components of the denervated heart include ventricular loading conditions, circulating catecholamine levels, myocardial contractile capabilities, donor/recipient size mismatch, and the effects of atrial contraction with the standard atrial cuff anastomosis surgery. These components may be responsible for abnormal hemodynamics including restrictive physiology early and late after transplantation and increased resting heart rate. Denervation of the cardiac allograft also leads to impaired renin-angiotensin-aldosterone regulation and impedes normal vasoregulatory response to changes in intracardiac filling pressures. These physiological factors and many others (Table 1) affect exercise tolerance in the heart transplant recipient, and will be discussed in this chapter.

Cardiac Denervation

Cardiac transplantation involves removing the diseased heart and leaving an atrial cuff[2] which results in the complete denervation of the donor heart, with loss of both afferent and efferent nerve connections (Figure 1).[3–5] Therefore, the donor heart rate will not respond to vagolytic muscle relaxants, anticholinergics, anticholinesterases, digoxin, nifedipine, phenylephrine, or nitroprusside. Afferent denervation alters cardio-

From: Balady GJ, Piña IL (eds). *Exercise and Heart Failure*. Armonk, NY: Futura Publishing Company, Inc.; ©1997.

Table 1

Factors Affecting Function of the Transplanted Heart

Hemodynamic
  Donor/recipient body size relation
  Donor/recipient atrial asynchrony
  Early postoperative restrictive physiology
  Late postoperative restrictive physiology

Denervation
  Afferent denervation
    Altered reflex control of peripheral vasoconstriction/vasodilation
    Altered NA^+/H_2O regulation via central nervous system—dependent
      vasopressin, renin, angiotensin, aldosterone secretion
  Efferent denervation
    Absent vagal nerve control
    Rapid heart rate at rest
    Attenuated heart rate response to exercise
  Hypersensitivity to circulating catecholamines

Altered hormonal milieu
  Atrial natriuretic peptide secretion changed
  Elevated exercise circulating catecholamines

Myocardial injury/maladaptation
  Organ preservation/recovery injury
  Intraoperative complications
  Rejection
  Ventricular hypertrophy
  Hypertension (increased ventricular wall stress)
  Allograft arteriopathy (ischemia)

From Reference 1.

vascular homeostasis by impairing renin-angiotensin-aldosterone regulation, impeding the normal vasoregulatory response to changing cardiac filling pressures,[6] eliminating the normal diurnal variation in blood pressure,[7] and eliminating the subjective experience of angina.[8] Braith et al[9] suggest that ablation of the cardiac afferent nerves may disinhibit the cardiorenal neuroendocrine reflex. This may result in the increase in renal nerve activity and renal vascular resistance, reduction of glomerular filtration rate, and the increase in vasopressin, plasma renin activity, angiotensin II, and aldosterone. The authors suggest that these effects would impair the ability to excrete salt, leading to abnormal blood pressure and fluid homeostasis in heart transplant recipients. Efferent denervation results in loss of sympathetic and parasympathetic nervous system effects. These include increasing the resting heart rate, eliminating the influence on the heart of vagal signaling from the central nervous sys-

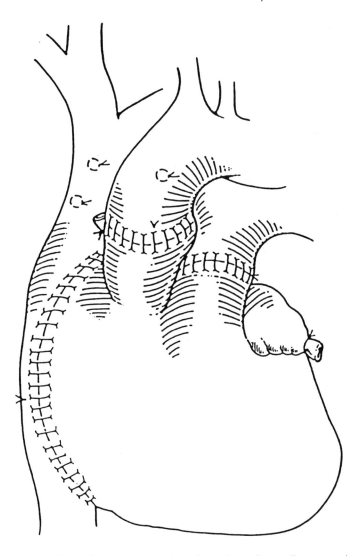

Figure 1: The mid-atrial surgical technique for orthotopic cardiac transplantation. The posterior walls of the recipient atria are left in place and sutured to the donor heart, which has had its posterior atrial walls removed. From Reference 2.

tem,[10] blunting the usual rapid changes in heart rate and contractility during exercise, hypovolemia, or vasodilation.[11]

Cardiac reinnervation has recently been demonstrated, but this phenomenon appears to be both delayed and incomplete. Stark et al[8] demonstrate a tyramine-induced cardiac epinephrine release response indicative of reinnervation in two patients with angina and transplant coronary artery disease. Wilson et al[12] studied norepinephrine release in heart transplant patients in response to tyramine and sustained handgrips, and suggest that reinnervation commonly occurs, but the pattern of reinnervation is extremely variable. Recently, Burke et al[13] report that stimulation of reinnervating sympathetic neurons with tyramine in transplant patients causes a significant but subnormal increase in left ventricular contraction and a transient decrease in coronary blood flow velocity. This suggests that reinnervation can produce physiologically meaningful changes in left ventricular function and coronary artery tone.

Electrophysiology

The mid-atrial cuff transplant surgical technique allows for the presence of two P waves on the electrocardiogram. The P wave from the remnant of the recipient atria does not transmit past the anastomosis suture lines, which accounts for one P wave being asynchronous. The resting heart rate of the denervated heart is usually between 90 beats and 110 beats per minute due to the loss of vagal tone. Alexopoulos et al[14] demonstrate through the use of 24-hour Holter monitoring that transplanted hearts compared to normal volunteers have higher average heart rates, similar maximum heart rate, significantly higher minimum heart rate, and reduced heart rate variability. The altered sinus node response in the denervated heart is consistent with a dominant effect of the autonomic nervous system on resting sinus node fluctuation. In contrast, there appears little autonomic nervous system influence on the atrioventricular and His-Purkinje conduction systems in the resting denervated heart.[15] Clinically significant atrial and ventricular arrhythmias are infrequent following cardiac transplantation, although atrial arrhythmias are associated with cardiac rejection. Prolonged bradyarrhythmias (>24 hours) were reported by Miyamoto et al[16] in 401 patients, with less than 5% of patients requiring a permanent pacemaker, but the majority of these patients returned to sinus rhythm within 1 year.

Neuroendocrine Response

Various studies have suggested an increased sensitivity to the effects of β-adrenergic agonists, particularly with respect to chronotropic actions, as a means to compensate for the lack of innervation.[17,18] The mechanisms for this increased sensitivity appear to involve increased

β_2-receptors[19,20] and/or presynaptic lack of neuronal uptake of catecholamines.[18] Brodde et al[21,22] report gradually increasing β_2-receptors with increasing time after transplant. The β_2-receptor is responsive to epinephrine and is therefore thought to be the "epinephrine receptor."[23] While plasma catecholamine levels are markedly elevated in patients with severe congestive heart failure, normalization of plasma levels of norepinephrine occurs at about 2 weeks following heart transplant. Norepinephrine levels are markedly elevated with exercise, as compared with healthy subjects, but are not chronically elevated at rest. Similarly, the hypersecretion of vasopressin and plasma renin activity is observed during exercise. This is believed to be a result of ablation of the cardiac mechanoreceptor afferents.[24]

Plasma volume generally increases about 15% in cyclosporine-treated transplant patients.[25] This is linked to cyclosporine and corticosteroid-mediated renal fluid retention and to an abnormal cardiorenal neuroendocrine reflex, which contribute to an increase in intracardiac filling pressures and to a diluted hematocrit. Atrial natriuretic peptide is reportedly increased in heart transplant patients.[26] However, the kidneys appear refractory to its effects although the mechanism is not clear.

Myocardial Function at Rest

The denervated heart requires mechanisms other than neural to function normally in daily activities. The Frank-Starling mechanism remains a major factor in the transplanted heart, and thus cardiac transplant patients are often referred to as "preload dependent." In the presence of hypotension or hypovolemia, the denervated heart cannot respond with a reflex tachycardia, but rather it responds primarily with an increase in stroke volume. Increases in venous return with a subsequent increase in left ventricular end-diastolic volume results in an increase in stroke volume and thus ejection fraction, by means of the Frank-Starling mechanism. Therefore, assurance of adequate preload is especially important in the heart transplant patient prior to the administration of anesthesia.[27]

Hemodynamics in heart transplant patients may be abnormal immediately after transplant due to inadequate preservation, acute withdrawal of sympathetic myocardial support, or afterload mismatch. However, ventricular function quickly recovers and the resting cardiac output is usually normal or low. Since the resting heart rate is usually elevated, the resting stroke volume is therefore small. Systolic and diastolic hypertension is seen in up to 90% of post-transplant patients as a result of cyclosporine therapy.[28] Left ventricular wall mass may be increased, possibly due to compensation for hypertension or due to the effects of cyclosporine or as a result of no lymphatic drainage in the donor heart.[29] Up to one third of the patients may exhibit an elevated pulmonary capillary wedge pressure, most likely due to a combination of depressed systolic function, decreased compliance, and hypervolemia.[30] However, the majority of cardiac transplant patients have stable hemodynamics longterm after transplant, as reported by Tischler et al in a 4-year longitudinal study.[31] The mid-atrial anastomosis between donor and recipient heart is reported to have an effect on cardiac function.[32] Since the native and donor atria do not contract synchronously, less than the expected 15% to 20% of the normal atrial contribution to the net stroke volume is seen, however, the clinical impact is not known.[1]

Systolic function of the denervated heart has been found to be relatively well preserved in longitudinal echocardiographic and radiopaque myocardial marker studies.[23,33,34] Von Scheidt et al[35] find normal contractility of the denervated transplanted heart in 30 of 34 patients with a mean post-transplant interval of 27 months. They conclude that the activity of cardiac autonomic nerves is not necessary to provide normal baseline contractility of the human heart.

A restrictive hemodynamic pattern has been documented early postoperatively that resolves within days or weeks.[31] A subclinical latent restrictive hemodynamic state may persist for much longer.[36] In approximately 10% to 15% of patients, a persistently impaired ventricular filling late after transplant may occur, usually due to graft rejection.[37] Donor/recipient heart size mismatch may also affect resting hemodynamics. At 3 months after transplant, there is a reported negative linear relationship between resting heart rate, right atrial pressure, pulmonary capillary wedge pressure, and the donor-to-recipient body weight ratio. However, by 1 year postoperative, the effect was not significant.

Myocardial Function During Exercise

The manner in which the denervated heart responds to exercise is similar to the normal heart except for the sequence of physiological mechanisms used.[50] In the transplanted heart, the initial response to exercise is an increased stroke volume secondary to increased venous return, which is due to a combination of muscle and thoracic pumping and to decreased peripheral vascular resistance. Through this mechanism, stroke volume can be increased by up to 20%, thus increasing cardiac output via the Frank-Starling mechanism. If exercise is more vigorous, further increases of cardiac output are mediated by chronotropic and inotropic responses to circulating catecholamines (Figure 2). This contrasts to the normal heart, where increased stroke volume and heart rate occur simultaneously rather than sequentially.

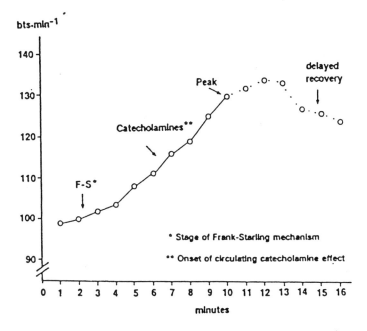

Figure 2: Typical transplanted denervated heart rate response to increasing effort. Note the high resting rate, the delayed rate of acceleration during effort, the delayed deceleration during recovery, and the tendency for the rate to continue to rise after the termination of effort (peak exercise). From Reference 50.

The response to exercise is abnormal in heart transplant patients,[7,35,46] but appears adequate to enable the patients to perform the activities of daily life. Table 2 summarizes the abnormal exercise physiology in heart transplant patients. Initiating physical activities is slower for heart transplant patients, who require 6 minutes to 10 minutes of steady work to increase heart rate compared with 2 minutes to 3 minutes in subjects without a denervated heart.[38] Over the first year after transplant, myocardial response to exercise improves, probably the result of increasing β_2-receptor density of the denervated donor heart. However, even with this β-adrenergic supersensitivity to the action of plasma epinephrine, the chronotropic response at the peak of effort is reduced.[39–41] Niset et al[42] report that at 1 month after transplant, during vigorous exercise, the heart rate may continue to climb after cessation of exercise for the next 2 minutes in the recovery period. However, at 1 year, this heart rate increase at the end of the effort is no longer present. This finding is also observed by Folino et al[43] who studied patients more than 3 years after transplant. Limited reinnervation may play a role in this observation.

The peak heart rate, cardiac output, and ventricular ejection fraction are subnormal when compared to healthy controls.[35] Since there is

---

Table 2

Abnormal Exercise Physiology in Heart Transplant Patients

Increased resting heart rate
Delayed heart rate increase at onset of exercise
Delayed return to resting heart rate after cessation of exercise
Decreased resting left ventricular ejection fraction
Decreased exercise right and left ventricular ejection fractions
Reduced exercise cardiac output
Increased exercise arterial-mixed venous oxygen difference
Decreased maximal oxygen uptake
Reduced maximal power output
Slower oxygen uptake kinetics during exercise
Reduced anaerobic threshold
Increased exercise ventilatory equivalents for oxygen and carbon dioxide
Increased exercise left ventricular end-diastolic pressure
Increased exercise pulmonary artery, pulmonary capillary wedge, and right
   atrial pressures
Increased exercise left ventricular end-systolic and diastolic volume indices

---

From Reference 2.

a normal or elevated rise in circulating catecholamines at peak exercise[6,44] and the responsiveness of the sinoatrial node to β-adrenergic stimulation is normal or increased, the most likely reason for the attenuated peak heart rate response to exercise after transplant is lack of direct innervation of the sinoatrial node.[45,46] Using blood pool radionuclide angiography in 28 heart transplant patients, Verani et al[47] report that during exercise there were significant increases in left and right ventricular ejection fractions; however, they were significantly lower than in normal subjects. Therefore, it appears that heart transplant patients have mildly impaired ventricular functional reserve at maximum exercise stress.

Hemodynamics in response to exercise are dependent on loading conditions. During exercise, intracardiac filling pressures (right atrium, pulmonary artery, pulmonary capillary wedge pressures) are elevated. In a study by Clark et al,[48,49] the left ventricular end diastolic pressure at 4 minutes to 6 minutes of exercise in heart transplant patients averaged 21 mm Hg compared with values of 12 mm Hg in normal volunteers. Elevation of intracardiac pressures during mild to moderate exercise, associated with a slightly lower cardiac output elevation, can unmask a latent persistent pulmonary hypertension limiting exercise stroke volume adaptation. This may be responsible for mild pulmonary congestion during exercise and, while stimulating pulmonary J-receptors, lead to the restrictive breathing pattern documented at exercise among some heart transplant recipients.

Niset et al[42] observe that oxygen uptake during exercise testing was low at 1 month and 1 year after transplant compared to expected values (Figure 3). In addition, peak oxygen consumption was 42% and 58% of predicted values at 1 month and 1 year after transplant, respectively. The immediate functional consequence of the low-peak oxygen consumption in transplant patients is that exercise is quickly halted by fatigue. Kavanaugh[50] reports that heart transplant patients during submaximal effort demonstrate normal oxygen uptake, higher minute ventilation, higher perceived exertion, higher ventilatory equivalent for oxygen, and lower absolute ventilatory threshold, thus implying an earlier onset of anaerobic metabolism. Savin et al[51] report that transplant patients had higher peak lactate levels and ventilatory effort but lower peak oxygen uptake and peak work rates compared with normal subjects, also suggesting an earlier onset of anaerobic metabolism. Therefore, anaerobic metabolism occurs at a lower power output in heart transplant recipients compared to normal volunteers. Lactate production is increased relative to normal controls, with a resultant increase in ventilation and ventilatory equivalent for oxygen. However, the oxygen consumption at anaerobic threshold is substantially lower relative to both normal subjects and to age-matched general surgery patients.[29] Table 3 illustrates the distribution of heart transplant patients according to functional class as measured by cardiopulmonary exercise testing at 1 month and 1 year after transplant. It is noteworthy that approximately

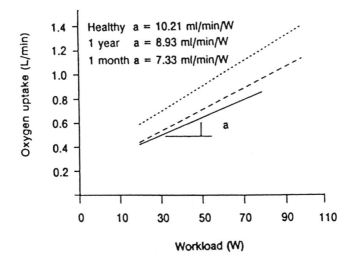

Figure 3: Oxygen uptake during incremental maximal exercise test: healthy subjects (short dashed line), heart recipients 1 month (solid line) and 1 year (long dashed line) postoperatively. From Reference 42.

Table 3

Heart Transplant Recipients Distribution in Functional Class
(as Measured by Cardiopulmonary Stress Testing)
1 Month and 1 Year After Transplant

Class	1 Month	1 Year
I	12.8%	42.5%
II	38.3%	48.1%
III	46.8%	5.6%
IV	2.1%	3.7%

Modified from Reference 42.

57% of heart transplant patients are still New York Heart Association functional Class II to Class IV at 1 year after transplant.

Isometric exercise in cardiac transplant patients results in no increase in cardiac output due to the denervated heart, however, there is the expected increase in blood pressure. This pressor response is most likely from an increase in α-adrenergic tone mediated by the central nervous system and not from increased circulating catecholamines.[7]

Other Factors Affecting Cardiac Performance

Early after heart transplantation, skeletal muscle atrophy may affect exercise, which may limit exercise capabilities.[52,53] In the immediate postoperative period, the transplant patient has a 10% to 50% reduction in lean body mass due to prolonged preoperative physical inactivity, together with high corticosteroid administration.[50,54] Consequently, maximal work output is reduced, and maximal oxygen uptake is only two-thirds of the normal age-matched population. Therefore, in early exercise testing of transplant patients, anaerobic metabolism commonly occurs before peak exercise levels are reached.[50] Many of these exercise parameters improve later after transplant, once muscle mass and physical condition is restored.

Acute rejection may affect both systolic and diastolic function. Moriguchi et al[55] reviewed 400 echocardiograms in 49 transplant patients and report a correlation of decreased left ventricular ejection fraction (measured by Simpson's rule) to acute rejection. The diastolic dysfunction associated with acute rejection is similar to that observed in restrictive cardiomyopathy, with reduced end-diastolic volume and peak filling. In a recent report, Chan et al[56] report decreased coronary flow reserve in heart transplant patients experiencing acute rejection, with return to baseline levels after successful antirejection therapy. This would imply that in the presence of acute rejection there may be impairment of ventricular function during exercise. The development of transplant coronary artery disease, which is observed in up to 50% of all heart transplant patients by 5 years after transplant, may affect both systolic and diastolic function. As the donor heart is denervated, angina is usually not experienced and silent myocardial infarctions may occur.

More recently, the bicaval anastomosis technique has been used to perform heart transplantation (Figure 4).[57] This differs from the standard

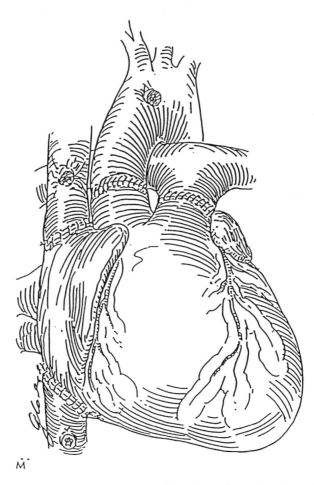

Figure 4: The bicaval surgical technique for orthotopic cardiac transplantation. Donor atria are intact and anastomoses are performed in both cava as well as the pulmonary veins. From Reference 7.

mid-atrial anastomosis by keeping both atria intact and performing anastomoses in both cava as well as the pulmonary veins. This avoids dyssynchronous atrial contractions and may improve cardiac performance by contributing more blood flow to the ventricles. Freimark et al[58] report that the bicaval technique produced more physiological atrial function compared with the mid-atrial technique, as evidenced by greater atrial ejection via Doppler echocardiography.

Exercise Training

Exercise training has been reported to be beneficial after heart transplantation;[2,29,42,50,] however, all studies involved selected patients. We performed a randomized trial[59] of 24 heart transplant patients randomized to either a structured cardiac rehabilitation program (11 patients) or to routine exercise at home (13 patients). The patients randomized to cardiac rehabilitation participated in an average of 20 sessions which included use of the exercise treadmill along with personalized exercise instruction. Cardiopulmonary exercise testing was performed within 4 weeks after transplant and repeated at 6 months after transplant in both groups. The patients in the cardiac rehabilitation group compared to the control group demonstrated a trend to greater exercise time (+2.6 minutes versus +1.0 minutes in the control group), significantly greater improvement in peak oxygen consumption (+6.4 mL/kg/min versus +2.6 mL/kg/min in the control group), and work load (+40 watts versus +12 watts in the control group), and a significantly improved reduction in ventilatory efficiency (−14 versus −5 ventilatory equivalent for carbon dioxide in the control group). We concluded that structured cardiac rehabilitation appeared to be beneficial in attaining a greater exercise capacity after heart transplantation.

Summary

Experience and success with heart transplantation has led to the understanding of the pathophysiology of the denervated heart. Understanding the importance of preload, the electrophysiology of the denervated heart, the altered response to exercise, and the potential complications after transplant will be necessary to provide appropriate care for the heart transplant patient. Finally, the finding that the donor heart does not respond normally to exercise permits us to appreciate the functional limitations of many heart transplant patients and perhaps suggest therapy that may improve their functional state.

References

1. Young JB, Winters WL, Bourge R, Uretsky BF. Task force four: Function of the heart transplant recipient. *J Am Coll Cardiol* 1993;22:31–41.
2. Squires RW. Exercise training after cardiac transplantation. *Med Sci Sports Exerc* 1991;23:686–694.
3. Willman VL, Cooper T, Cian LG, et al. Neural responses following auto-transplantation of the canine heart. *Circulation* 1963;27:713–716.
4. Donald DE, Shephard JT. Response to exercise in dogs with cardiac dener-vation. *Am J Physiol* 1963;205:393–400.
5. Gilmore JP, Daggett WN. Response of the chronic cardiac denervated dog to acute volume expansion. *Am J Physiol* 1966;210:509–512.
6. Schuler S, Thomas D, Thebken M, et al. Endocrine response to exercise in cardiac transplant patients. *Transplant Proc* 1987;19:2506–2509.
7. Gaer J. Physiological consequences of complete cardiac denervation. *Br J Hosp Med* 1992;48:220–224.
8. Stark RP, McGinn AL, Wilson RF. Chest pain in cardiac transplant recipi-ents. Evidence of sensory reinnervation after cardiac transplantation. *N Engl J Med* 1991;324:1791–1794.
9. Braith RW, Mills RM, Wilcox CS, et al. Breakdown of blood pressure and body fluid homeostasis in heart transplant recipients. *J Am Coll Cardiol* 1996;27:375–383.
10. Uretsky BF. Physiology of the transplanted heart. *Cardiovasc Clin* 1990;20: 23–56.
11. Tsakiris AG, Donald DE, Rutishaver WJ, et al. Cardiovascular responses to hypertension and hypotension in dogs with denervated hearts. *J Appl Phys-iol* 1969;27:817–821.
12. Wilson RF, Christensen BV, Olivari MT, et al. Evidence for structural sym-pathetic reinnervation after orthotopic cardiac transplantation in humans. *Circulation* 1991;83:1210–1220.
13. Burke MN, McGinn AL, Homans DC, et al. Evidence for functional sym-pathetic reinnervation of left ventricle and coronary arteries after ortho-topic cardiac transplantation in humans. *Circulation* 1995;91:72–78.
14. Alexopoulos D, Yusuf S, Johnson JA, et al. The 24-hour heart rate behavior in long-term survivors of cardiac transplantation. *Am J Cardiol* 1988;61:880–884.
15. Bextonn RS, Nathan AW, Hellestrand KJ, et al. The electrophysiologic char-acteristics of the transplanted human heart. *Am Heart J* 1984;107:1–7.
16. Miyamoto Y, Curtiss EI, Kormos RL, et al. Bradyarrhythmia after heart transplantation. *Circulation* 1990;82(suppl IV):IV-313–IV-317.
17. Borow KM, Neumann A, Arensman FW, et al. Left ventricular contractility and contractile reserve in humans after cardiac transplantation. *Circulation* 1985;71:866–872.
18. Gilbert EM, Eiswirth CC, Mealey PC, et al. Beta-adrenergic supersensitiv-ity of the transplanted human heart is presynaptic in origin. *Circulation* 1989;79:344–349.
19. Steinfath M, von der Leyen H, Hecht A, et al. Decrease in beta-1- and in-crease in beta-2-adrenoreceptors in long-term follow-up after orthotopic cardiac transplantation. *J Mol Cell Cardiol* 1992;24:1189–1198.
20. Farrukh HM, White M, Port JD, et al. Up-regulation of beta-2-adrenergic re-ceptors in previously transplanted, denervated nonfailing human hearts. *J Am Coll Cardiol* 1993;22:1902–1908.
21. Brodde OE, Khamssi M. Development of beta-adrenoceptor number in the

transplanted human heart. *Naunyn Schmiedebergs Arch Pharmacol* 1991;343 (suppl)R60(abstr).
22. Brodde OE, Khamssi M, Zerkowski HR. Beta-adrenoceptors in the transplanted human heart: Unaltered beta-adrenoceptor density, but increased proportion of beta-adrenoceptors with increasing posttransplant time. *Naunyn Schmiedegbergs Arch Pharmacol* 1991;344:430–436.
23. Carlsson E, Hedberg A. Are the cardiac effects of noradrenaline and adrenaline mediated by different beta adrenoreceptors? (Abst) *Acta Physiol Scand* 1976:440–441.
24. Braith RW, Wood CE, Limacher MC, et al. Abnormal neuroendocrine responses during exercise in heart transplant recipients. *Circulation* 1992;86: 1453–1463.
25. Bellet M, Carbol C, Sassano P, et al. Systemic hypertension after cardiac transplantation: Effect of cyclosporine on the renin-angiotensin-aldosterone system. *Am J Cardiol* 1985;56:927–931.
26. Singer DRJ, Buckley MG, MacGregor CA, et al. Increased concentration of plasma atrial natriuretic peptides in cardiac transplant recipients. *Br Med J* 1986;293:1391–1392.
27. Stover EP, Siegel LC. Physiology of the transplanted heart. In Royston D, Freeley TW eds: *Anesthesia for the Patient with a Transplanted Organ.* Boston: Little, Brown and Company; 1995:33:11–20.
28. Miller LW, Schlant RC, Kobashigawa JA, et al. 24th Bethesda Conference: Cardiac Transplantation (Task Force 5: Complications). *J Am Coll Cardiol* 1993;22(1):1–64.
29. Shephard RJ. Responses to acute exercise and training after cardiac transplantation: A review. *Can J Spt Sci* 1991;16:1:9–22.
30. Tamburino C, Corcos T, Feraco E, et al. Hemodynamic parameters one and four weeks after cardiac transplantation. *Am J Cardiol* 1989;63:635–637.
31. Tischler MD, Lee RT, Plappert T, et al. Serial assessment of left ventricular function and mass after orthotopic heart transplantation: A four-year longitudinal study. *J Am Coll Cardiol* 1992;19:60–6.
32. Valantine HA, Appleton CP, Hatle LK, et al. Influence of recipient atrial contraction on left ventricular filling dynamics of the transplanted heart assessed by Doppler echocardiography. *Am J Cardiol* 1987;59:1159–1163.
33. McLaughlin PR, Kleiman JH, Martin RP, et al. The effect of exercise and atrial pacing on left ventricular volume and contractility in patients with innervated and denervated hearts. *Circulation* 1978;58:476–483.
34. Ingels NB Jr., Hansen DE, Daughters GT, et al. Relation between longitudinal, circumferential, and oblique shortening and torsional deformation in the left ventricle of the transplanted human heart. *Circ Res* 1989;64:915–927.
35. von Scheidt W, Neudert J, Erdmann E, et al. Contractility of the transplanted, denervated human heart. *Am Heart J* 1991;121:1480–1488.
36. Young JB, Leon CA, Short HD III, et al. Evolution of hemodynamics after orthotopic heart and heart/lung transplantation: Early restrictive patterns persisting in occult fashion. *J Heart Transplant* 1987;6:34–43.
37. Valantine HA, Fowler MB, Hunt SA, et al. Changes in Doppler echocardiographic indexes of left ventricular function as potential markers of acute cardiac rejection. *Circulation* 1987;76(suppl V):V86–92.
38. Stinson EB, Caves PK, Griepp RB, et al. Hemodynamic observations in the early period after human heart transplantation. *J Thorac Cardiovasc Surg* 1975;69:264–270.
39. Campeau L, Pospisil L, Grondin P, et al. Cardiac catheterization findings at

rest and after exercise in patients following cardiac transplantation. *Am J Cardiol* 1970;25:523–528.

40. Hosenpud JD, Morton MJ, Wilson RA, et al. Abnormal exercise hemodynamics in cardiac allograft recipients 1 year after cardiac transplantation: Relation to pre-load reserve. *Circulation* 1989;80:525–532.

41. Quigg R, Rocco MG, Gauthier DF, et al. Mechanism of the attenuated peak heart rate response to exercise after orthotopic cardiac transplantation. *J Am Coll Cardiol* 1989;14:338–344.

42. Niset G, Hermans L, Depelchin P. Exercise and heart transplantation. A review. *Sports Medicine* 1991;12(6):359–379.

43. Folino AF, Buja G, Miorelli M, et al. Heart rate variability in patients with orthotopic heart transplantation: Long-term follow-up. *Clin Cardiol* 1993; 16:539–542.

44. Degre SF, Niset GL, Desmet JM, et al. Cardiorespiratory response to early exercise testing after orthotopic cardiac transplantation. *Am J Cardiol* 1988; 60:926–928.

45. Hartmann A, Maul FD, Huth A, et al. Serial evaluation of left ventricular function by radionuclide ventriculography at rest and during exercise after orthotopic heart transplantation. *Eur J Nucl Med* 1993;20: 146–150.

46. Quigg RJ, Rocco MB, Gauthier DF, et al. Mechanism of the attenuated peak heart rate response to exercise after orthotopic cardiac transplantation. *J Am Coll Cardiol* 1989;14:338–344.

47. Verani MS, George SE, Leon CA, et al. Systolic and diastolic ventricular performance at rest and during exercise in heart transplant recipients. *J Heart Transplant* 1988;7:145–151.

48. Clark DA, Quint RA, Mitchell RL, Angell WW. Coronary artery spasm. Medical management, surgical denervation and autotransplantation. *J Thorac Cardiovasc Surg* 1976;73:332–339.

49. Clark DA, Schroeder JS, Griepp RB, et al. Cardiac transplantation in man. Review of the first three years' experience. *Am J Med* 1973;54:563–576.

50. Kavanaugh T. Exercise training in patients after heart transplantation. *Herz* 1991;16:243–250.

51. Savin WM, Haskell WL, Schroeder JS, Stinson EB. Cardiorespiratory responses of cardiac transplant patients to graded, symptom limited exercise. *Circulation* 1980;62:55–60.

52. Mancini DM, Walter G, Reichek N, et al. Contribution of skeletal muscle atrophy to exercise intolerance and altered muscle metabolism in heart failure. *Circulation* 1992;85:1364–1373.

53. Drexler H. Skeletal muscle failure in heart failure. *Circulation* 1992;85: 1621–1622.

54. Kavanaugh T, Yacoub M, Mertens DJ, et al. Cardiorespiratory responses to exercise training after orthotopic cardiac transplantation. *Circulation* 1988;77: 162–171.

55. Moriguchi J, Stevenson L, Kobashigawa J, et al. Decrease in 2-dimensional echocardiographic ejection fraction during transplant rejection: A study of 400 biopsies. (Abst) *J Am Coll Cardiol* 1988;11:121A.

56. Chan SY, Kobashigawa JA, Stevenson LW, et al. Myocardial blood flow at rest and during pharmacologic vasodilation in cardiac transplant patients with acute rejection using positron emission tomography. *Circulation* 1994; 90:204–212.

57. Laks H, Martin SM, Grant PW. Techniques of cardiac transplantation. In

Kapoor AS, Laks H eds: *Atlas of Heart-Lung Transplantation:* New York: Mc-Graw-Hill, Inc.; 1994:51–73.

58. Freimark D, Czer LS, Aleksic I, et al. Improved left atrial transport and function with orthotopic heart transplantation by bicaval and pulmonary venous anastomoses. *Am Heart J* 1995 Jul;130(1):121–126.

59. Kobashigawa JA, Leaf DA, Gleeson JP, et al. Benefit of cardiac rehabilitation in heart transplant patients: A randomized trial. *J Heart Lung Transplant* 1994;13:S77.

Therapeutic Approaches to Heart Failure and Their Impact on Exercise Tolerance

Chapter 7

Overview of Medical Therapy in Heart Failure:
The Challenge of Rational Polypharmacy

James B. Young, MD

Overview

Traditionally, pharmacological treatment of heart failure focused on ameliorating a dropsical state with diuretics or increasing cardiac contractility using various cardiac glycoside preparations.[1-3] Contemporary insight into the variegate clinical and pathophysiological manifestations of heart failure has now, however, allowed a much more eclectic approach to the milieu, utilizing quite a broad spectrum of drugs.[4-9] Indeed, polypharmacy has become the rule as opposed to the exception in patients with significant ventricular dysfunction.[10] Because heart failure is now an epidemic, and patients present with variable pictures, an overview of the latest state-of-the-art drug treatment philosophy is in order. Aggressive pharmacotherapeutic management of patients with heart failure hopefully can prevent deterioration of ventricular function, which invariably results in worsening congestive heart failures, frequent hospitalization, and high mortality. Because polypharmacy is often encountered (and may be necessary) in these patients, a rational approach to this practice is important.

Recently released Clinical Practice Guidelines by the United States Department of Health and Human Services Agency for Health Care Policy and Research,[11] as well as a report of the Joint American College of Cardiology/American Heart Association Task Force on Practice Guidelines for the Evaluation and Management of Heart Failure[12] focused on appropriate diagnostic strategies and care of patients with a variety of ventricular dysfunction states leading to heart failure and cir-

From: Balady GJ, Piña IL (eds). *Exercise and Heart Failure.* Armonk, NY: Futura Publishing Company, Inc.; ©1997.

culatory inadequacy. These reports stressed the importance of a well reasoned diagnosis based on an appropriate definition of the heart failure syndrome and subsequent tailored treatment programs.

Definition

Heart failure has been viewed mainly as a circulatory situation, developing when the cardiac pump inadequately perfuses peripheral organ beds because of decrement in cardiac output and subsequent alteration in myocyte loading characteristics.[4-6] Formerly, heart failure was always associated with increased venous pressure, fluid retention, and dropsical states. This definition focused more on late-stage clinical settings, characterizing congestive heart failure when symptoms and physical findings are obvious, readily diagnosed, and usually secondary to volume overload and fluid congestion. Insight into the complicated pathophysiology of myocardial and circulatory failure subsequently required clinicians to view heart failure in quite a different light. It is now well accepted that this condition is a multifactorial milieu with perturbation of multiple neuroendocrine, humoral, and inflammatory feedback loops precipitated by one sort or another of myocardial injury, which causes hemodynamic and myocyte loading abnormalities.[4,13,14] The earliest stages of heart failure can, therefore, be quite subtle. Importantly, because initial homeostatic compensation is generally quite effective, symptoms and physical findings traditionally associated with congestive heart failure are not often present in the syndrome's earliest stages. Though compensatory mechanisms initially ameliorate peripheral flow disturbances to some organs, these feedback loop systems themselves eventually become problematic, creating inherent myocyte and circulatory difficulties of their own, which lead to problematic cardiac remodeling.[13] Clinicians today are moving toward a more encompassing definition of heart failure that focuses upon abnormalities noted at a very basic physiological, humoral, cellular, subcellular organelle, and molecular biodynamic level long before hemodynamic alterations traditionally associated with congestive heart failure are apparent.

Table 1 lists several considerations essential to creating a contemporary definition of heart failure. It is important to consider these issues because staged and tailored drug therapy is based upon these points. As might be anticipated from the preceding comments, heart failure should not be defined solely as "congestive" heart failure, but should include a broad spectrum of adjective characterization, such as acute or chronic, right-sided or left-sided, systolic or diastolic, and dilated or hypertrophic. As further clarification of pathophysiological systems important in the heart failure milieu come apparent, new adjectives will

Table 1

Heart Failure Definition

Considerations

- Heart failure is a milieu or syndrome rather than a specific disease.
- Myocardial injury from variagate causes results in altered myocyte loading characteristics and diminished peripheral vascular red blood flow.
- Mechanical, neurohormonal, humoral and inflammatory responses create initial circulatory compensation but contribute subsequently to cardio/circulatory injury.
- The earliest stages of heart failure are at molecular biodynamic levels with noxious cardiac injury inducing reversion to fetal genotypic programs resulting in myocyte hypertrophy and myocardial remodeling.
- Patients may be asymptomatic or have varying degrees of fatigue, dyspnea, or dropsical states that fluctuate in severity based on premorbid aerobic conditioning, diet, medications, and disease causing myocyte injury.

be included in the description, and undoubtedly therapeutics will become even more complicated as they become directed towards very specific system perturbation.

Diagnosis

Obviously, to most effectively treat heart failure populations, an appropriate diagnosis must be made.[5,6] Suspected heart failure patients no longer simply present with pulmonary rales, edema, gallop rhythms, and complaints of dyspnea. Patients may have a wide spectrum of presentations based on the predominance of systolic or diastolic dysfunction, selective cardiac chamber enlargement, and underlying diseases. It is extremely important to note that many, if not most, patients with heart failure are actually asymptomatic the majority of the time.[15–18] Heart failure is common in patients with ischemic heart disease, hypertension, diabetes mellitus, or combinations of these difficulties. Also, not every patient with a dropsical state has heart failure. Many other diseases frequently cause fluid retention. Questions, therefore, that should be asked whenever heart failure is considered, and an evaluation planned, include: (1) Is myocyte, myocardial, and circulatory failure actually present? (2) What caused the difficulty in the first place? (3) What are the patient's short- and long-term prognoses? (4) In asymptomatic patients can deterioration of ventricular function be prevented? (5) In symptomatic patients, can symptoms be eliminated or attenuated? (6) What can be done to cure or treat the underlying diseases? (7) Can factors precipitating sudden deterioration be eliminated?

Any patient evaluation must be planned so that information obtained will address these questions and allow tailoring of appropriate therapeutic maneuvers to prevent, cure, or treat the heart failure syndrome. Obviously, it is becoming important to identify patients with heart failure early, before substantive symptoms develop, if a major impact on morbidity and mortality is to be expected.[19, 20] Indeed, Table 2 summarizes important considerations to make while diagnosing heart failure, and one cannot over emphasize the importance of suspecting significant left ventricular systolic dysfunction in asymptomatic patients. These individuals often present with complicated hypertensive states or difficulties engendered by atheroscerlotic heart disease, including myocardial infarction or anginal states.

Pharmacotherapy and the Pathophysiology of Heart Failure

Diuretics, mainstays for treatment of congestive heart failure for decades, relieve congestion and decrease symptoms and physical findings caused by volume overload. It should be obvious that these drugs are most useful in the late stages of heart failure rather than during incipient syndrome development.[21] Cardiac glycosides have been used for centuries to increase contractility, but subsequently have been associated with amelioration of neurohumoral perturbations as well. Still, a diuretic-digitalis glycoside based protocol created the mainstay of heart failure therapeutics for many years because of the fact that heart failure was generally diagnosed during stages of congestion.[22]

A variety of different therapeutic strategies have been used more recently to attenuate pathophysiological difficulties now known to be

---

Table 2

Diagnosing Heart Failure

Considerations

- Recognize the milieu
- Determine etiology of syndrome
- Clarify factors precipitating deterioration
- Stage severity of syndrome
- Establish prognosis
- Tailor therapy to pathophysiology observations

important. Acutely hemodynamic changes should be considered. Drugs which ameliorate these abnormalities generally will increase cardiac output with concomitant decrement in ventricular filling pressure. Short-term clinical trial end points focus on increased exercise tolerance and symptomatic improvement and, interestingly, drugs that attenuate abnormal hemodynamics do not always translate into improved quality of life or mortality reduction. Clinical trial experience with a spectrum of agents emphasizes this point. Prazosin, for example, is very effective in lowering preload and afterload with subsequent increase in cardiac output in severe heart failure, but these effects do not appear sustained, nor does this drug decrease mortality.[23] Flosequinan, a phosphodiesterase inhibitor with inotropic and vasodilating properties, improved heart failure patients' quality of life and exercise times significantly, but increased mortality.[24]

Clinical Trials

Clinical trials, indeed, have been extraordinarily important in helping clinicians design appropriate and rational heart failure treatment protocols. The initial large-scale mortality endpoint clinical trial that suggested an approach other than simply digitalis and diuretics is the first Veterans Administration Cooperative Vasodilator Heart Failure Trial (VHeFT-I).[23] This hallmark study indicated that the direct-acting arterial and venous vasodilating combination of hydralazine and isosorbide dinitrate decreased morbidity and mortality in patients with severe congestive heart failure when these drugs were added to a baseline digoxin and diuretic therapeutic protocol. Equally important was the concomitant observation that the above-mentioned peripheral α-adrenergic-blocking agent prazosin had no significant effect on mortality or morbidity. This emphasizes the important fact that although many vasodilators are capable of ameliorating hemodynamic perturbation seen in heart failure, these drugs do not always translate into morbidity and mortality diminution.[23,25] The second pivotal heart failure mortality endpoint clinical trial to address the vasodilator paradigm is the Cooperative North Scandinavian Enalapril Survival Study (CONSENSUS),[26] which studied the use of enalapril, an angiotensin-converting enzyme (ACE) inhibitor in New York Heart Association (NYHA) Class IV patients. A rather dramatic 40% reduction in mortality was noted, as well as improvement in heart failure signs and symptoms, decrement in heart size, improvement in functional class, and reduction of subsequent hospital admissions for heart failure.

An example of a clinical trial not specifically focused on heart failure, but ultimately providing a great deal of insight into drug therapy in the setting of ventricular dysfunction, is the Multicenter Diltiazem Postmyocardial Infarction Trial (MDPIT).[27] MDPIT gave insightful information regarding the calcium channel blocker diltiazem's detrimental effect in patients suffering myocardial infarction and having heart failure. The Cardiac Arrhythmia Suppression Trial (CAST)[28] convincingly demonstrates that potent Class I antiarrhythmic drugs substantially increase mortality when given to suppress minimal ventricular arrhythmia observed after acute myocardial infarction. Although not specifically selecting patients with clinical heart failure or left ventricular dysfunction, 80% of the trial participants had an ejection fraction less than 50%.

Not all medications theoretically beneficial in the heart failure milieu have proved effective when specific clinical heart failure studies were designed. Xamoterol (Corwin) was studied because of the belief that positive inotropic effects would benefit heart failure patients.[29] Unfortunately, a marked increase in mortality was observed, pointing out that certain aspects of positive inotropism must be detrimental. The initial report of the Studies Of Left Ventricular Dysfunction (SOLVD) program[30] detail experience with the ACE inhibitor, enalapril, in patients with mild to moderate congestive heart failure (symptoms in the face of left ventricular systolic ejection fraction less than 35%). Substantive reduction in morbidity and mortality was noted. A second Veterans Administrative Cooperative Vasodilator Heart Failure Trial (VHeFT-II) further investigates the "vasodilator and heart failure" hypothesis with a comparison of the ACE inhibitor enalapril to the direct acting drug combination of hydralazine and isosorbide dinitrate.[31] As in VHeFT-I, observations suggested that not all vasodilators are alike, since the ACE inhibitor, enalapril, promoted further reduction in mortality than the active drug control group, hydralazine-isosorbide dinitrate.

Phosphodiesterase inhibitors have also been evaluated in heart failure patients because of their combined inotropic and vasodilating effects. Unfortunately, the Prospective Randomized Milrinone Survival Evaluation (PROMISE) had to be terminated early because of excessive drug treatment-linked mortality (a 34% increase in cardiovascular death). Milrinone given in this fashion appeared to be proarrhythmic.[32]

The SOLVD prevention trial was important because it was the first heart failure clinical study to suggest that the treatment of asymptomatic patients with left ventricular systolic dysfunction is extremely important.[33] Furthermore, it was the first study to suggest that initial drug therapies in heart failure were not diuretics and digitalis glycosides, but rather ACE inhibitors. In this study, patients with asymptomatic, or minimally symptomatic, nonovert, heart failure manifested by an ejection fraction less than 35% had less morbidity and mortality reduction when treated with enalapril. These patients were not generally on either an ACE inhibitor or digitalis preparation. This study was the first to suggest that treatment strategies for heart failure should be tailored to the severity of a patient's clinical state, and that an ACE inhibitor should be considered firstline therapeutics in heart failure patients with systolic left ventricular dysfunction.

The Survival And Ventricular Enlargement Trial (SAVE) randomized patients with an ejection fraction of 40% or less after an acute myocardial infarction to captopril or placebo, in addition to usual therapy 3 to 17 days after the acute event.[34] Patients generally did not exhibit classic evidence of congestive heart failure, and other than the time of trial entry, closely resembled the SOLVD prevention trial population. Substantial morbidity and mortality reduction, including the diminution of recurrent major ischemic events such as myocardial infarction, was noted in the captopril treatment group. These findings have been reproduced in similar clinical settings with ramipril and Accupril®, newer ACE inhibitors. This strongly suggests that some beneficial effects of ACE inhibitors in the heart failure milieu, and particularly in the acute postmyocardial infarction setting, represent a class effect.[35] These observations should be compared to the previously mentioned MDPIT trial with diltiazem, as well as a postinfarction study using nifedipine in a trial design similar to MDPIT. The Second Prevention Israeli Nifedipine Trial (SPRINT) demonstrated no benefit for the nifedipine group, and indeed, early mortality was higher in patients assigned to the calcium channel blocker group.[36,37] The disparate results noted in clinical heart failure trials using various vasodilating compounds serves to reemphasize the fact that seemingly logical therapies must be critically tested prior to their endorsement.[38,39]

Along these lines, amiodarone has recently been evaluated in two large multicenter clinical trials using mortality endpoints.[40,41] Because sudden cardiac death and significant ventricular arrhythmias are common in heart failure patients, conventional wisdom suggests that elimination of these arrhythmias might translate into morbidity and mortality reduction.[42–45] The GESICA Trial was a randomized, although unblinded, mortality endpoint clinical study of amiodarone in severe chronic congestive heart failure with substantive ventricular systolic dysfunction and dilation.[40] A reduction in morbidity and mortality was noted and may have been independent of amiodarone's antiarrhythmic actions. These observations are in sharp contrast to the results of antiarrhythmic use in heart failure, generally,[46] and the CAST trial, specifically.[28] A subsequently published Veterans Administration Cooperative Trial also studying amiodarone does not demonstrate similar efficacious results.[41] The two trials were quite different in their patient populations with the GESICA study having a preponderance of dilated cardiomyopathy and presumably Chagas disease patients.

Finally, a growing portfolio of evidence is accruing that some newer and experimental therapies may further add to our heart failure treatment armamentarium. Studies focusing on traditional and new β-blocking drugs will be detailed separately, as will specific calcium channel blocking agents thought not detrimental in heart failure. Importantly however, a new clinically unavailable compound, vesnarinone, may be one of use.[47] Vesnarinone seemingly produces beneficial effects in novel fashion, although some inotropic and vasolidating effects are apparent. The first multicenter clinical Vesnarinone trial demonstrates the greatest mortality reduction yet seen in a severe clinical heart failure population. A dosing paradox, however, may be present, with the 120 mg dose of vesnarinone in the initial clinical trial leading to an increased mortality (while the 60 mg dose had a beneficial effect on mortality.) A second, much larger endpoint study has abruptly ended, and preliminary observations indicate that 60 mg doses could also increase mortality. Interestingly, hemodynamics are not greatly affected, but interdiction of cyotokine perturbation seems apparent with vesnarinone.[14]

The spectrum of clinical trials and heart failure gives insight regarding appropriate and inappropriate therapies. It is common sense that recommendations regarding clinical use of these drugs be based on experience in clinical trials, that patients treated with these compounds should represent the type of patient entered into the clinical study, and that drugs used should be prescribed in fashion similar to the way they were used in these studies.[11, 48–51]

Specific Drug Classes Used in Heart Failure

Because the concept of tailoring drug therapy to specific clinical situations has become widely endorsed, treatment of patients with heart failure must be highly individualized. Representative drugs from those drug classes available should be used judiciously and treatment protocols should be carefully thought through.

Diuretics

Dropsy is often a troublesome component of heart failure. When pulmonary or peripheral edema is noted, diuretics can be invaluable agents to alleviate salt and water retention, which is characteristic of more advanced heart failure syndromes.[21] Generally, thiazides such as hydrochlorothiazide or chlorothaladone are prescribed in the lowest dose necessary to create effective diuresis during initial attempts at amelioration of volume overload. As congestion worsens, more potent loop diuretics such as furosemide, bumetanide, or torsemide can be prescribed. Occasionally, for particular refractory edematous conditions, combinations of different diuretic classes may be effective.[51] A thiazide combined with a potassium sparing agent, or a thiazide and a loop diuretic can be particularly efficacious, though electrolyte disturbances will be profound on occasion. High doses of pulsed oral agents or intermittent intravenous diuretics can help resolve particularly troublesome dropsical conditions.[52]

By reducing blood volume, diuretics lower cardiac filling pressure with subsequent reduction in ventricular wall stress, pulmonary edema, and peripheral congestion. These agents, however, are associated with significant concomitant difficulties.[53–55] Electrolyte abnormalities can be life-threatening (hypokalemia with metabolic alkalosis or hypomagnesemia), and reduction in plasma volume is known to reflexly activate the renin-angiotensin aldosterone system as well as increase sympathetic nervous system drive. These can paradoxically promote further sodium and water retention while increasing left ventricular afterload.

Diuretic therapy alone is not justified in the heart failure milieu. These agents must be combined with vasodilating compounds and in particular, ACE inhibitors. Patients with congestive heart failure in the setting of low systolic function should also receive concomitant digoxin therapy.[22] Interestingly, stopping the diuretics or creating interval diuretic holiday should be considered in patients who have been congestion-free for a period.[56]

Direct Acting Vasodilators

A well-accepted observation in patients with heart failure is that dilation of the peripheral arteriolar bed produces beneficial effects. Relaxing venous capacitance vessels also diminishes preload, which will contribute to a reduction in pulmonary artery and left ventricular end diastolic pressures. Venous capacitance vessels can be dilated by nitrates while arteriolar dilation is affected by hydralazine. Combination of arterial and venous dilation occurs with ACE inhibitors and some α-adrenergic blockers (prazosin, for example). Although calcium channel-blocking drugs are peripheral arteriolar dilators, concern continues to exist regarding their safety in patients with congestive heart failure.[57–59] It is important to remember that dilation of the arterial bed alone, without concomitant venous dilation, will likely fail to achieve the sustained benefits desired in patients with chronic dropsical conditions due to left ventricular dysfunction. Likewise, although acute dyspnea can be alleviated with ad hoc administration of short-acting sublingual nitroglycerin, long-term attenuation of neurohormonal perturbation or mechanical responses to heart failure may not be observed. It is important to remember that combinations of hydralazine and isosorbide dinitrate in doses that provide balanced vasodilatory effect (approximately 100 mg of hydralazine daily and 40 mg of isosorbide dinitrate daily) improved mortality by 38% in moderate congestive heart failure patients when added to digoxin and diuretic therapy in the VHeFT-I trial.[23]

Angiotensin-Converting Enzyme Inhibitors

Based on observations made in large mortality endpoint clinical trials, ACE inhibitors have now assumed the role of firstline drug therapy in patients with heart failure. These drugs have multifactorial benefits, including attenuation of renin-angiotensin aldosterone system activation and vasodilation. Although these drugs block the conversion of angiotensin I to angiotensin II, a potent vasoconstrictor and aldosterone release stimulator, ACE inhibitors may have additional benefit by promoting activation of vasodilating prostaglandins. The broadest spectrum of heart failure patients has been studied with this class of drugs.[19, 35] Clinical trials evaluating asymptomatic patients with systolic left ventricular dysfunction, as well as terminally ill NYHA Class IV dropsical individuals justify their use in such a broad spectrum.[7–9,19] Many double-blind, placebo-controlled clinical trials have demonstrated the ability of ACE inhibitors to relieve dyspnea and improve exercise tolerance, decrease hospitalizations for heart failure, and prevent development of symptomatic congestive heart failure in those patients with asymptomatic left ventricular systolic dysfunction.[7,20] In patients without symptomatic congestive heart failure, ACE inhibitors should be considered firstline therapy, even if used only as single-drug therapy.[20] As congestive symptoms develop, combining ACE inhibitors with digoxin and diuretics becomes important.[7, 22]

Angiotensin II Receptor Blocking Drugs

Two types of angiotensin II receptors have been identified, the ATI receptors and the ATII receptors, with all known effects mediated by the ATT receptor subtype.[60,61] These effects include direct vasoconstriction, stimulation of the adrenal cortex to secrete aldosterone, and stimulation of the pituitary gland to secrete adrenal corticotrophin hormone, oxytocin, and vasopressin. As noted above, the importance of the renin-angiotensin-aldosterone system in the pathophysiology of hypertension and heart failure is uncontested today. Although ACE inhibitors are generally well tolerated, they do have some adverse effects such as cough and angioedema.[62] These are considered to be due to at-tenuated bradykinin metabolism as a result of ACE inhibitor inhibition, rather than as an effect of the interference with renin-angiotensin-al-dosterone system. Furthermore, ACE inhibitors may not completely block production of angiotensin II. Alternative pathways mediated by chymase enzyme located in tissues, can be attenuated by specific an-giotensin II receptor blockers. Using these agents either singly or in conjunction with an ACE inhibitor may more completely block adverse angiotensin II effects, while being devoid of ACE inhibitor-specific side effects (cough and angioedema), since they will not interfere with the bradykinin system. On the other hand, these agents may not offer ben-efits induced by bradykinin mediated vasoactive effects.

Losartan has been shown to lower preload and afterload, and in-crease cardiac output both after initial dosing and during long-term therapy.[61] However, when comparing the magnitude of these effects with ACE inhibitors, the hemodynamic changes are more modest. Still, however, symptomatic relief accrues in heart failure patients. Antici-pated alterations in neurohormonal abnormalities characterizing heart failure are seen with angiotensin II receptor blocking drugs. Although these compounds resemble the effects of ACE inhibitors, no long-term data are available regarding impact on mortality or major morbidity. An intriguing hypothesis is that angiotensin II receptor blocking com-pounds can be used in patients who are intolerant of ACE inhibitors be-cause of cough, angioneurotic edema, or other idiosyncratic reactions. Alternatively, combined use of angiotensin-II receptor blockers and ACE inhibitors is an intriguing hypothesis.

Digitalis Glycosides

Cardiac glycosides, specifically digoxin, are the only positive in-otropic agents currently available for long-term, oral, outpatient ad-ministration.[22] Digoxin acts via several mechanisms. This drug inhibits the myocyte's sodium pump, which increases intracellular calcium concentration and subsequent force of myocardial contraction. Higher levels of intracellular sodium produce a shortened refractory period, and heightened cell excitability as a result of reduced muscle cell mem-brane potential. Improved ventricular contractility leads to increased stroke volume, decreased filling pressure, decreased ventricular vol-ume, and decreased vascular resistance. Digoxin also inhibits baro-receptor-induced adrenergic nervous system augmentation with its sub-sequent renin-angiotensin-aldosterone system activation. Digoxin is, therefore, helpful in ameliorating fluid retention states.

Debate has raged for many years over the utility of digitalis glycosides in patients with heart failure and normal sinus rhythm.[22,63] Concern has been raised regarding digoxin toxicity. Furthermore, no large scale mortality endpoint clinical trial data are yet completely available with respect to digoxin. The question of at least clinical utility has been answered satisfactorily by two recently completed clinical trials: the Prospective Randomized Study Of Ventricular Failure and the Effect of Digoxin (PROVED) and the Randomized Assessment of Digoxin on Inhibitors of the ACE (RADIANCE).[64,65] These sister studies were designed to assess the contribution of digoxin treatment to patients' clinical status when used in a setting of either diuretic therapy alone or combination diuretic/ACE inhibitor. Both trials entered patients having mild to moderate congestive heart failure with left ventricular ejection fractions less than 35%. PROVED studied the combination of digoxin and diuretics, while RADIANCE evaluated the combination of digoxin diuretic and ACE inhibitors. Both studies demonstrate that withdrawal of digoxin therapy in similar congestive heart failure patient populations lead to significant increase in the probability that heart failure would worsen over time, with concomitant reduction in exercise tolerance and increase in hospitalization rates. Digoxin therapy was also related to better ventricular performance. When comparing the PROVED and RADIANCE patient populations, it is also evident that triple therapy is superior to an ACE inhibitor and diuretic combination alone.[22,64,65] Results of the Digitalis Investigators Group (DIG) Trial, a multicenter, multinational mortality endpoint clinical study, with over 6000 patients enrolled, are eagerly awaited. Preliminary results suggest that digoxin does not have an impact on mortality, but significantly reduces hospitalization for worsening heart failure. Furthermore, digoxin appears to be generally safe and well-tolerated.[65a]

β-Blockers

The use of β-blockers in the treatment of congestive heart failure has been of considerable controversy.[66–68] The first reports that patients with congestive heart failure due to idiopathic dilated cardiomyopathy having resting tachycardia, improved markedly after long-term β-blocker treatment, appeared over 2 decades ago.[66,67] Many subsequent studies confirmed the fact that patients with even severe congestive heart failure seemed to improve when careful upward dose titration of metoprolol occurred. Still, many patients were made worse with β-blocker therapy. Indeed, it has become a truism that severe heart failure patients undergo periods of substantive clinical deterioration before benefits begin to accrue. Despite the growing dossier suggesting benefit of β-blockers, data are controversial regarding major morbidity and mortality reduction with these agents.

The Metoprolol and Dilated Cardiomyopathy (MDC) Trial[69] did suggest a decrement in morbidity when metoprolol was prescribed, when a combined endpoint of mortality and need for cardiac transplantation was analyzed. In this clinical trial, however, absolute death rate was higher in the metoprolol treated group than the placebo patients. Intriguing is the fact that when β-blockers are given to patients having recently suffered a myocardial infarction, morbidity and mortality is reduced. In fact, in the Beta Blocker Heart Attack Trial (BHAT), the group benefiting most was that group suffering clinical heart failure in the peri-infarction period.[70]

More recently, carvedilol and bucindilol, two drugs having both traditional β-blocking effects and peripheral arteriolar vasodilating activity, have been suggested to be beneficial in heart failure patients.[71–74] In particular, a clinical trial of carvedilol indicated mortality reduction in moderately severe heart failure patients when this drug was added to standard therapy.[73] Although all of the data are not yet available, it is likely that β-blocker therapy will become more routine if the dossier continues to suggest benefit without substantive toxicity. Clarification of exact populations likely to benefit from this strategy as well as specific agents effective, their dose, and administration technique, remain incomplete to date. Still, however, as with ACE inhibitors, β-blockers interdict many aspects of the activated adrenergic neurohormonal pathways known to be detrimental in heart failure patients. The effect of β-blockers on exercise capacity in heart failure is discussed in detail in Chapter 8.

Calcium Channel Blockers

As mentioned earlier, calcium channel blockers are examples of drugs, or a drug class, that may create problems in patients with substantive ventricular dysfunction and heart failure. Although these agents can be peripheral vasodilators (lowering afterload and systemic vascular resistance), they have significant negative inotropic effects that are offset, usually, by reflex activation of adrenergic systems and tachycardia. It has been suggested that newer drugs in this class (amlodipine and felodopine) seem to have less negative inotropism and more potent selective peripheral vasodilatory actions; to date, however, sustaining symptomatic benefit has not been entirely clear.[7] In patients who have had acute myocardial infarction with left ventricular systolic dysfunction, some of the calcium channel blockers have proved detrimental with a greater chance of adverse effects noted in patients randomized to calcium channel blocker groups.[36,37] The VHeFT-III trial, which compared felodipine to placebo (on top of digoxin, diuretics, and ACE inhibitors) in patients with moderately severe congestive heart failure, showed no substantive toxicity, however no benefit could be documented either.[75] A multicenter Prospective Randomized Study of Amlodipine (PRAISE), demonstrates that significant reduction in morbidity and mortality did occur, however this was only noted in patients with nonischemic, dilated cardiomyopathy.[76] Neither the VHeFT-III nor PRAISE Trials have been published in final form. A follow-up amlodipine (PRAISE-II) Trial, to further characterize potential benefit of amlodipine in this patient population is underway.

Since patients with heart failure frequently have concomitant ischemic heart disease or hypertension, calcium channel blockers might be an attractive option as concomitant therapy. This strategy might be best readdressed on an individual-patient basis in heart failure, and particularly in those with congestive heart failure. Control of hypertension with ACE inhibitors or hydralazine, and treatment of angina pectoris with aggressive nitrate prescription or β-blockade could be considered more reasonable substitutes for calcium channel blocker use.

Antiarrhythmic Drugs

The prevalence of substantive ventricular dysrhythmia in heart failure patients is high.[45] The temptation to use antiarrhythmic drugs is, therefore, great. Unfortunately, the vast majority of clinical trials have demonstrated an inverse relationship between ventricular function and antiarrhythmic drug benefit. In fact, as left ventricular ejection fraction falls, the likelihood of arrhythmia control diminishes, with risk of proarrhythmia and adverse events substantially increasing.[46] Amiodarone may possibly be the one exception.[40,41] The two clinical trials previously mentioned have studied this drug in compulsive fashion with one demonstrating that low dose amiodarone was safe and efficacious in heart failure, particularly in dilated cardiomyopathy patients.[40] A second trial did not confirm significant mortality reduction and benefit with this drug, however the drug was well tolerated.[41] The drug is a very expensive compound and can have substantive toxicity. Amiodarone use must be governed by prudence and care. Furthermore, optimal dosing of amiodarone is yet to be defined in heart failure patients, with one study demonstrating that very low doses of this drug (50 mg or 100 mg daily without loading) can increase ejection fractions and ameliorate dysrhythmia.[77]

Atrial fibrillation presents a particularly vexing problem in heart failure with many pharmacotherapeutic approaches considered. Amiodarone may, in this circumstance, provide particularly advantageous benefits in patients with this atrial dysrhythmia and depressed ejection fraction. Heart rate control with digoxin remains, however, the prime treatment technique. Pacemaker therapy with atrial-ventricular node ablation might provide more physiological control of dysrhythmias than pharmacological therapy. Electrical cardioversion may be preferable to the use of Vaughn-Williams Class IA or IC antiarrhythmic agents, in view of potential proarrhythmic disasters with these compounds.[46]

Anticoagulation

The use of coumadin in a routine fashion in patients with congestive heart failure not having atrial fibrillation is not recommended.[11,12,48] Patients with substantive congestive heart failure also frequently have significant hepatic congestion, which may render anticoagulation difficult to achieve safely. Additionally, with the large number of drugs taken by patients with heart failure, an important tenant is to continue only those medications with demonstrable effectiveness. Routine anticoagulation in heart failure patients has never been demonstrated to be beneficial by well-designed clinical trials.[78–80] Still, heart failure patients with a history of systemic or pulmonary embolism, atrial fibrillation, or mobile left ventricular thrombi might be considered candidates for anticoagulation with a goal of an international normalization ratio of 2.0:3.0.

Other Therapies

Long-term parenteral infusion of dobutamine or milrinone, both potent inotropic and vasodilating drugs, can be beneficial in decompensated patients with dilated ventricles and severe congested states coupled to low output symptomatology.[80–83] Care must be used in patient selection because dobutamine has been suggested to increase mortality in severely ill, advanced, end-stage heart failure patients when infused chronically in the outpatient setting.[83] Occasionally, these patients can benefit from left ventricular assist device placement or cardiac transplantation.[84]

General Principles of
Heart Failure Pharmacotherapy

Table 3 and Figure 1 summarize an approach to managing patients with heart failure, with a focus on pharmacotherapeutic strategy. It is

Table 3

Heart Failure Therapeutics

Principles

- Use appropriate drugs to treat underlying diseases
  - Control hypertension
  - Alleviate cardiac ischemia
  - Address diabetes mellitus
  - Normalize thyroid function
  - Correct anemia
- Stop, if possible, potentially harmful drugs
  - Antiarrthymic agents
  - Calcium channel blockers
  - Nonsteroidal antiinflammatory agents
- Review carefully drugs of unproven benefits
  - Anticoagulants
  - Amiodarone
- Begin drugs to prevent deterioration/reduce mortality
  - Angiotension-converting enzyme inhibitor
  - Hydralazine/isosorbide dinitrate combination
- Use drugs to control symptoms
  - Diuretics
  - Digoxin
  - Nitrates
  - Parenteral inotropes (dobutamine/milrinone)
- Protect against drug induced metabolic perturbation
  - Treat hypokalemia
  - Consider magnesium replishment
- Consider "experimental" agents
  - Beta-blockers (metoprolol, carvedilol, bucindolol)
  - Calcium channel blockers (amlodipine, felodipine, mebipradil)
  - Nonglycoside inotropes (flosequinon, vesnarinone)
- Prescribe rationale polypharmacy
  - Fewest side effects possible
  - Program designed to ensure compliance
  - Consider cost of drugs used

important to note that drug prescription should not be done in isolation, and the principles listed in Table 3 should be adhered to. It must be emphasized that, first, an appropriate diagnosis of heart failure should be made. Staging the syndrome severity is extraordinarily important because pharmacotherapy is based on severity of syndrome presentation, as well as underlying diseases or comorbid conditions. Obviously, detecting substantive left ventricular dysfunction at its earliest, such that preventative strategies can be employed, is optimal. Indeed, the discovery of asymptomatic left ventricular systolic dysfunc-

Tailored Therapy for Heart Failure

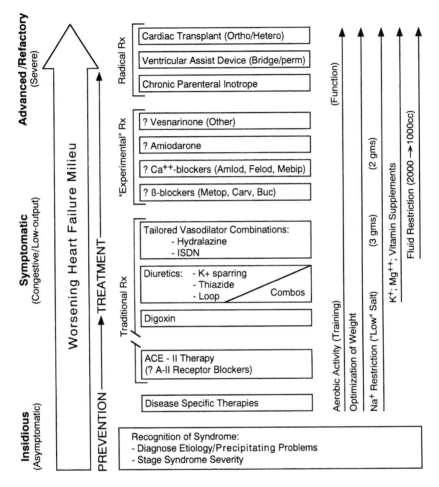

Figure 1: The tailored approach to heart failure is based upon appropriate recognition of the syndrome with protocols keeping the milieu's severity in perspective. Traditional, experimental, and radical therapies all have an appropriate place. Some drugs are controversial with respect to whether or not benefits occur (eg, amiodarone, calcium channel blockers). In other situations, some drugs may decrease aspects of heart failure morbidity at the expense of increasing mortality (eg, flosequinon, vesnarinone). Attention must be paid to sodium and fluid restriction, as well as exercise and electrolyte replenishment. Treating patients with heart failure is no longer the simple task of prescribing bed rest, diuretics and digitalis glycoside. Therapeutic principles delineated in Table 3 should be considered. (Amlod = amlodipine; felod = felodipine; mebip = mebipridil; metop = metoprolol; carv = carvedilol; Buc = bucindolol; ISDN = isosorbide dinitrate; ACE-I = angiotensin-converting enzyme inhibitor; A-II = angiotensin-II).

tion is extraordinarily important, so that timely intervention with ACE inhibitors can be accomplished with the hope of preventing functional deterioration and promoting beneficial remodeling. Importantly, staging the severity of heart failure will ultimately relate to the number of drugs prescribed, because a diagnosis of heart failure does not always mean congestive failure is present. Only those patients with a congestive state, and possibly hypertension, should receive diuretic therapy. Obviously, treatment of underlying diseases or precipitating problems is essential. Although heart failure per se, cannot be cured, frequently the underlying disease state (such as hyperthyroidism) can be eliminated. Treating coronary heart disease, which is causing myocardial ischemia, can be particularly beneficial.

Because patients with heart failure frequently take many drugs, discontinuation of those which are potentially harmful or of unproven benefit can be important. One should always question whether antiarrhythmic drugs, calcium channel blockers, and nonsteroidal inflammatory compounds have played a role in any given patient's deterioration, or are in fact, necessary. Remember, stopping certain drugs can often be as important as starting others. The use of β-blockers and anticoagulants is more controversial. However, the portfolio suggesting that β-blockers are beneficial has grown substantially, and it is likely that we soon will turn more often to these compounds. Certain subsets of patients are likely to benefit from anticoagulation, however, this approach on a routine basis is discouraged.

Regimens with proven efficacy and benefit should surround ACE inhibitor prescription. These agents have been demonstrated over and again to prevent functional deterioration, particularly in asymptomatic patients with left ventricular systolic dysfunction. These drugs should be used as first line therapy in any patient with reduced left ventricular ejection fraction. When they cannot be tolerated, one might consider the combination of hydralazine and isosorbide dinitrate or, possibly, the substitution of an angiotensin II receptor blocking compound. The latter approach is somewhat speculative at the present time. When symptomatic congestive heart failure presents, particularly with substantive depression of left ventricular ejection fraction and cardiomegaly, diuretics and digoxin become extraordinarily important. Indeed, taken together, the PROVED and RADIANCE Trials demonstrate that patients with congestive heart failure do best with triple therapy consisting of digoxin, an ACE inhibitor, and a diuretic.

The fact that polypharmacy is so frequent in heart failure patients means that rationale prescription of multiple drugs is mandatory. When many drugs are simultaneously dispensed, each compound prescribed should affect pathophysiological processes via different and complimentary mechanisms. The one possible exception to this might be combined prescription of an ACE inhibitor with an angiotensin II receptor blocking drug. Ideally, compounds used should have different sites of metabolism or excretion, the toxicity of one drug should not be increased by another drug, and each drug's beneficial effect should be enhanced when combinations are used. Also important is the fact that a program designed to ensure optimal compliance is essential, as is consideration of the costs of drugs employed. Thought must also be given to how drugs for heart failure have been prescribed in clinical trials. Drugs should be given to patient populations and in doses defined by clinical trials.

Activity recommendations and dietary restriction are also important in patients with heart failure. There is now reasonable agreement that regular aerobic exercise is beneficial and should be encouraged for all patients with stable heart failure.[86] Dietary recommendations are important with particular attention to sodium restriction. A low-salt diet is reasonable even in patients with asymptomatic left ventricular systolic dysfunction. A 2 g salt diet is somewhat difficult to attain and many have recommended a compromise of 3 g sodium restriction.[11,12] As the heart failure milieu worsens, and in particular, as serum sodium falls with increased total body water volume, restriction of salt consumption becomes extraordinarily important. Free water and fluid volume restriction also become important as the syndrome worsens. Because alcohol depresses myocardial contractility, patients should be careful about the quantity of alcohol ingested. This may be particularly significant in some patients who have dilated cardiomyopathy with normal coronaries. Complete alcohol abstinence is critical in those with a diagnosis of alcohol-induced heart failure or cardiomyopathy. Also important is adequate magnesium and potassium consumption as well as reasonable protein intake. Since patients with severe heart failure may suffer from cardiac cachexia, adequate protein and vitamin consumption should be encouraged. Still, there is no proven role for high-dose antioxidant vitamin therapy or co-Q10 ingestion to treat heart failure.[7,11,12]

Common Pitfalls in Treating Heart Failure

Epidemiological data assessing therapeutic strategies for heart failure patients characterize the fact that ACE inhibitors are under-used in this situation.[10–12] This may be because of excessive fear regarding blood pressure lowering or renal dysfunction. Clinical trials reaffirm the safety of these drugs even when patients have relative hypotension and modest impairment of renal function. Other common pitfalls are listed in Table 4 and include inadequate ACE inhibitor dose. It is not uncommon to see doses of captopril in the range of 6 mg to 12 mg used twice daily

---

Table 4

Pitfalls While Treating Heart Failure

Issues

- Excessive fear of blood pressure-lowering
- Not aggressively treating hypertension
- Overconcern about renal function when using angiotensin-converting enzyme inhibitors
- Nonsteroidal anti-inflammatory agents
- Inadequate angiotension-converting enzyme inhibitor doses
- Incorrectly ascribing cough as an angiotensin-converting enzyme inhibitor side effect and stopping the drugs
- Lack of adequate sodium restriction
- Inappropriate limitation of aerobic exercise
- Incomplete K^+ and Mg^{++} replenishment
- Conservative management of atrial fibrillation
- Unwarranted ventricular arrhythmia therapy
- Use of dobutamine/milrinone in patients with hypertension or inadequately treated congestive heart failure

---

in patients with normal blood pressures and low ejection fraction. Clinical trials generally used 100 mg, on average, of this drug. Additionally, lack of attention to sodium restriction is commonly apparent. Also, incorrectly ascribing a cough to an ACE inhibitor and stopping the drug because of this may be problematic. Many factor can cause cough in heart failure patients, and one needs to be cautious when attributing this to ACE inhibitor therapy. Furthermore, even though the cough may clearly be related to one of these drugs, careful explanation of the drug's benefit may convince patients to tolerate this nuisance side effect. Inappropriate limitation of aerobic exercise is also noted. In fact, exercise training and aerobic conditioning may ameliorate many aspects of the heart failure syndrome. Compulsive attention to potassium and magnesium replenishment must be emphasized in patients on diuretics. It should be noted that normal serum magnesium levels do not exclude the possibility of total body magnesium deficiency. Some recommend routine administration of magnesium supplementation in any patient on a diuretic. It should be pointed out that magnesium supplementation often helps maintain adequate potassium levels. The finding of persistent hyponatremia and hypokalemia may reflect inadequate salt and water restriction in patients, and must be addressed. Another common mistake is very conservative management of atrial fibrillation when successful conversion to normal sinus rhythm by electrical cardioversion would be greatly beneficial. Unwarranted antiarrhythmic therapy, and use of dobutamine or milrinone infusion in patients not likely to benefit (mild to moderate heart failure with hypertension or inadequately treated congestive heart failure), should be avoided.

Successful treatment of appropriately diagnosed and staged heart failure and avoidance of common pitfalls will result in improved morbidity and mortality in this large and growing population of severely ill patients.

References

1. Fishberg AM. *Heart Failure*, 2nd Ed. Philadelphia: Lea & Febiger; 1940.
2. Selzer A. Fifty years of progress in cardiology: A personal perspective. *Circulation* 1988;77:955–963.
3. Braunwald E, Mock MB, Watson JT. *Congestive Heart Failure. Current Research and Clinical Applications*. New York: Grum & Stratton; 1982.
4. Young JB, Pratt CM. Hemodynamic and hormonal alterations in patients with heart failure: Toward a contemporary definition of heart failure. *Semin Nephrol* 1994;14:5,427–440.
5. Young JB, Farmer JA. The diagnostic evaluation of patients with heart failure. In Hosenpud JD, Greenberg GH eds: *Congestive Heart Failure; Pathophysiology, Diagnosis and Comprehensive Approach to Management*. New York: Springer-Verlag; 1994;597–621.
6. Young JB. Assessment of heart failure. In Colluci WS, Braunwald E eds: *Heart Failure: Cardiac Function and Dysfunction. Atlas of Heart Diseases*. 1995; 79:1171–1190.
7. Young JB. Contemporary management of patients with heart failure. *Med Clin North Am* 1995;79:1171–1190.
8. Braunwald E. ACE inhibitors—A cornerstone of the treatment of heart failure. *N Engl J Med* 1991;325:351–353.
9. Cohn JN. The prevention of heart failure—A new agenda. *N Engl J Med* 1992;327:725–727.
10. Young JB, Weiner DH, Yusuf S, et al. Patterns of medication use in patients with heart failure: A report from the Registry Of Studies of Left Ventricular Dysfunction (SOLVD). *South Med J* 1994;88:423–514.
11. Konstam M, Dracup K, Baker D, et al. *Heart Failure: Evaluation and care of patients with left ventricular systolic dysfunction.Clinical Practice Guideline #11*. AHCPR Publication 94-0612. Rockville, MD: Agency for Health Care Policy and Research, Public Health Service, U.S. Department of Health and Human Services. June, 1994.
12. Committee on Evaluation and Management of Heart Failure. Guidelines for the Evaluation and Management of Heart Failure. Report of the American College of Cardiology/American Heart Association Task Force on Practice Guidelines. *J Amer Coll Cardiol* 1995;6:5:1376–1398.
13. Young JB. Heart failure, ventricular remodelling and the renin-angiotensin system: Insights from recently completed clinical trials. *Eur Heart J* 1993; (suppl C)14:14–17.
14. Mann DL, Young JB. Basic mechanisms in congestive heart failure: Recognizing the role of proinflammatory cytokines. *Chest* 1994;105:897–904.
15. Kannel WB. Epidemiology aspects of heart failure. *Cardiol Clin* 1989;7:1–9.

16. Ghali JK, Cooper R, Ford E. Trends in hospitalization rates for heart failure in the United States 1973–1986. *Arch Intern Med* 1990;150:769–772.
17. Kannel WB, Belanger AJ. Epidemiology of Heart Failure. *Am Heart J* 1991; 121:951–957.
18. Schocken DD, Arrieta MI, Leaverton PE. Prevalence of mortality rate of congestive heart failure in the United States. *J Amer Coll Cardiol* 1992;20: 301–306.
19. Young JB. Angiotensin converting enzyme inhibitors in heart failure: New strategies justified by recent clinical trials. *Int J Cardiol* 1994;43:151–163.
20. Young JB. Asymptomatic left ventricular dysfunction: To treat or not to treat? *J Heart Lung Transplant* 1994;13:S135–S140.
21. Cody RJ, Kubo SH, Pickworth KK. Diuretic treatment for the sodium retention of congestive heart failure. *Arch Intern Med* 1994;154:1905–1914.
22. Young JB. Do digitalis glycosides still have a role in congestive heart failure? *Cardiol Clin* 1994;12:1.
23. Cohn JN, Archibald DG, Ziesche S, et al. Effect of vasodilator therapy on mortality in chronic congestive heart failure: Results of a Veterans Administration Cooperative Study. *N Engl J Med* 1986;314:1547–1552.
24. Young JB. Evolving concepts in the treatment of heart failure: Should new inotropic agents carry promise or paranoia? *Pharmacotherapy* 1996;16:78–84.
25. Sueta CA, Gheorghiade M, Adams KF, et al. for the Epoprostenol Multicenter Research Group. Multicenter randomized trial of epoprostenol in patients with severe heart failure. *Am J Cardiol* 1995;75:34A–43A.
26. The CONSENSUS Trial Study Group. Effects of enalapril on mortality in severe congestive heart failure: Results of the Cooperative North Scandinavian Enalapril Survival Study (CONSENSUS). *N Engl J Med* 1987;316:1429–1435.
27. Held PH, Yusuf S. Calcium antagonists in the treatment of ischemic heart disease: Myocardial infarction. *Coron Artery Dis* 1994;5:21–26.
28. Hallstrom A, Pratt CM, Green HL, et al. Relations between heart failure ejection fraction, arrhythmia suppression and mortality: Analysis of the cardiac arrhythmia suppression trial. *J Am Coll Cardiol* 1995;25:1250–1270.
29. Xamoterol in Severe Heart Failure Study Group: Xamoterol in severe heart failure. *Lancet* 1990;336:1–6.
30. The SOLVD Investigators. Effect of enalapril on survival in patients with reduced left ventricular rejection fractions and congestive heart failure. *N Engl J Med* 1991;325:293–302.
31. Cohn JN, Johnson G, Ziesche S, et al. A comparison of enalapril with hydralazine-isosorbide dinitrate in the treatment of chronic congestive heart failure. *N Engl J Med* 1991;325:303–310.
32. Packer M, Carver JR, Rodeheffer RJ, et al. for the PROMISE Study Research Group. Effect of oral milrinone on mortality in severe chronic heart failure. *N Engl J Med* 1991;325:468–475.
33. The SOLVD Investigators. Effect of enalapril on mortality and the development of heart failure in asymptomatic patients with reduced left ventricular ejection fractions. *N Engl J Med* 1992;327:685–691.
34. Pfeffer MA, Braunwald E, Moye LA, et al. on behalf of the SAVE Investigators. Effect of captopril on mortality and morbidity in patients with left ventricular dysfunction and myocardial infarction: Results of the Survival and Ventricular Enlargement Trial. *N Engl J Med* 1992;327:669–677.
35. Young JB. Reduction of ischaemic events with angiotensin converting inhibitors: Lessons and controversy emerging from recent clinical trials. *Cardiovasc Drugs Ther* 1995;8:89–131.

36. The Israeli SPRINT Study Group: The Secondary Prevention Israeli Nifedipine Trial (SPRINT): A randomized intervention trial of nifedipine in patients with acute myocardial infarction. *Eur Heart J* 1989;9:354–364.

37. Goldbourt U, Bahar S, Reicher-Reiss H, et al. for the SPRINT Study Group. Early adminstration of nifedipine in suspected myocardial infarction. *Arch Intern Med* 1993;153:345–353.

38. Packer M. Calcium channel blockers in chronic heart failure: The risks of physiologically rational therapy. *Circulation* 199;82:2254–2257.

39. Francis GS. Calcium channel blockers and congestive heart failure. *Circulation* 1991;83:336–8.

40. Doval HC, Nul DR, Grancelli HO, et al. Randomized trial of low-dose amiodarone in severe congestive heart failure: Grupo de Estudio de la Sobrevida en la Insuficiencia Cardiaca en Argentina (GESICA). *Lancet* 1994; 344:493–498.

41. Singh SN, Fletcher RD, Risher SG, et al. Amiodarone in patients with congestive heart failure and asymptomatic ventricular arrhythmia: Survival Trial of Antiarrhythmic Therapy in Congestive Heart Failure. *N Engl J Med* 1995;333:77–82.

42. Packer M. Sudden unexpected death in patients with congestive heart failure: A second frontier. *Circulation* 1985;72:681–685.

43. Francis GS. Development of arrhythmias in the patient with congestive heart failure: Pathophysiology, prevalence and prognosis. *Am J Cardiol* 1986;57:3B–7B.

44. Francis GS. Should asymptomatic ventricular arrhythmias in patients with congestive heart failure be treated with antiarrhythmic drugs? *J Am Coll Cardiol* 1988;12:274–283.

45. Stevenson WG, Stevenson LW. (Eugene Braunwald E. ed:) Sudden death in heart failure: Mechanism and prevention in heart disease; Update I. Philadelphia: WB Saunders Co.; 1995.

46. Pratt CM, Eaton T, Francis M, et al. The inverse relationship between left ventricular ejection fraction and outcome of antiarrhythmic therapy: A dangerous imblance in the risk-benefit ratio. *Am Heart J* 1989;118:433–440.

47. Feldman AM, Bristow MR, Parmley WW, et al. Effects of vesnarinone on morbidity and mortality in patients with heart failure. *N Engl J Med* 1993; 329:149–155.

48. Baker DW, Konstam MA, Bottorff M, Pitt B. Management of Heart Failure. I. Pharmacology Treatment. *JAMA* 1994;272:1361–1366.

49. Dracup K, Baker DW, Dunbar SB, et al. Management of Heart Failure. II. Counseling, Education, and Lifestyle Modifications. *JAMA* 1994;262:1442–1446.

50. Baker DW, Jones R, Hodges J, et al. Management of Heart Failure. III. The Role of Revascularization in the Treatment of Patients with Moderate or Severe Left Ventricular Systolic Dysfunction. *JAMA* 1994;272:1528–1534.

51. Parmley WW. Clinical Practice Guidelines: Does the Cookbook Have Enough Recipes? *JAMA* 1994;272:1374–1375.

52. Ellison DH. The physiologic basis of diuretic synergism: Its role in treating diuretic resistance. *Ann Intern Med* 1991;114:886–894.

53. Ikram H, Chan W, Espiner EA, Nicholls MG. Hemodynamic and hormone responses to acute and chronic furosemide therapy in congestive heart failure. *Clin Sci* 1980;59:443–449.

54. Francis GS, Siegel RM, Goldsmith SR, et al. Acute vasoconstrictor response to intravenous furosemide in patients with chronic congestive heart failure: Activation of the neurohumoral axis. *Ann Intern Med* 1985;103:1–6.

55. Bayliss J, Norell M, Canepa-Anson R, et al. Untreated heart failure: Clinical and neuroendocrine effects of introducing diuretics. *Br Heart J* 1987;57: 17–22.
56. Grinstead WC, Francis MJ, Marks GF, et al. Discontinuation of chronic diuretic therapy in stable heart failure patients. *Am J Cardiol* 1994;73:881–886.
57. Elkayam U, Shotan A, Mehra A, Ostrzega E. Calcium channel blockers in heart failure. *J Am Col Cardiol* 1993;(A):139–144.
58. Prameshwar J, Pool E, Wilson PA. The role of calcium antagonist in the treatment of chronic heart failure. *Eur Heart J* 1993;14 (A):38–44.
59. Conti CR. Use of calcium antagonist to treat heart failure. *Clin Cardiol* 1994;17:101–102.
60. Gottlieb SS, Dickstein K, Fleck E, et al. Hemodynamic and neurohormonal effects of the angiotensin II antagonist losartan in patients with congestive heart failure. *Circulation* 1993;88(pt 1):1602–1609.
61. Crozier I, Ikram H, Awan N, et al. for the Losartan Hemodynamic Study Group. Losartan in heart failure: Hemodynamic effects and tolerability. *Circulation* 1995;91:691–697.
62. Kostis JB, Shelton MS, Gosselin G, et al. for the SOLVD Investigators. Adverse effects of enalapril in the Study of Left Ventricular Dysfunction (SOLVD). *Am Heart J* 1996;131:2:350–355.
63. Jaeschke R, Oxman AD, Guyatt GH. To what extent do congestive heart failure patients in sinus rhythm benefit from digoxin therapy? A systematic overview and meta-analysis. *Am J Med* 1990;88:279–286.
64. Packer M, Gheorghiade M, Young JB, et al. Withdrawal of digoxin from patients with chronic heart failure treatment with angiotensin-converting enzyme inhibitors. RADIANCE Study. *N Engl J Med* 1993;329:1–7.
65. Uretsky BF, Young JB, Shahidi FE, et al. Randomized study assessing the effect of digoxin withdrawal in patients with mild to moderate chronic congestive heart failure: Results of the PROVED trial. *J Am Coll Cardiol* 1993;22: 955–962.
65a. The Digitalis Investigators Group. Rationale, implementation and baseline characteristics of patients in the DIG trial: A large simple trial to evaluate the effects of digitalis on mortality in heart failure. *Clin Trials* (in press).
66. Waagstein F, Hjalmarson A, Varnauskas E, Wallentin I. Effect of chronic beta-adrenergic receptor blockade in congestive cardiomyopathy. *Br Heart J* 1975;37:1022–1036.
67. Engelmeier RS, O'Connell JB, Walsh R, et al. Improvement in symptoms and exercise tolerance by metoprolol in patients with dilated cardiomyopathy: A double-blind, randomized, placebo-controlled trial. *Circulation* 1985;72:536–546.
68. Eichhorn EJ. The paradox of beta adrenergic blockade for the management of congestive heart failure. *Am J Med* 1992;92:527–538.
69. Waggstein F, Bristow MR, Swedberg K, et al. Beneficial effects of metoprolol in idiopathic dilated cardiomyopathy: Metoprolol in Dilated Cardiomyopathy (MDC) Trial Study Group. *Lancet* 1993;342:1441–1446.
70. Chadda K, Goldstein S, Byington R, Curb JD. Effect of propranolol after acute myocardial infarction in patients with congestive heart failure. *Circulation* 1986;73:503–510.
71. Metra M, Nardi M, Giubbini R, Dei Cas L. Effects of short and long-term carvedilol administration on rest and exercise capacity and clinical conditions in patients with idiopathic dilated cardiomyopathy. *J Am Coll Cardiol* 1994;24:1678–1687.

72. Krum H, Sackner-Bernstein JD, Goldsmith RL, et al. Double-blind placebo-controlled study of the long-term efficacy of carvedilol in patients with severe chronic heart failure. *Circulation* 1995;92:1499–1506.
73. Packer M, Bristow MR, Cohn J, et al. Effect of carvedilol on morbidity and mortality in patients with chronic heart failure. *N Engl J Med* 1996;334:1349–1355.
74. Woodley SL, Gilbert EM, Anderson JL, et al. β-blockade with bucindolol in heart failure due to ischemic vs. idiopathic dilated cardiomyopathy. *Circulation* 1991;84:2426–2441.
75. Cohn JN, Ziesche SM, Loss LE, Anderson GF, and the VHeft Study Group. Effect of felodipine on short-term exercise and neurohormone and long-term mortality in heart failure: Results of VHeFT-III. *Circulation* 1995;92:I-143.
76. O'Connor CM, Belkin RN, Carson PE, et al. Effect of amlodipine on mode of death in severe chronic heart failure: The PRAISE Trial. *Circulation* 1995;92;I-143.
77. Mahmarian JJ, Smart FW, Moye LA, et al. Expoloring the minimal dose of amiodarone with antiarrhythmic and hemodynamic activity. *Am J Cardiol* 1994;74:681–686.
78. Meltzer RS, Visser CA, Fuster V. Intracardiac thrombi and systemic embolization. *Ann Intern Med* 1986;104:689–698.
79. Cohn JN, Benedict CR, LeJemtel TH, et al. and the SOLVD Investigators. Risk of thromboembolism in left ventricular dysfunction [abstract]. *Circulation* 1992:86(suppl I):I-252.
80. Dunkman WB, Johnson GR, Carson PE, et al. Incidence of thromboembolic events in congestive heart failure. The VHeFT VA Cooperative Studies Group. *Circulation* 1993;87(suppl IV):IV-94–101.
81. Applefeld MM, Newman KA, Sutton FJ, et al. Outpatient dobutamine and dopamine infusions in the management of chronic heart failure: Clinical experience in 21 patients. *Am Heart J* 1987;144:589–595.
82. Miller LW, Mirkle EJ, Hermann V. Outpatient dobutamine for end-stage congestive heart failure. *Crit Care Med* 1990;18(PT 2):530–533.
83. Dies F, Krell MJ, Whitlow P, et al. Intermittent dobutamine in ambulatory outpatients with chronic cardiac failure [abstract]. *Circulation* 1986;74 (suppl II):II-38.
84. McCarthy PM, Sabik J. Implantable circulatory support devices as a bridge to heart transplantation. *Semin Thorac Surg* 1991;6:174–180.
85. Coats AJS, Adamopoulos S, Radaelli A, et al. Controlled trial of physical training in chronic heart failure: Exercise performance hemodynamics, ventilation, and autonomic function. *Circulation* 1992;85:2119–2131.
86. Wenger NK, Froelicher ES, Smith LK, et al. *Cardiac Rehabilitation as Secondary Prevention. Clinical Practice Guideline. Quick Reference Guide for Clinicians, No. 17.* Rockville, MD: U.S. Department of Health and Human Services, Public Health Service, Agency for Health Care Policy and Research and National Heart, Lung, and Blood Institute. AHCPR Pub. No. 96-0673. October 1995.

Chapter 8

Effects of Long-Term Beta-Adrenergic Blockade on Exercise Capacity in Patients with Chronic Heart Failure

Eugene E. Wolfel, MD and
Michael R. Bristow, MD, PhD

Introduction

The syndrome of chronic heart failure is associated with heightened adrenergic activity manifested by elevation of systemic and cardiac norepinephrine levels.[1,2] Increased adrenergic activation has even been shown to be associated with asymptomatic left ventricular dysfunction prior to the onset of clinical heart failure.[3] The current "adrenergic hypothesis" of heart failure is that long-term alterations in hemodynamics lead to deactivation of baroreceptors and perhaps activation of excitatory reflexes, resulting in a vicious cycle of excessive neurohumoral stimulation that leads to deterioration in myocardial function.[4] This increase in adrenergic activity leads to alterations in myocardial β-adrenergic receptor signal transduction, including downregulation of the β_1-adrenergic receptor, leading to an increase in the β_2/β_1 ratio.[5] In addition, there is uncoupling of the myocardial β_2-adrenergic receptor from the receptor-G protein-adenylyl cyclase complex and an upregulation of the inhibitory G protein (G_i). These changes lead to a blunting of contraction in response to specific β-agonists.[5] These findings are somewhat dependent on the cardiomyopathic phenotype, with more β_1-adrenergic receptor downregulation in nonischemic cardiomyopa-

This work was supported by NIH RO1 HL 48013–05.

From: Balady GJ, Piña IL (eds). *Exercise and Heart Failure.* Armonk, NY: Futura Publishing Company, Inc.; ©1997.

thy and more receptor uncoupling in ischemic cardiomyopathy. These alterations in myocardial β-adrenergic receptor gene expression and function lead to pharmacological desensitization, with a blunted response to acute sympathetic* stimulation, as occurs with exercise.

Patients with chronic heart failure have reduced aerobic exercise performance related to multiple factors, including cardiac, peripheral circulatory, and skeletal muscle maladaptations.[6] The downregulation of β_1-adrenergic receptors and other less prominent β-adrenergic signal transduction abnormalities observed in the failing myocardium may play a significant role in the cardiac inotropic and chronotropic responses to exercise. In a recent study in patients with nonischemic cardiomyopathy there was a strong correlation between the myocardial β_1-adrenergic receptor density (B_{max}) obtained from endomyocardial biopsies and maximal oxygen consumption ($\dot{V}O_{2max}$) (Figure 1, top).[7] There was also a significant correlation between B_{max} and the increase in heart rate from rest to maximal exercise (Δ heart rate), suggesting a limitation in cardiac chronotropic response with the observed downregulation of the myocardial β_1-adrenergic receptor (Figure 1, bottom). Lisinopril, an angiotensin converting enzyme (ACE) inhibitor has also been shown to increase β-receptor density in the failing myocardium[8] and to improve maximal exercise responses,[9] again suggesting a potential role for the myocardial β-adrenergic receptor in exercise tolerance in patients with chronic heart failure. Therefore, pharmacological reduction of sympathetic stimulation may correct the alterations in myocardial β-adrenergic receptor signal transduction and result in improved exercise capacity in chronic heart failure patients.

β-adrenergic blockade has been used for over 20 years to inhibit sympathetic activity in chronic heart failure.[10] Early studies with metoprolol, a β_1-selective blocker, resulted in a favorable clinical response, an apparent improvement in left ventricular function, and perhaps a trend toward reduced mortality.[11] To be an efficacious therapy in the management of chronic heart failure, β-adrenergic blockers should reduce symptoms, alleviate fluid retention, improve left ventricular function and cardiac hemodynamics, improve functional capacity, and improve survival.[12] Although acute β-adrenergic blockade in patients with left ventricular dysfunction resulted in a deterioration in resting hemodynamics,[13] long-term therapy often led to improvements in hemodynamics and alleviation of symptoms.[13–18] Studies with several β-adrenergic blockers with different pharmacological properties have resulted in improvements in resting left ventricular function and improved functional class in patients with both ischemic and nonischemic cardiomy-

---

*The term "adrenergic" refers to sympathetic nerve activity, the marker of which is increased neurotransmitter (norepinephrine) measurements. "Sympathetic" refers to a combination of neurotransmitter and hormonal (epinephrine) activity.

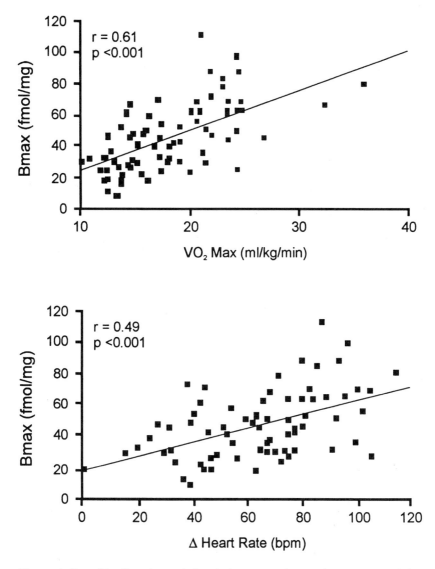

Figure 1: Top: Significant correlation between peak exercise oxygen uptake (VO_{2max}) and β-adrenoreceptor density (B_{max}) from endomyocardial biopsy samples in 72 patients with idiopathic dilated cardiomyopathy. Bottom: Significant correlation between the change in heart rate from rest to peak exercise (Δ heart rate) and β-adrenreceptor density in the same patients. (Data from Reference 7).

opathy.[14–16] A more recent placebo-controlled study with metoprolol in dilated cardiomyopathy demonstrated a 34% reduction in the need for the combined endpoints of cardiac transplantation and death.[15] Even more recent placebo-controlled data with carvedilol, a vasodilating β-adrenergic blocker, revealed a 65% reduction in mortality risk in patients with either ischemic or nonischemic cardiomyopathy.[17,18] Despite these favorable responses to long-term β-adrenergic blockade in chronic heart failure, there have been conflicting results on the ability of these agents to improve exercise capacity. In view of the pharmacological heterogeneity of these agents, the results of the various clinical trials must be interpreted based on knowledge of the type and dose of β-adrenergic blocker, the type of exercise evaluation, and the known effects of β-adrenergic blockade on exercise capacity in normal subjects.

Pharmacological Properties of Various β-Adrenergic Blockers

Before discussing the effects of β-adrenergic blockade on exercise capacity in heart failure patients, it is important to recognize that there is substantial diversity in the pharmacological profile of the various β-adrenergic blockers that have been used to treat chronic heart failure patients. Metoprolol, bucindolol, and carvedilol, the three major β-adrenergic blockers used in clinical heart failure trials, differ in several fundamental pharmacological properties (Table 1). Propranolol is shown, since it is the prototype β-adrenergic blocker that was used in the Beta Blocker Heart Attack (BHAT) Trial. BHAT showed a significant decrease in the risk of total cardiovascular mortality, sudden death, and recurrent myocardial infarction when used as a secondary prevention therapy in patients after myocardial infarction, especially in patients with left ventricular dysfunction.[19] Propranolol is the classic nonselective β-adrenergic blocker with no vasodilator or α-adrenergic blocking properties. Propranol is not well tolerated by subjects with heart failure because it blocks both β_1 and β_2 receptors and actually elevates systemic vascular resistance. This leads to myocardial de-

Table 1

Properties of Different β-Adrenoreceptor Blocking Agents

β-blocker	β_1/β_2 Selectivity	Vaso-dilator	Alpha-blocker	Inverse Agonism	Atypical Binding*	β-receptor Effects
metoprolol	74:1	−	−	+++	−	upregulates
bucindolol	1:1	+	−	+	+	downregulates
carvedilol	7:1	+	+	++	+	downregulates
propranolol	1:1	−	−	+++	−	upregulates

*guanine nucleotide modulatable binding

pression from withdrawal of myocardial support and increases in afterload. Metoprolol, a β_1-selective agent with a 75-fold affinity for β_1-adrenergic compared to β_2-adrenergic receptors, has been used successfully in several chronic heart failure trials. It has been shown to upregulate the β_1-adrenergic receptor and improve the responsiveness to β-agonist stimulation.[20] It does not produce a reduction in plasma norepinephrine levels due to the blocking of norepinephrine clearance. Because it does not block β_2-receptors and it increases cardiac adrenergic activity acutely, metoprolol produces less myocardial depression than propranolol, and has been tolerated by 79% of patients with Class II to Class III chronic heart failure. It also has substantial *inverse agonist* properties, where it inactivates active-state unoccupied receptors. Because of its upregulation of the β_1-adrenergic receptor, metoprolol would be expected to increase exercise capacity if reductions in β_1-adrenergic receptor density are partially responsible for decreased exercise capacity.[7] However, since β_2-receptors are unblocked chronically and there is no reduction in cardiac or systemic norepinephrine, there may be less favorable effects on left ventricular function and prevention of sudden death and all cardiac death, compared to the newer third-generation β-adrenergic receptor blockers, bucindolol and carvedilol.

In contrast, bucindolol, a new third-generation β-adrenergic blocker, is a nonselective blocker and has the additional property of vasodilation by a direct effect on vascular smooth muscle. Bucindolol has no agonist (ISA) properties in human cardiac systems, but it has *atypical* pharmacological characteristics, which include guanine nucleotide modulatable binding and downregulation of β-adrenergic receptors.[21] Bucindolol also causes a reduction in circulating norepinephrine levels, which results in a reduced adrenergic state.[22] Bucindolol's mild inverse agonist profile also likely contributes to its excellent tolerability.[23] Perhaps because of the degree of antiadrenergic effects related to a combination of its typical and atypical properties, bucindolol may produce more favorable effects on left ventricular function and hemodynamics than the second-generation β-adrenergic blocker, metoprolol.[24] These features impart a potential survival benefit to this drug, which is currently being evaluated in the Beta Blocker Evaluation of Survival Trial (BEST).[25] However, these features would also be expected to limit the ability of the drug to increase exercise capacity.

Carvedilol is the other new third-generation β-adrenergic blocker with vasodilator properties. It has strong α-adrenergic blocking ability with its affinity for the α_1-adrenergic receptor, one-third of its affinity for β-adrenergic receptors. It is mildly selective with a $\beta1/\beta_2$ affinity of approximately 7:1.[26] It also has atypical binding features and has been shown to downregulate myocardial β-adrenergic receptors in cultured cells [27] and to not upregulate the downregulated β_1-receptors in the failing human heart.[28] Carvedilol produces favorable effects on clinical outcome[17,18] and cardiac function[28] which, again, may be greater than those produced by metoprolol. However, as for bucindolol, the limited ability to respond to an acute sympathetic stimulus such as exercise may limit its ability to improve exercise capacity in heart failure patients.

Based on the unique features of several of these β-adrenergic blockers, it is impossible to conclude that the effect of these agents on exercise capacity is a class effect. The effects of long-term therapy with these drugs on exercise capacity in chronic heart failure patients must be evaluated according to their β-receptor subtype selectivity, effects on myocardial β-receptor expression, effects on circulating norepinephrine, and inverse agonist properties. These features will determine their effect on mortality, cardiac function, and exercise capacity.[29]

Effects of β-Adrenergic Blockers on Peak Exercise Capacity

Improvements in exercise capacity are usually determined by an increase in maximal exercise oxygen uptake ($\dot{V}O_{2max}$), as measured on either a treadmill or cycle ergometer.[30] Patients with chronic heart failure are often limited by dyspnea and fatigue and usually do not fulfill the physiological criteria for $\dot{V}O_{2max}$, therefore the highest attainable $\dot{V}O_2$ at the end of exercise (peak $\dot{V}O_2$) is used to quantify exercise capacity.[31]

Unless careful attention is paid to other determinants of peak exercise performance such as the respiratory exchange ratio (RER, $VCO_2/\dot{V}O_2$) or blood lactate levels, this measurement can be affected to a large degree by patient motivation. The lack of a gold standard for peak exercise capacity in patients with chronic heart failure contributes to the difficulty in determining the effect of long-term β-adrenergic blockade on exercise capacity. Most of the available data consist of either peak exercise $\dot{V}O_2$, estimated $\dot{V}O_2$ described in METS (1 MET = 3.5 mL/kg/min or resting $\dot{V}O_2$), or most commonly, exercise duration.

Metoprolol

Most of the available clinical studies on long-term β-adrenergic blockade and exercise capacity in heart failure have used the β_1-selective blocker metoprolol. Although there are several studies available that evaluated peak exercise capacity as one of the endpoints of therapy, most studies have consisted of small numbers of patients with a short (<2 months) treatment period. However, there are several studies that present compelling data that metoprolol improves peak exercise capacity in patients with chronic heart failure.[15,32-34]

The first study that demonstrates an improvement in peak exercise duration involves both a double-blind, placebo-controlled trial and a crossover study in 20 patients with nonischemic, dilated cardiomyopathy.[32] Patients received an average daily dose of 92 mg of metoprolol for 12 months. Peak exercise capacity, as reported with a MET score, doubled in the randomized study and increased by 50% in the crossover phase of the study (Figure 2). Accompanying the increase in peak exercise capacity were a 58% increase in resting left ventricular ejection fraction (LVEF) in the randomized phase and 35% increase in the crossover phase, when compared to placebo. Patients who were initially NYHA Functional Class II to Class III (2.4±0.9 SEM) also improved their status to Class I to Class II (1.5±0.6 SEM) after 12 months of metoprolol therapy. Mortality could not be evaluated due to the small number of patients in the trial. This was the first study to definitively demonstrate that long-term β-adrenergic blockade with the β_1-selective blocker metoprolol could increase peak exercise capacity in heart failure. The results are limited, however, because of the lack of objective physiological measurements of $\dot{V}O_2$. The heart rate responses to peak exercise were also an interesting aspect of this trial, as these responses may relate to the observed improvement in peak exercise capacity. The mean peak exercise heart rates in the metoprolol-treated patients were identical to those at the onset of therapy, prior to drug administration, but occurred at a higher estimated MET level of exercise. Heart rates during submaximal exercise were mildly reduced after 12 months of metoprolol therapy, with a 11% decrease in the randomized phase and a 23% decrease in the crossover phase. These heart rate reductions were less than reported with other β-adrenergic blocker studies in chronic heart failure. This effect of heart rate on peak exercise performance will be dramatically demonstrated in studies using the newer third-generation vasodilating β-adrenergic blockers, bucindolol and carvedilol. The results do support the hypothesis that upregulation of myocardial β-adrenergic receptors can improve exercise capacity in chronic heart failure.[7]

Several other studies support the concept that therapy with metoprolol in chronic heart failure can improve peak exercise capcity. In a small study using open-labeled metoprolol for 2 months in patients with chronic heart failure secondary to both ischemic and nonischemic cardiomyopathy, there was a significant 9% increase in directly measured peak $\dot{V}O_2$ (14.8±1.1 to 16.1±0.9 mL/kg/min).[33] The average daily dose was 97 mg of metoprolol, which was comparable to the doses in the previous described trial[32] and is consistent with a high degree of β-adrenergic blockade. In this trial there was a 21% reduction in heart rate at peak exercise after the 2 month treatment period. These

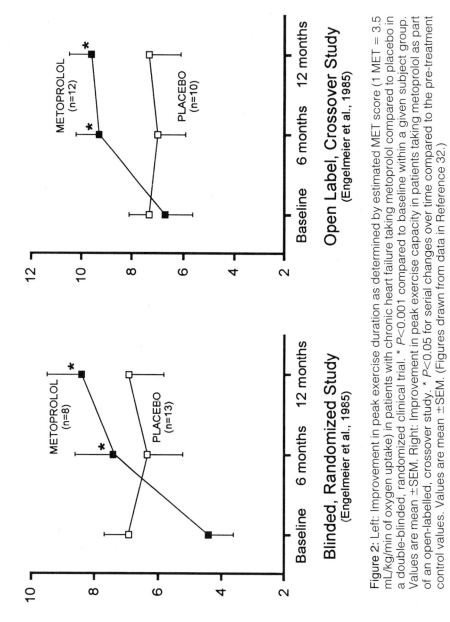

Figure 2: Left: Improvement in peak exercise duration as determined by estimated MET score (1 MET = 3.5 mL/kg/min of oxygen uptake) in patients with chronic heart failure taking metoprolol compared to placebo in a double-blinded, randomized clinical trial. * $P<0.001$ compared to baseline within a given subject group. Values are mean ±SEM. Right: Improvement in peak exercise capacity in patients taking metoprolol as part of an open-labelled, crossover study. * $P<0.05$ for serial changes over time compared to the pre-treatment control values. Values are mean ±SEM. (Figures drawn from data in Reference 32.)

data suggest that an increase in peak exercise capacity can occur with metoprolol even with a substantial reduction in heart rate at peak exercise. Accompanying the increase in peak $\dot{V}O_2$ was a modest increase in workload on the cycle ergometer (90±8 watts to 95±7 watts) and a definite 67% increase in resting LVEF. Despite the use of objective physiological techniques during exercise, this study was compromised by the lack of a placebo group. Long-term therapy with metoprolol also appears to maintain the benefit in exercise capacity. After 19 months of therapy with an average daily dose of 61 mg of metoprolol, patients with nonischemic dilated cardiomyopathy had a greater peak exercise duration (9.4±1.2 min) on a treadmill than patients receiving placebo (8.2±0.7 min).[34]

Despite the favorable benefits reported in these studies, the overall numbers of patients receiving metoprolol were small and the durations of therapy and doses of drug varied between the various studies. To address the issue of the efficacy of long-term metoprolol therapy in nonischemic cardiomyopathy, 383 patients were randomized to either placebo or metoprolol, as part of the Metoprolol in Dilated Cardiomyopathy Trial (MDC).[15] In the 194 patients receiving an average daily dose of 108 mg of metoprolol, there was a 34% reduction in the combined endpoints of death and need for cardiac transplantation. There was a 14% improvement in total exercise duration on either a treadmill or cycle ergometer after 6 months of therapy, and a 13% increase at 12 months (Figure 3). In contrast, patients on placebo demonstrated a significant improvement (8%) at 6 months, but lost this effect with no increase in exercise capacity compared to entry into the trial, at 12 months. Thus, for the first time, an improvement in exercise capacity with long-term metoprolol therapy was demonstrated in a large multicenter clinical trial in patients with nonischemic cardiomyopathy. Accompanying this increase in exercise capacity was a 54% increase in resting LVEF at 12 months and improvement in quality-of-life measures. No heart rate data at peak exercise are available for the entire trial, but a substudy reported a 9% decrease in exercise heart rate at 50% of maximal exercise capacity.[35] At rest there were significant decreases in heart rate and pulmonary capillary wedge pressure (PCWP) and increases in systolic blood pressure, stroke volume, and stroke work index only in the metoprolol-treated patients at 12 months.

Favorable hemodynamic responses during exercise accompany the improvement in peak exercise capacity reported with metoprolol.[35,36] In an open-labelled study of high-dose (127 mg) metoprolol in 21 patients with both ischemic and nonischemic cardiomyopathy, treated for 14 months, there was a 25% increase in peak exercise workload on a cycle ergometer (104±9 watts to 130 ±9 watts).[36] Resting LVEF improved by 52%, and invasive hemodynamic measurements at a workload equiva-

Metoprolol in Dilated Cardiomyopathy Study

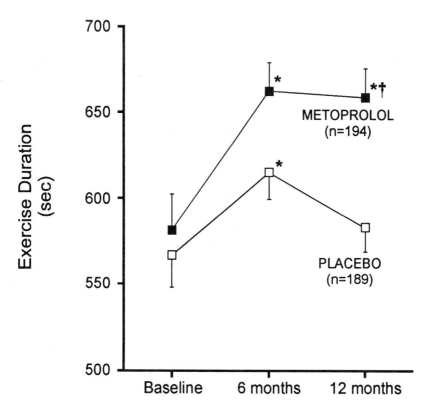

Figure 3: Improvement in exercise duration in patients taking metoprolol as part of the Metoprolol in Dilated Cardiomyopathy (MDC) Study. * $P<0.01$ for comparison with baseline values. † $P<0.05$ for comparisons between the metoprolol and placebo groups. Values are mean $\pm$SEM. (Figure drawn from data in Reference 15.)

lent to 50% peak $\dot{V}O_2$ demonstrated a 13% increase in mean arterial pressure (MAP), a 21% increase in cardiac index, a 30% increase in stroke volume index, and a 64% increase in stroke work index. There was no change in exercise heart rate at this submaximal workload after 14 months of metoprolol therapy. Arteriovenous oxygen content difference decreased somewhat (14.5 ± 2.5 vol % to 13.1 ± 3.1 vol %) after long-term metoprolol therapy. There were no significant changes in right atrial pressure (RAP), PCWP, or either myocardial or total body $\dot{V}O_2$ at this submaximal workload. Myocardial metabolic measurements using arterial and coronary sinus sampling demonstrated that long-term metoprolol therapy led to no change in coronary sinus blood flow during exercise, no myocardial lactate production with exercise, a decrease in myocardial norepinephrine spillover during exercise, and no change in myocardial $\dot{V}O_2$. These data suggest that metoprolol allows a greater myocardial workload without higher metabolic costs in chronic heart failure patients. Because this study did not have a placebo group, similar measurements were performed as part of a hemodynamic substudy of the MDC trial.[35] Forty patients with nonischemic cardiomyopathy were studied at baseline and after 6 months and 12 months of therapy. Twenty patients received an average daily dose of 130 ± 6 mg of metoprolol, with an 11% improvement in peak exercise duration after 12 months of therapy. There was a 62% increase in resting LVEF in the subjects receiving metoprolol, with no change in the placebo group. At a submaximal workload representing 50% of maximal capacity, there were several favorable hemodynamic changes after 12 months of metoprolol therapy (Figure 4). There were no comparable changes seen in the placebo group. Heart rate was decreased by 9% at both 6 months and 12 months of therapy. There were significant increases in cardiac index, stroke volume index, and stroke work index after 6 months of metoprolol therapy, with further increases at 12 months. Although there were trends toward reductions in all intracardiac filling pressures with metoprolol, only PCWP was significantly lower at 12 months. Coronary sinus blood flow and myocardial $\dot{V}O_2$ were unchanged, while net myocardial lactate extraction increased with metoprolol. Thus, in a subset of patients in a large clinical trial of metoprolol in nonischemic cardiomyopathy, improved hemodynamic status during submaximal exercise was shown to accompany the increases in peak exercise capacity.

Thus, long-term therapy with the β_1-selective blocker metoprolol has been shown to improve peak exercise capacity in several well-controlled clinical trials. These data support the role of the reduction in the myocardial β-receptor in the decreased exercise capacity in chronic heart failure patients, since therapy with a drug that increases β-receptor density improved exercise capacity. Despite these results, there is still some question about the role of peak exercise heart rate in ability of these patients to improve peak exercise performance with long-term β-adrenergic blockade. Clearly this is an issue in normal subjects who have been shown to have masking of improvements in peak exercise capacity after exercise training with β-adrenergic blockade, if tested while still taking β-blockers.[37,38] There are minimal data available to address this question in these studies with metoprolol in chronic heart failure patients. This will become an important issue when the exercise responses of the newer third-generation vasodilating β-blockers with atypical receptor binding are evaluated. Despite the favorable benefits of metoprolol on exercise capacity and resting LVEF, there has been no favorable benefit on cardiac survival and prevention of sudden death.

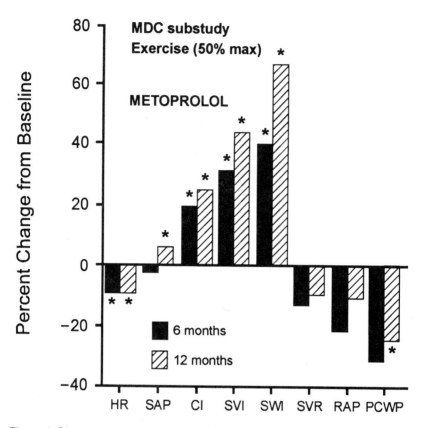

Figure 4: Changes in hemodynamics during an exercise load of 50% maximal intensity after 6 and 12 months of therapy with metoprolol as part of a substudy of the MDC study.There were no significant changes in the placebo group (data not shown). HR = heart rate, SAP = systolic arterial pressure, CI = cardiac index, SVI = stroke volume index, SWI = stroke work index, SVR = systemic vascular resistance, RAP = right atrial pressure, PCWP = pulmonary capillary wedge pressure. * $P<0.05$ compared to baseline, pre-treatment values. (Figure drawn from data in Reference 35.)

This lack of benefit in these important clinical areas may be related to the lack of blockade of the myocardial β_2-adrenergic receptors, which are relatively increased in patients with chronic heart failure. This theoretical consideration, along with the favorable benefit of propranolol, a nonselective β-adrenergic blocker, on total and sudden cardiac death after myocardial infarction, has led to the development and testing of new third-generation β-adrenergic blockers with different pharmacological properties that make them amenable to therapy in chronic heart failure patients.

Bucindolol

Bucindolol is a nonselective β-adrenergic blocker with a 10-fold more potent affinity for the β_1-adrenergic receptor than metoprolol; in addition, it blocks the remaining β_2-adrenergic receptors. It also has "atypical" GTP-dependent or "guanine nucleotide modulatable" binding, which is associated with a downregulation of myocardial cell β-receptor density.[26] During exercise, the reduced total β-receptor number associated with chronic heart failure and the failure of bucindolol to restore the β-receptors to more normal levels may be important in determining the effect of this drug on exercise capacity. In addition, circulating levels of norepinephrine are decreased in the resting state with bucindolol, and although there are no data available on plasma norepinephrine during exercise, decreased levels seem plausible[39] and would lead to decreased stimulation. Finally, bucindolol has intrinsic vasodilating activity that might lead to an increase in cardiac output during exercise. Thus, there are several reasons to suggest that the exercise responses to long-term bucindolol therapy may be different from those of metoprolol.

Bucindolol has been compared to metoprolol in regard to hemodynamic and energetic effects on the failing heart.[24,40] In a study comparing 3 months of therapy with either 100 mg of metoprolol per day or 190 mg of bucindolol per day in 30 patients with nonischemic cardiomyopathy, there were comparable increases in resting LVEF, stroke volume, and peak dP/dt in both treatment groups.[40] Both β-adrenergic blockers also produced comparable improvements in isovolumic relaxation and reductions in ventricular volume. Bucindolol therapy resulted in a greater increase in resting cardiac index and a greater reduction in left ventricular end-diastolic pressure than did therapy with metoprolol. In contrast, there were greater reductions in coronary blood flow and myocardial $\dot{V}O_2$ with metoprolol than with bucindolol. A more recent study reviewed the experience of long-term therapy with 6 months of metoprolol, at 128 ± 37 mg/day, and with bucindolol, at 192 ± 27 mg/day, in a total of 34 patients with chronic heart failure secondary to nonischemic cardiomyopathy.[24] There was slightly greater β-adrenergic blockade with bucindolol, since there was greater reduction in peak exercise heart rate with bucindolol compared to metoprolol, although the mean daily heart rates on ambulatory monitoring were similar with both drugs. Despite the shorter duration of therapy with bucindolol (3 months) versus metoprolol (6 months), there were greater increases in resting stroke volume and stroke work indices with bucindolol. In addition, only bucindolol therapy was associated with a significant decrease in resting systemic vascular resistance and an upward and leftward shift in the relation of stroke volume index to PCWP, suggesting improved intrinsic myocardial function. Both drugs produced a comparable and significant increase in resting LVEF, but decreases in left ventricular end-diastolic size were seen only with bucindolol. Overall, these results suggested that bucindolol has a similar or slight advantage over metoprolol in the effects on left ventricular function and resting cardiac hemodynamics. These differences may be explained by the pharmacological differences between these two β-adrenergic blockers.

Despite all of the potential hemodynamic benefits of bucindolol in chronic heart failure, there have been no reported increases in peak exercise VO_2 with this nonselective β-adrenergic blocker (Figure 5, left). In fact, peak exercise VO_2, as well as exercise duration, tend to decrease with long-term bucindolol therapy. In a double-blind, placebo-controlled study of 23 patients with nonischemic cardiomyopathy, 14 of which received a mean daily dose of 170 mg of bucindolol, there were no significant increases in either peak exercise VO_2 or exercise duration after 3 months of therapy.[22] There was a 26% reduction in peak exercise heart rate after 3 months of bucindolol therapy. Despite the lack of a significant change in objectively measured peak exercise capacity, there was a 35% mean increase in resting LVEF, significant increases in resting cardiac index and left ventricular stroke work index, and reductions in resting intracardiac filling pressures. None of these changes were seen in the placebo group. NYHA Functional Class also improved with long-term bucindolol therapy (2.5 ± 0.1 to 1.6 ± 0.1, $P<0.05$) which placed most patients in Class I and Class II after 3 months of therapy. A larger study evaluating the effects of bucindolol in ischemic versus nonischemic cardiomyopathy patients also found no improvement in either peak exercise VO_2 or exercise duration.[39] After 3 months of therapy with 180 mg of bucindolol daily, there was a 10% decrease in peak exercise VO_2 accompanied by a 27% reduction in peak exercise heart rate. There were no differences in exercise responses to long-term bucindolol therapy between the ischemic and nonischemic cardiomyopathy groups. Despite the lack of improvement in peak exercise performance, bucindolol therapy was associated with a 33% increase in resting LVEF, a significant increase in resting stroke work index, a reduction in left ventricular size, and a decrease in PCWP. Except for the reduction in left ventricular size, all the favorable hemodynamic benefits occurred exclusively in the patients with nonischemic cardiomyopathy. However, the ischemic group appeared to have more advanced disease with a lower resting LVEF, a lower peak exercise VO_2, and a higher dose of diuretic than the nonischemic group. Hemodynamic, symptomatic, and functional class improvement occurred, despite the lack of an increase in peak exercise capacity on the treadmill. Similar results were seen with prolonged therapy with open-labelled bucindolol in 20 patients with nonischemic cardiomyopathy.[41] After 23 months of bucindolol at a mean daily dose of

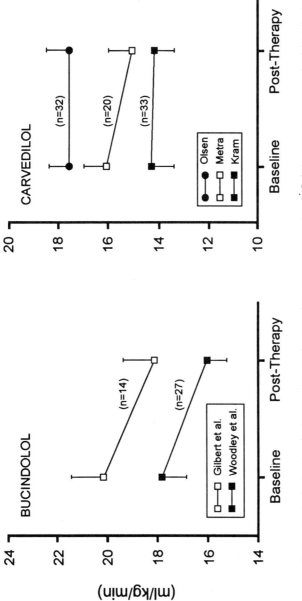

Figure 5: Left: Lack of change in peak exercise oxygen uptake ($\dot{V}O_2$) in two separate double-blinded, placebo-controlled clinical trials using bucindolol in patients with chronic heart failure. Duration of therapy was 12 weeks in both studies. (Figure drawn from data in Reference 22 and Reference 39.) Right: Lack of change in peak exercise $\dot{V}O_2$ in three separate double-blinded, placebo-controlled clinical trials using carvedilol in patients with chronic heart failure. Duration of therapy was 3–4 months in all studies. (Figure drawn from data in Reference 16, Reference 43, and Reference 44.) Values are mean ±SEM.

176 mg there were no changes in peak exercise V̇O$_2$ (19.2±4.9 to 18.8±5.1 mL/kg/min). Functional class improved in 60% of the patients and worsened in 15%. Compared to entry values, resting LVEF increased by 40%. Since there was no placebo group, it is impossible to determine if long-term bucindolol therapy could have maintained peak exercise capacity, while exercise capacity may have declined in the untreated group.

Not all studies have shown a lack of improvement in peak exercise capacity with long-term bucindolol therapy. In a small study of 20 patients with both ischemic and nonischemic cardiomyopathy, 12 of whom received a mean daily dose of 200 mg of bucindolol for 3 months, there was a 19% increase in exercise duration during treadmill testing (Figure 6).[42] Peak exercise heart rate was reduced by 24% in the bucindolol-treated patients, although the peak heart rate at entry was lower than in other clinical trials (127±7 bpm). This improvement in peak exercise capacity was accompanied by a 21% increase in resting LVEF, an increase in resting cardiac output, an improved quality-of-life score, and a reduction in peak exercise PCWP. These patients had poorer functional capacity than in previous studies with no NYHA Functional Class II patients, 83% Class III and 17% Class IV patients. Despite the presence of a placebo group that demonstrated none of the favorable outcomes seen with bucindolol, the results of the study have a weakened impact due to the small number of patients evaluated.

The most definitive study to date on the effects of bucindolol in patients with chronic heart failure evaluated the dose-response of bucindolol on both hemodynamic and exercise responses in both ischemic and nonischemic cardiomyopathy patients in a multicenter trial.[14] In this double-blind, placebo-controlled trial, 38 patients received a low dose (12.5 mg/day), 32 patients received a medium dose (50 mg/day), and 35 patients received a high dose (200 mg/day) of bucindolol. Patients were either functional Class II or Class III, and 71% had nonischemic cardiomyopathy, while the remaining 29% had ischemic cardiomyopathy. There was a direct correlation between the dose of bucindolol and the effects of resting LVEF. The higher the dose of bucindolol administrated, the greater the improvement in LVEF was, with a 7.8% increase in the high dose group. Overall, there were no changes in exercise duration on the treadmill in all patients receiving bucindolol (Figure 6). There was an inverse relationship between the dose of bucindolol and peak exercise duration, with the highest dose of bucindolol causing a small reduction in exercise duration when compared to placebo. These reductions in exercise duration with increasing doses of bucindolol were directly related to the decrease in peak exercise heart rate seen with the high degree of total β-adrenergic blockade seen with this drug (Figure 7). At the highest dose of bucindolol, 200 mg/day, there was a 26% reduction in peak exercise heart rate, compared to a 15% reduction in patients receiving the low

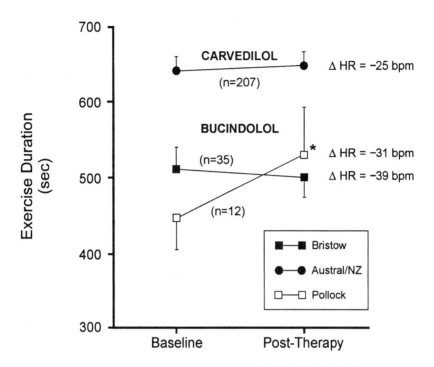

Figure 6: Change in peak exercise duration in doubled-blinded, placebo-controlled trials with bucindolol and carvedilol with special reference to the reduction in peak exercise heart rate by both drugs after chronic therapy. Values are mean ±SEM. *P*<0.05 by paired t-test. (The bucindolol data are taken from patients on the highest dose of 200 mg per day in Reference 14 and from patients in Reference 42. The carvedilol data is taken from Reference 45.)

dose, 12.5 mg/day. Although the study was underpowered to evaluate both fatal and nonfatal outcomes, there were fewer adverse clinical events in the high dose as compared to the low dose of bucindolol. There were no favorable changes seen in the placebo group. These results suggested a paradox in the outcome of therapy with bucindolol in patients with chronic heart failure. The highest dose of the drug was associated with the most benefit in improved left ventricular function, a decrease in left ventricular size, and a possible reduction in both fatal and nonfatal events. In comparison, the lowest dose of bucindolol was associated with the least adverse effects on exercise capacity, and at the highest dose of bucindolol, exercise capacity appeared to be reduced in comparison with the placebo. The progressive reduction in peak exercise heart rate with increasing doses of bucindolol appeared to be responsible for the negative effects on

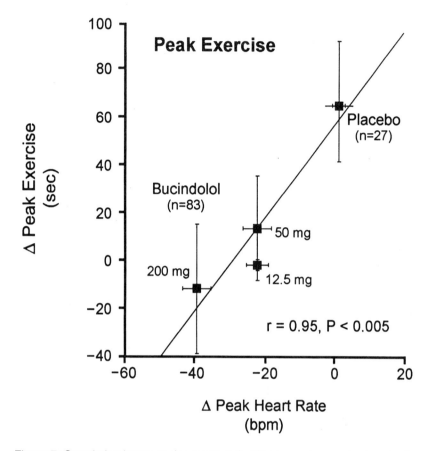

Figure 7: Correlation between the mean reduction in peak exercise heart rate and the mean change in peak exercise duration as a function of the dose of bucindolol. Higher doses of bucindolol were associated with a greater reduction in peak exercise heart rate and a decrease in peak exercise duration. Values are mean ±SEM. (Figure drawn from data in Reference 14.)

exercise capacity. This blunting of peak exercise heart rate due to the high degree of total β-adrenergic receptor blockade with bucindolol may prevent any determination of improved exercise capacity at peak exercise, as seen with other β-adrenergic blockers in normal subjects.[37,38]

Carvedilol

Carvedilol is a unique, slightly selective β_1-adrenergic blocker, which has vasodilating properties due to α-adrenergic blockade.[26] Its affinity for myocardial α-receptors is one-third of its affinity for β-adrenergic receptors.[26] It also has atypical binding, and results in downregulation of myocardial β-adrenergic receptors.[26,27] Based on these receptor binding characteristics, there may be a diminished response to the acute stimulation of exercise, similar to that seen with bucindolol. However, since carvedilol is a slightly selective β-adrenergic blocker, not all myocardial β_2-receptors will be blocked by lower doses of this drug. In addition, the vasodilating properties, secondary to α-adrenergic blockade, are more pronounced than those of bucindolol and can result in an increase in cardiac output and enhanced peripheral vasodilation during exercise, as occurs acutely with all α_1-adrenergic receptor blockers that can enhance exercise capacity. Thus, the differences between carvedilol and bucindolol, α_1-adrenergic blockade with moderate vasodilator activity and β-receptor subtype selectivity differences, can influence exercise capacity in chronic heart failure patients.

There have been three studies that have evaluated the effects of carvedilol on peak exercise $\dot{V}O_2$ as part of a double-blind, placebo-controlled design in patients with both ischemic and nonischemic cardiomyopathy.[16,43,44] In a total of 89 patients receiving an average daily dose of 50 mg of carvedilol for 4 months, there were no significant increases in peak exercise $\dot{V}O_2$ (Figure 5, right). In two of these studies, peak exercise heart rates were decreased with carvedilol by 21%[43] and 24%[16] respectively, and these heart rate data are similar to the clinical studies with bucindolol. Despite the lack of an improvement in peak exercise capacity, there were significant increases in resting LVEF compared to placebo in all carvedilol-treated patients. In a study of 60 patients with both ischemic and nonischemic cardiomyopathy, 36 of which were randomized to carvedilol, there was a 53% increase in resting LVEF accompanied by significant increases in resting stroke volume and stroke work, and a decrease in resting PCWP after 4 months of carvedilol therapy.[43] Despite the lack of improvement in peak exercise $\dot{V}O_2$ and exercise duration, carvedilol had a favorable impact on NYHA Functional class with 47% in Class II and 53% in Class III prior to randomization, and 12% in Class I, 79% in Class II, and only 9% in Class III after 4 months of therapy. Thus, there was a discrepancy between a measure of total functional capacity, NYHA Functional Class, and an objective measure of peak exercise capacity $\dot{V}O_2$, raising an issue of a limitation in peak exercise testing in the definition of exercise capacity in patients on β-adrenergic blockers. Similar findings were seen in a study of 46 patients with chronic heart failure, where the 33 patients receiving carvedilol also had an improvement in functional class (2.8 ± 0.1 to 1.9 ± 0.2, $P<0.05$).[44] In this study, carvedilol had a lower incidence of adverse events compared to placebo (8% versus 44%) and there was an associated 38% increase in resting LVEF, an increase in resting stroke volume index, and reductions in intracardiac filling pressures, all related to carvedilol therapy. Similar findings were also seen in a European study, where 20 patients randomized to carvedilol had improvements in resting LVEF, resting hemodynamics, and improved quality-of-life scores, despite no increase in peak exercise $\dot{V}O_2$.[16] A larger, multicenter, clinical trial with carvedilol in patients with only ischemic cardiomyopathy also confirmed the results of several of these smaller trials.[45] In 207 patients receiving an average daily dose of 50 mg of carvedilol for 6 months, there were no increases in exercise duration as measured with a treadmill protocol (Figure 6). Carvedilol-treated subjects did have a 20% reduction in peak exercise heart rate and a 23% reduction in peak exercise rate-pressure product, findings not seen in the placebo group. Despite the potential benefits of this reduction in myocardial $\dot{V}O_2$ in patients with ischemic heart disease, there was no prolongation of exercise time. However, carvedilol did have positive therapeutic effects: a 19% increase in resting LVEF and a reduction in heart size. When compared to the other smaller therapeutic trials with carvedilol in patients with primarily nonischemic cardiomyopathy, there were no significant improvements in functional class in these ischemic patients receiving carvedilol.

Despite the lack of improvement in peak exercise capacity with carvedilol in patients with chronic heart failure, favorable hemodynamic changes at peak exercise have been reported.[16] In 20 patients who received carvedilol as part of a 4-month, double-blind, placebo-controlled trial, there were significant increases in cardiac index, stroke volume index, and stroke work index, accompanied by reductions in systemic vascular resistance, pulmonary vascular resistance, and both right and left heart filling pressures at peak exercise (Figure 8). Peak exercise heart rate was decreased by 24% after long-term carvedilol therapy, and this pharmacological effect of β-adrenergic blockade may have prevented the expected increase in exercise capacity that would have been expected to occur as a result of the other favorable hemodynamic changes at peak exercise.

Effects of β-Adrenergic Blockers on Submaximal Exercise Capacity

Reductions in peak exercise heart rate occur in all studies using long-term β-adrenergic blockade in the treatment of chronic heart failure. This pharmacological effect of β-adrenergic blockade may prevent the expected increase in exercise capacity, since many other favorable outcomes have been reported in these patients. Determination of submaximal exercise performance has been used as an alternate means of evaluating exercise capacity after long-term β-adrenergic blockade.

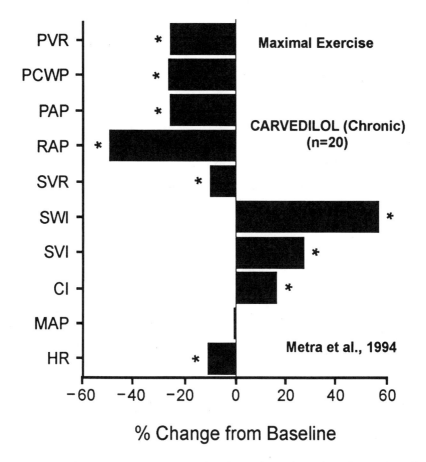

% Change from Baseline

Figure 8: Changes in peak exercise hemodynamics after 4 months of carvedilol in a double-blinded, placebo controlled trial. There were no significant changes in the placebo group (data not shown). * $P < 0.05$ compared to pre-treatment values. (Figure drawn from data in Reference 16.)

Submaximal exercise is less dependent on heart rate responses and thereby may be less influenced by the heart rate effects of long-term β-adrenergic blockade. Also, submaximal exercise performance may be a better reflection of a patient's daily activity level and could better correlate with the improvements in resting cardiac function (LVEF), cardiac hemodynamics, and functional class.

There have been several approaches to the determination of submaximal exercise capacity in heart failure patients. The 6-minute walk test has been shown to be a sensitive and reproducible determination of exercise capacity in patients with chronic heart failure.[46] Patients are asked to walk as great a distance as possible in 6 minutes with limited hemodynamic and other measurements. The distance walked, after several tests to familiarize the patient with the procedure, is used to describe exercise capacity. There have been no studies using the 6-minute walk test with metoprolol in patients with chronic heart failure, probably because of the reported increase in peak exercise capacity in several studies. There have been several studies with both bucindolol and carvedilol that have evaluated exercise capacity with the 6-minute walk test after a variable period of β-blocker therapy (Table 2). In a small study of 12 patients who received a mean daily dose of 200 mg of bucindolol as part of a double-blind, placebo-controlled trial, there was a minimal, although statistically significant, increase in the 6-minute walk test.[42] This study was also the only one to show an improvement in peak exercise capacity with bucindolol. Because of the small number of patients and the minimal increase in walking time, the effects of bucindolol on the 6-minute walk test was uncertain. In a larger trial evaluating the dose-response effects of bucindolol in chronic heart failure, there were no increases in walking time with either low, medium, or high dose bucindolol.[14] At the highest dose of bucindolol, 200 mg/day, at which the most improvement in resting LVEF was observed, there was no significant improvement in walking time. There also appeared to be worsening of walking time with increasing doses of buncidolol similar to the response at peak exercise. Similar findings were observed with carvedilol. In a smaller study of chronic heart failure patients, there was

Table 2

Submaximal Exercise: Results of 6-Minute Walk Tests with Bucindolol and Carvedilol

Bucindolol	N	Baseline	Post-Therapy	
Pollock et al. (3 mo)	12	377 ± 54	389 ± 48	p < 0.05
Bristow et al. (3 mo)*	35	493 ± 16	527 ± 11	p = ns
Carvedilol				
Australia-New Zealand (3 mo)	207	390 ± 6	396 ± 6	p = ns
Krum et al. (3 mo)	33	391 ± 19	444 ± 18	p < 0.01
MOCHA (6 mo)**	80	356 ± 14	361 ± 12	p = ns

Results are expressed in meters with mean ± SEM. *Dose of bucindolol was 200 mg per day.

**Dose of carvedilol was 50 mg per day. There were no significant changes in walk time in any placebo group in these trials.

ns = not significant; MOCHA = Multicenter Oral Carvedilol Heart Failure Assessment.

a significant 14% increase in walking time after 4 months of carvedilol therapy.[44] This improvement in the 6-minute walk test occurred despite no significant increase in peak exercise $\dot{V}O_2$. Other larger studies with carvedilol in chronic heart failure do not support this finding. In the Australia-New Zealand Study, 207 patients with ischemic cardiomyopathy randomized to carvedilol did not demonstrate an improvement in the 6-minute walk test.[45] The distances walked prior to randomization were similar in both this study and the previous discussed smaller clinical trial. Recent data from the Multicenter Oral Carvedilol Heart Failure Assessment (MOCHA) Trial also fail to demonstrate an improvement in walking time.[18] This trial investigated the dose-response effects of carvedilol at low (12.5 mg), medium (25 mg) and high (50 mg) daily doses on exercise capacity, resting LVEF, and mortality. Both the 6-minute walk test and the 9-minute self-activated treadmill test were used to quantify exercise capacity. The latter test has been shown to be another method to evaluate exercise at a submaximal level.[47] There were no increases in exercise time with either test with any dose of carvedilol (Figure 9, left). In fact, distance walked during either test decreased with increasing doses of carvedilol. In addition, an inverse relationship was seen between carvedilol dose and both resting LVEF and mortality. Resting LVEF increased and mortality declined progressively with higher doses of carvedilol (Figure 9, right). Thus, a paradox again existed between the dose-response effects of a third-generation β-adrenergic blocker on cardiac function and outcome and exercise capacity. Cardiac function was improved and, in this case, mortality was reduced at the highest dose of carvedilol, at the expense of exercise tolerance. This situation is similar to that seen with peak exercise and the 6-minute walk test results with bucindolol.[14] Recent data suggest that patients approach their peak exercise $\dot{V}O_2$ on the 9-minute self-activated treadmill test[48] and that a similar situation may occur with the 6-minute walk test. Thus, the exercise responses mimic those with peak exercise testing, and it is not surprising that heart rate may again be a limiting factor in patients taking β-blockers during these tests. In general, these tests have failed to show consistent improvement in exercise capacity in heart failure patients on long-term β-blocker therapy and, in fact, are poor measures of submaximal exercise performance.

A recent approach to quantifying submaximal exercise capacity is to determine the walking time during a fixed level of submaximal work, defined as a given percentage of peak exercise $\dot{V}O_2$. Two small clinical trials have evaluated the effects of carvedilol on exercise tolerance at 80% and 85% peak $\dot{V}O_2$ respectively (Figure 10). In the first study of 20 patients randomized to carvedilol as part of a double-blind, placebo-controlled trial, there was a significant 147% improve-

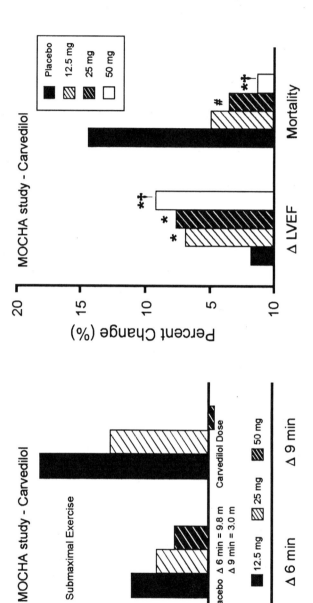

Figure 9: Left: Changes in exercise capacity during submaximal exercise as measured in the 6-minute walk test and the 9-minute self-activated treadmill test as a function of the dose of carvedilol in the Multicenter Oral Carvedilol Heart Failure Assessment (MOCHA) Trial. There were no significant increases in distance walked in either test with any dose of carvedilol compared to placebo. Right: Improvement in resting left ventricular ejection fraction (LVEF) and reduction in mortality as a function of the dose of carvedilol in the MOCHA trial. * $P < 0.005$ versus placebo; #$P < 0.05$ versus placebo; †$P < 0.01$ for dose-response relation. (Figures drawn from data in Bristow M, Gilbert E, Abraham W, et al. *Circulation* 1995;92(suppl I):I-142.)

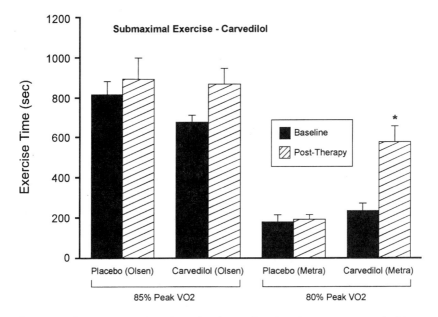

Figure 10: Improvement in submaximal exercise duration as measured with a fixed workload test with carvedilol in two double-blinded, placebo-controlled trials. (Olsen, n = 36; Metra, n = 20). Values are mean ±SEM. * *P*<0.05 compared to pre-treatment values. (Figure drawn from data in Reference 16 and Reference 43.)

ment in exercise time at 80% peak V̇O$_2$ after 4 months of therapy.[16] This increase in exercise time during submaximal exercise occurred despite no improvement in peak exercise capacity. The other study showed a trend toward improved submaximal exercise capacity, with a 27% increase in exercise capacity at 85% peak V̇O$_2$.[43] Despite the higher exercise intensity in this study, patients had a greater baseline exercise duration than in the previous study, suggesting that these patients may have been healthier or less deconditioned. This could have explained the lack of a significant increase in submaximal exercise time in this relatively small study. This type of testing is difficult since the workload is chosen after a peak exercise test is performed, and there is significant variability in the response in individual patients. However, this type of submaximal exercise testing has been the only method that has shown an improvement in exercise capacity with long-term β-adrenergic blockade, and it does not appear to be dependent on exercise heart rate. Further testing of this method in large multicenter, clinical trials will be required to determine if this is the method of choice for evaluating exercise performance in heart failure patients on β-blockers.

Lessons from β-Adrenergic Blockade in Normal Subjects

β-Adrenergic blockade has been shown to affect exercise performance in normal subjects.[49] In general, nonselective β-adrenergic blockade has a greater effect on limiting exercise capacity than β_1-selective drugs. There is a reduction in peak exercise cardiac output, mainly due to the decrease in maximal heart rate, with a subsequent mild decrease in $\dot{V}O_{2max}$. In addition to the cardiovascular effects of β-adrenergic blockade, there are also effects on muscle substrate use, with a 30% reduction in fatty acid use. The effects on skeletal muscle blood flow and carbohydrate metabolism in skeletal muscle are less clear. These findings in normal subjects may be relevant to patients with chronic heart failure. Although much of the lack of improvement in peak exercise performance with β-adrenergic blockade in heart failure patients appear to be related to the reduction in peak exercise heart rate, the effects of this therapy on skeletal muscle blood flow and skeletal muscle metabolism have not been investigated. These peripheral effects may be extremely relevant in the deconditioned heart failure patient.

Summary

β-Adrenergic blockade has been shown to be a potentially important therapy in the management of chronic heart failure related to both ischemic and nonischmeic cardiomyopathy. Newer drugs, such as carvedilol and bucindolol, have been shown to have a greater effect on improving cardiac function than the second-generation β-blocker, metoprolol, and recent data with carvedilol suggest that there may also be a substantial survival benefit from using these agents.[17,18] Despite these favorable clinical outcomes, with these agents, there has been minimal evidence for improved exercise performance. Peak exercise performance has been shown to improve only with long-term metoprolol therapy, probably because of its effects on increasing β_1-receptor density, its lack of blockade of the β_2-receptor, and perhaps the longer duration of treatment compared to the studies with the third-generation agents. However, these pharmacological properties may also explain the lack of survival benefit and perhaps smaller degrees of improvement in cardiac function with this β-blocker. The newer agents, carvedilol and bucindolol, downregulate the β-receptor, block some or all of the β_2-receptor population, and lower systemic or cardiac norepinephrine levels.[24,28,39] These properties may explain the greater increases in cardiac function and a potential improvement in survival with these drugs. This hypothesis is currently being tested with bucindolol in the BEST Trial[25] and has been strongly suggested by data from the U.S. Carvedilol Heart Failure Trial Program.[17,18] Because of the higher degree of blockade of all β-receptors as well as the lack of increase in myocardial β-receptor density, exercise capacity, especially at peak exercise, has not improved with these third-generation agents. A large component of this limitation may be related to the blunting of heart rate at peak exercise by these β-blockers. However, the possibility of peripheral circulatory, metabolic, and skeletal muscle effects of these drugs cannot be excluded. Recent data suggest that submaximal exercise performance may be a more ideal method of evaluating exercise capacity in these patients. There is still some controversy about the optimal method of recording submaximal exercise performance. Ultimately, β-adrenergic blockade may improve cardiac performance, but not the peripheral deconditioning seen in most chronic heart failure patients. Therapeutic modalities such as exercise conditioning[50] may also be required in conjunction with long-term β-adrenergic blockade to improve exercise capacity and favorably influence clinical outcome in these patients.

References

1. Thomas JA, Marks BH. Plasma norepinephrine in congestive heart failure. *Am J Cardiol* 1978;41:233–243.
2. Hasking GJ, Esler MD, Jennings GL, et al. Norepinephrine spillover to plasma in patients with congestive heart failure: Evidence for increased overall and cardiorenal sympathetic nervous activity. *Circulation* 1986;73:615–621.
3. Francis GS, Benedict C, Johnstone DE, et al. for the SOLVD Investigators. Comparison of neuroendocrine activation in patients with left ventricular dysfunction with and without congestive heart failure: A substudy of the Studies of Left Ventricular Dysfunction (SOLVD). *Circulation* 1990;82:1724–1729.
4. Bristow, MR. Pathophysiologic and pharmacologic rationales for clinical management of chronic heart failure with beta-blocking agents. *Am J Cardiol* 1993;71:12C–22C.
5. Bristow, MR. Changes in myocardial and vascular receptors in heart failure. *J Am Coll Cardiol* 1993;22(suppl A):61A–71A.
6. Hanson P. Exercise testing and training in patients with chronic heart failure. *Med Sci Sports Exer* 1994;26:527–537.
7. White M, Yanowitz F, Gilbert EM, et al. Role of beta-adrenergic receptor down-regulation in the peak exercise response in patients with heart failure due to idiopathic dilated cardiomyopathy. *Am J Cardiol* 1995;76:1271–1276.
8. Gilbert EM, Sandoval A, Larrabee P, et al. Lisinopril lowers cardiac adrenergic drive and increases β-receptor density in the failing human heart. *Circulation* 1993;88:472–480.
9. Giles TD, Katz R, Sullivan JM, et al. Short- and long-acting angiotensin-con-

verting enzyme inhibitors: A randomized trial of lisinopril versus captopril in the treatment of congestive heart failure. *J Am Coll Cardiol* 1989;13: 1240–1247.

10. Waagstein F, Hjalmarson A, Varnauskas E, et al. Effect of chronic β-adrenergic receptor blockade in congestive cardiomyopathy. *Br Heart J* 1975; 37:1022–1036.

11. Swedberg K, Hjalmarson A, Waagstein F, et al. Prolongation of survival in congestive cardiomyopathy by β-receptor blockade. *Lancet* 1979;1:1374–1377.

12. Packer M. How should we judge the efficacy of drug therapy in patients with chronic congestive heart failure? The insights of six blind men. *J Am Coll Cardiol* 1987;9:433–438.

13. Waagstein F, Caidahl K, Wallentin I, et al. Long-term β-blockade in dilated cardiomyopathy: Effects of short- and long-term metoprolol treatment followed by withdrawal and readministration of metoprolol. *Circulation* 1989; 80:551–563.

14. Bristow MR, O'Connell JB, Gilbert EM, et al. Dose-response of chronic β-blocker treatment in heart failure from either idiopathic dilated or ischemic cardiomyopathy. *Circulation* 1994;89:1632–1642.

15. Waagstein F, Bristow MR, Swedberg K, et al. Beneficial effects of metoprolol in idiopathic dilated cardiomyopathy. *Lancet* 1993;342:1441–1446.

16. Metra M, Nardi M, Giubbini R, et al. Effects of short- and long-term carvedilol administration on rest and exercise hemodynamic variables, exercise capacity, and clinical conditions in patients with idiopathic dilated cardiomyopathy. *J Am Coll Cardiol* 1994;24:1678–1687.

17. Packer M, Bristow MR, Cohn JN, et al. The effect of carvedilol on morbidity and mortality in patients with chronic heart failure. *N Engl J Med* 1996;334:1349–1355.

18. Bristow MR, Gilbert EM, Abraham WT, et al. Carvedilol produces dose-related improvements in left ventricular function and survival in subjects with chronic heart failure. *Circulation* 1996 (in press).

19. Chadda K, Goldstein S, Byington R, et al. Effect of propranolol after acute myocardial infarction in patients with congestive heart failure. *Circulation* 1986;73:503–510.

20. Heilbrunn SM, Shah P, Bristow MR, et al. Increased β-receptor density and improved hemodynamic response to catecholamine stimulation during long-term metoprolol therapy in heart failure from dilated cardiomyopathy. *Circulation* 1989;79:483–490.

21. Hershberger RE, Wynn JR, Sundberg L, et al. Mechanism of action of bucindolol in human ventricular myocardium. *J Cardiovasc Pharmacol* 1990;15: 959–967.

22. Gilbert EM, Anderson JL, Deitchman D, et al. Long-term β-blocker vasodilator therapy improves cardiac function in idiopathic dilated cardiomyopathy: A double-blind, randomized study of bucindolol versus placebo. *Am J Med* 1990;88:223–229.

23. Lowes BD, Chidiac P, Olsen S, et al. Clinical relevance of inverse agonism and guanine nucleotide modulatable binding properties of β-adrenergic blocking agents. *Circulation* 1994;90(suppl I):I-543.

24. Bristow MR, Abraham WT, Yoshikawa T, et al. Comparison of second- and third-generation β-blocking agents in the treatment of chronic heart failure. *Cardiovasc Drugs Ther* 1996 (in press).

25. The BEST Steering Committee. Design of the Beta-Blocker Evaluation Survival Trial (BEST). *Am J Cardiol* 1995;75:1220–1223.

26. Yoshikawa T, Port JD, Asano K, et al. Cardiac adrenergic receptor effects of carvedilol. *Eur Heart J* 1996;17(suppl B):8–16.
27. Bristow MR, Larrabee P, Muller-Beckman B, et al. Effects of carvedilol on adrenergic receptor pharmacology in human ventricular myocardium and lymphocytes. *Clin Invest* 1992;70:S105–S113.
28. Gilbert EM, Abraham WT, Olsen S, et al. Comparative hemodynamic, LV functional, and anti-adrenergic effects of chronic treatment with metoprolol vs. carvedilol in the failing heart. *Circulation* 1996 (in press).
29. Bristow MR, Gilbert EM. Improvement in cardiac myocyte function by biological effects of medical therapy: A new concept in the treatment of heart failure. *Eur Heart J* 1995; 16(suppl F):20–31.
30. Weber KT, Kinasewitz GT, Janicki JS, et al. Oxygen utilization and ventilation during exercise in patients with chronic cardiac failure. *Circulation* 1982;65:1213–1223.
31. Le Jemtel TH, Mancini D, Gumbardo D, et al. Pitfalls and limitations of "maximal" oxygen uptake as an index of cardiovascular functional capacity in patients with chronic heart failure. *Heart Failure* 1985;1:112–124.
32. Engelmeier RS, O'Connell JB, Walsh R, et al. Improvement in symptoms and exercise tolerance by metoprolol in patients with dilated cardiomyopathy: A double-blind, randomized, placebo-controlled trial. *Circulation* 1985;72:536–546.
33. Nemanich JW, Veith RC, Abrass IB, et al. Effects of metoprolol on rest and exercise cardiac function and plasma catecholamines in chronic congestive heart failure secondary to ischemic or idiopathic cardiomyopathy. *Am J Cardiol* 1990;66:843–848.
34. Anderson JL, Lutz JR, Gilbert EM, et al. A randomized trial of low-dose beta-blockade therapy for idiopathic dilated cardiomyopathy. *Am J Cardiol* 1985;55:471–475.
35. Andersson B, Hamm C, Persson S, et al. Improved exercise hemodynamic status in dilated cardiomyopathy after beta-adrenergic blockade treatment. *J Am Coll Cardiol* 1994;23:1397–1404.
36. Andersson B, Blomstrom-Lundqvist C, Hedner T, et al. Exercise hemodynamics and myocardial metabolism during long-term beta-adrenergic blockade in severe heart failure. *J Am Coll Cardiol* 1991;18:1059–1066.
37. Wolfel EE, Hiatt WR, Brammell HL, et al. Effects of selective and nonselective β-adrenergic blockade on mechanisms of exercise conditioning. *Circulation* 1986;74:664–674.
38. Sweeney ME, Fletcher BJ, and Fletcher GF. Exercise testing and training with β-adrenergic blockade: Role of the drug washout period in "unmasking" a training effect. *Am Heart J* 1989;118:941–946.
39. Woodley SL, Gilbert EM, Anderson JL, et al. β-blockade with bucindolol in heart failure caused by ischemic versus idiopathic dilated cardiomyopathy. *Circulation* 1991;84: 2426–2441.
40. Heesch CM, Marcoux L, Hatfield RN, et al. Hemodynamic and energetic comparison of bucindolol and metoprolol for the treatment of congestive heart failure. *Am J Cardiol* 1995;75:360–364.
41. Anderson JL, Gilbert EM, O'Connell JB, et al. Long-term (2 year) beneficial effects of beta-adrenergic blockade with bucindolol in patients with idiopathic dilated cardiomyopathy. *J Am Coll Cardiol* 1991;17:1373–1381.
42. Pollock SG, Lystash J, Tedesco C, et al. Usefulness of bucindolol in congestive heart failure. *Am J Cardiol* 1990;66:603–607.
43. Olsen SL, Gilbert EM, Renlund DG, et al. Carvedilol improves left ventric-

ular function and symptoms in chronic heart failure: A double-blind randomized study. *J Am Coll Cardiol* 1995;25:1225–1231.

44. Krum H, Sackner-Bernstein JD, Goldsmith RL, et al. Double-blind, placebo-controlled study of the long-term efficacy of carvedilol in patients with severe heart failure. *Circulation* 1995;92:1499–1506.
45. Australia-New Zealand Heart Failure Research Collaborative Group. Effects of carvedilol, a vasodilator-β-blocker, in patients with congestive heart failure due to ischemic heart disease. *Circulation* 1995;92:212–218.
46. Guyatt GH, Sullivan MJ, Thompson PJ, et al. The six-minute walk test: A new measure of exercise capacity in patients with chronic heart failure. *Can Med Assoc J* 1985;132:919–923.
47. Sparrow J, Parameshwar J, Poole-Wilson PA. Assessment of functional capacity in chronic heart failure: time-limited exercise on a self-powered treadmill. *Br Heart J* 1994;71:391–394.
48. Yamani MH, Wells L, Massie BM. Relation of the nine-minute self-powered treadmill test to maximal exercise capacity and skeletal muscle function in patients with congestive heart failure. *Am J Cardiol* 1995;76:788–792.
49. Van Baak MA. β-adrenoceptor blockade and exercise: An update. *Sports Med* 1988;4:209–225.
50. McKelvie RS, Teo KK, McCartney N, et al. Effects of exercise training in patients with congestive heart failure: A critical review. *J Am Coll Cardiol* 1995;25:789–796.

Chapter 9

Cardiac Transplantation:
Current Concepts and Future Directions

Michael Argenziano, MD and Eric A. Rose, MD

Introduction

In the year following the first successful human heart transplant in Capetown in 1967,[1] worldwide enthusiasm for this new procedure led to the establishment of over 60 cardiac transplant centers.[2] Despite the technical advances that had been achieved over the prior decade, the enthusiasm soon waned, as poor survival rates led to the abandonment of cardiac transplantation at all but a few centers. For the next decade, these centers would struggle to balance the high risk of allograft rejection with the adverse effects of nonspecific immunosuppressive regimens, leading to important advances such as the introduction, at Stanford, of endomyocardial biopsy techniques[3] and the use of rabbit antithymocyte globulin.[4] Finally, in 1980, the introduction of cyclosporine brought about a revolution in clinical cardiac transplantation, allowing improved survival rates and attenuation of immunosuppression-related side effects.

Since 1980, heart transplantation has been performed successfully in hundreds of centers worldwide.[5] Although the results of cardiac transplantation in the cyclosporine era have been impressive, with 1- and 5-year survival rates approaching 80% and 70%, respectively,[6] continued success has depended on a variety of advances made in response to new problems encountered as this modality has been applied to increasingly diverse patient populations. At the Columbia-Presbyterian Medical Center, where three orthotopic heart transplants were performed in 1977 and over 850 have since taken place, a 19-year experience in cardiac transplantation has witnessed many of these developments. These have included refinement of donor and recipient screen-

From: Balady GJ, Piña IL (eds). *Exercise and Heart Failure.* Armonk, NY: Futura Publishing Company, Inc.; ©1997.

ing and selection procedures, establishment of alternative immuno-suppressive strategies, and improvements in the hemodynamic management of high-risk patients. Finally, significant restrictions imposed by a limited donor organ supply, allograft rejection, and the sequelae of long-term immunosuppression have led to progress in alternative cardiac replacement modalities, the application of which is almost certain to alter the current role of allogeneic heart transplantation in the treatment of end-stage heart disease.

Indications

Given the prevalence and increasing worldwide frequency of end-stage heart disease, the over 2000 cardiac transplants performed in 1995 represent only a minor proportion of the potential recipient pool. The consequent discrepancy between supply and demand dictated by a shortage of usable donor organs has led to the formulation of guidelines for selection of recipients as well as donors. Initially stringent, recipient selection guidelines have evolved over the years and have generally been relaxed as experience has been gained with complex medical conditions.[7]

Selection Criteria

At Columbia-Presbyterian Medical Center, a well-defined set of inclusion and exclusion criteria have been established (Table 1 and Table 2). Eligible candidates must have end-stage heart failure with a life expectancy of less than 1 year, inoperable coronary artery disease with intractable anginal symptoms, or malignant ventricular arrhythmias unresponsive to medical or surgical therapy. Additionally, patients with

---

Table 1

Cardiac Transplantation Inclusion Criteria at Columbia-Presbyterian Medical Center

---

1. Patients with end-stage cardiac disease and a life expectancy of < 1 year
2. NYHA Class III or IV congestive heart failure refractory to maximal medical therapy and: (1) left ventricular ejection fraction $\leq$ 20% or
   (2) reduced functional capacity with $VO_{2max} \leq 14$ ml/kg/minute
3. Inoperable coronary artery disease with intractable anginal symptoms
4. Malignant ventricular arrhythmias unresponsive to medical or surgical therapy

---

NYHA = New York Heart Association.

Table 2

Cardiac Transplantation Exclusion Criteria at Columbia-Presbyterian Medical Center

1. Severe pulmonary hypertension with fixed pulmonary vascular resistance ($\geq$ 6 Wood units/m^2)
2. Pulmonary infarction within 6 to 8 weeks
3. Active infection
4. Significant chronic end-organ dysfunction:
   (1) serum creatinine > 2.5 mg/dL or creatinine clearance < 50 mL/min
   (2) serum total bilirubin > 2.5 mg/dL or serum AST > 2 times control values
   (3) significant coagulopathy or bleeding diathesis
5. Excessive obesity (> 130% ideal weight)
6. Evidence of drug, tobacco, or alcohol use
7. Active mental illness or psychosocial instability
8. Active or recent malignancy
9. Antibodies to HIV

AST = aspartate transaminase.

New York Heart Association (NYHA) Class III or Class IV heart failure refractory to maximal medical therapy are considered eligible if left ventricular ejection fraction is less than 20% and functional capacity is severely impaired, as assessed by determination of $\dot{V}O_{2max}$. Studies performed at our institution[8] have demonstrated the utility of this latter measure in the selection of appropriately disabled candidates, predicting a survival benefit in patients with a pretransplant $\dot{V}O_{2max} \leq 14$ mL/kg/min. Although an infrequent indication, we have also reported the successful transplantation of eight patients with cardiac tumors.[9] Given current advances in the medical management of heart failure, hemodynamic support by mechanical ventricular assistance and dynamic cardiomyoplasty, and myocardial revascularization techniques such as TMR[10] and recombinant growth factor therapy,[11] it is clear that the definitions of medically and surgically refractory end-stage heart failure have evolved and will continue to do so.

Exclusionary criteria used at our center (Table 2) have been formulated in an attempt to identify patients in whom the risk of death from transplant failure or from comorbid conditions does not justify the use of a scarce and valuable organ. Significant end-organ dysfunction, evidenced by reductions in creatinine clearance, elevations of serum creatinine and total bilirubin, or significant coagulopathy, is considered a contraindication to transplantation, as are active infection, recent pulmonary infarction, excessive obesity, evidence of drug, tobacco, or alcohol abuse, and active mental illness or psychosocial instability. Based on the well-established association of severe pulmonary hypertension with post-transplant right heart failure and death,[12,13] demonstration of pharmacological reversibility of pulmonary hypertension is considered an absolute requirement. Finally, because of rigorous immunosuppressive regimens and the potential need for intensification of this therapy during episodes of acute rejection, transplantation is not considered an option for patients with active or recent malignancy or the presence of antibodies to HIV.

Given the current definition of left ventricular assist devices (LVADs) as bridges-to-transplantation, all potential LVAD recipients are required to meet pretransplant inclusion and exclusion criteria. However, the proven ability of LVAD support to reverse acute deteriorations in peripheral organ function,[14] the high rate of successful transplantation in patients with infections prior to and during LVAD support,[15,16] and the successful diagnostic[17] and therapeutic[18] use of inhaled nitric oxide in patients with refractory pulmonary hypertension will likely require reformulation of these criteria, which may be yet further influenced by the initiation of trials of long-term LVAD support as a definitive therapy for end-stage heart disease.[19]

Donor Selection

Acceptance criteria for donor organs include: age under 65 years and no evidence of malignancy, septicemia, or antibodies to HIV, HBV, or HCV. Estimations of cardiac function are made by electrocardiography and echocardiography, and potential donors with prolonged cardiac dysfunction or a low cardiac output state are excluded. Finally, in male donors over age 45 and female donors over age 50, cardiac catheterization is recommended. Although the use of the "borderline" donor heart is a controversial topic, especially in the face of donor organ shortages, we and others[20] have successfully transplanted donor organs that do not strictly conform to these criteria.

Immunosuppression

While early immunosuppressive regimens were founded on double therapy with azathioprine and steroids, the majority of clinical success in heart transplantation has occurred in the years since the introduction of cyclosporine. Although cyclosporine was initially used in combination with steroids alone, azathioprine was added as a third agent at our institution in 1985.[2] In our current protocol, oral azathioprine and intravenous steroids are given preoperatively, and oral cyclosporine is given in proportion to creatinine clearance. Postoperatively, these agents are given intravenously, unless creatinine clearance is depressed, in which case cyclosporine is substituted with OKT3 until renal function improves. Subsequently, cyclosporine dosing is adjusted by monitoring of serum levels, azathioprine administration is guided by avoidance of significant myelosuppression, and steroids are tapered over the first 6 months to 1 year.

Outcomes

Survival

Actuarial survival for the first 16 years of cardiac transplantation at Columbia Presbyterian Medical Center is represented in Figure 1, and in Figure 2, it is shown to have improved during the cyclosporine era. The current actuarial survival at 1 year is 85% and approaches 70% at 5 years, comparing favorably with worldwide data of the Registry of

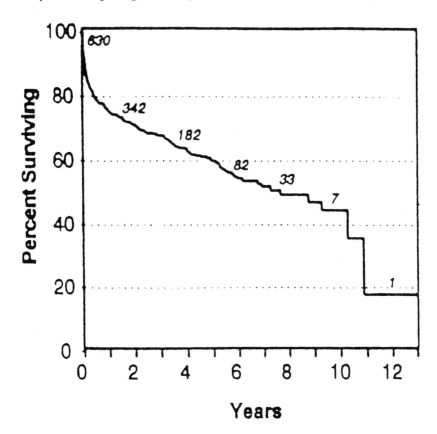

Figure 1: Kaplan-Meier actuarial survival for all heart transplant patients at the Columbia-Presbyterian Medical Center from 1977 to 1993. The probability of surviving 1 year approaches 80% and that of 5 years approaches 65%.

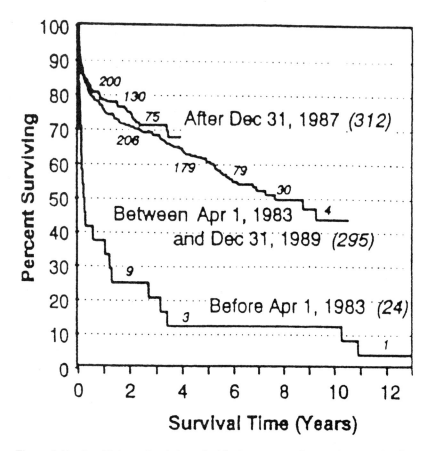

Figure 2: Kaplan-Meier actuarial survival for heart transplant patients at the Columbia-Presbyterian Medical Center according to the date of transplantation. The three time periods represent the pre-cyclosporine, early cyclosporine, and late cyclosporine eras at Columbia. The current probability of surviving 1 year approaches 85%.

the International Society for Heart and Lung Transplantation, which indicate 1- and 5-year survival estimates of 78% and 67%, respectively.[6] As in other series, the most frequent causes of death within the first year of cardiac transplantation are acute rejection and infection, while graft coronary artery disease (CAD), or allograft vasculopathy, are the leading cause of death after the first year.

Rejection

Episodes of acute rejection, diagnosed by routine endomyocardial biopsy and/or the new onset of clinical symptoms or alterations in cardiac function, are a common occurrence in the first year after transplantation.[12] Although the prevalence of rejection has declined in the era of immuno-suppressive triple-therapy,[12] a recent analysis of our experience[7] revealed an actuarial freedom from rejection of 45% at 1 year (Figure 3), with nearly 80% of first year rejections occurring within the first 3 months after transplantation. Interestingly, there were no significant differences in rejection frequency and actuarial freedom from rejection between primary transplant and retransplanted patients. Our algorithm for treatment of rejection has been published previously.[3] Briefly, low-grade (Grade I or Grade II) and clinically asymptomatic Grade III rejection is treated with oral steroid boost therapy, which is followed by weekly endomyocardial biopsy until histological resolution is confirmed. In cases of persistent rejection, a second steroid boost is given intravenously. Patients not responding to a second steroid dose, and all patients manifesting hemodynamic instability receive intravenous OKT3 or antithymocyte globulin, if hypersensitive to OKT3. In our reported experience, 52% and 36% of rejection episodes have responded to oral and intravenous steroid therapy, respectively, the remainder being treated with specific anti-T cell or anti-B cell modalities.

Graft Atherosclerosis

Accelerated graft coronary artery disease (CAD) remains a major complication and is the leading cause of late death after cardiac trans-

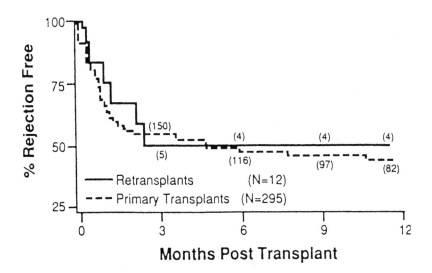

Figure 3: Actuarial freedom from rejection for 295 and 12 patients who underwent primary transplantation and retransplantation, respectively. Differences in actuarial freedom from rejection between these groups were not statistically significant.

plantation.[21-23] Angiographic evidence of graft CAD has been reported in as many as 45% of cardiac transplant patients surviving more than 3 years, and is associated with a five-fold increased risk of other cardiac events such as myocardial infarction, heart failure, or sudden death.[23,24] Although the exact pathogenic basis of graft CAD is not known, both immunologic and nonimmunologic mechanisms have been proposed for the development of the diffuse concentric myointimal proliferation that is characteristic of this process.[25] The observation that patients with graft CAD possess elevated plasma levels of the IL-2 receptor, a marker of acute allograft rejection,[26,27] suggests that acute allograft rejection and graft CAD may be related immune processes. However, since improvements in the immunologic control of acute rejection have not yielded a decreased incidence of graft CAD, and because clinical studies investigating this question[24,28,29] have produced conflicting results, this association has remained a matter of controversy.[30] In other studies, several nonimmunologic risk factors for the development of graft CAD have been identified,[31] including donor age and gender and recipient obesity and hyperlipidemia. These observations, together with the known effects of cyclosporine and steroids on weight gain and lipid metabolism, suggest a mechanism by which patients with frequent episodes of acute rejection might be at higher risk for graft CAD. Finally, cytomegalovirus (CMV) infection has been identified as a risk factor for graft CAD in two clinical studies,[32,33] and although precise mechanisms are unclear, it has been suggested that CMV infection promotes graft CAD via endothelial cell activation,[34] modulation of lipid metabolism[35] and/or immunologic stimulation.

Current approaches in the prevention of graft CAD include aggressive therapy of acute rejection episodes as well as risk factor modification through weight loss and lipid-lowering strategies, even though no objective data exist demonstrating the beneficial impact of these interventions on graft vasculopathy. Pharmacological therapies proposed for the prevention and treatment of graft CAD have included platelet modifying agents[36] and calcium channel blockers.[37] Although early enthusiasm for the use of aspirin and dipyridamole has been tempered by equivocal long-term results, short-term studies using quantitative angiography[37] and intravascular ultrasound[23] have confirmed the ability of diltiazem to prevent and even induce regression of graft CAD. Finally, percutaneous coronary atherectomy and angioplasty have been successfully performed for discrete proximal stenoses in cardiac transplant patients,[23] but it is presently unclear whether these techniques will have a significant impact in the treatment of graft CAD, which is usually diffuse and involves both proximal and distal coronary vessels.

Cardiac Retransplantation

Unfortunately, until the long-term benefits of these and other promising therapies can be established, cardiac retransplantation remains the only definitive treatment of graft CAD and other causes of graft failure. In a previous communication,[38] we reported 14 cases of cardiac retransplantation, including one patient who received a third transplant, among 431 patients transplanted over a 14-year period. Indications for retransplantation included graft CAD in eight cases, acute rejection in five cases, and one intraoperative graft failure. Despite reports of inferior survival rates in retransplanted patients,[23] we found no differences in linearized acute rejection rates or actuarial survival in retransplanted patients when compared to patients receiving a primary transplant, and we have encountered similar results in our experience with cardiac retransplantation in pediatric patients.[39]

Lymphoproliferative Disorders

Neoplasia is a recognized risk of chronic immunosuppression,[40] and malignancies not infrequently encountered after transplantation include malignant lymphoma, Kaposi's sarcoma, renal cell carcinoma, and hepatobiliary tumors. In addition, in as many as 5% of thoracic transplant recipients, a heterogeneous class of post-transplantation lymphoproliferative disorders (PTLDs) with a propensity for extranodal involvement have been reported.[41,42] Ranging in severity from atypical lymphoid hyperplasia, associated with a mononucleosis-like syndrome, to malignant lymphoma with metastatic potential, PTLDs have been shown to respond to reductions in immunosuppression as well as systemic chemotherapy.[43,44] As reported in a recent retrospective analysis,[41] 19 of 516 (4%) patients receiving cardiac allografts over a 9-year period developed PTLDs involving the lungs, gastrointestinal tract, lymph nodes, or multiple extranodal sites. Although no correlation was found between immunosuppression dosing and PTLD incidence or site of involvement, patients with PTLDs involving the lungs and gastrointestinal tract showed superior responses and improved survival after reduction of immunosuppression when compared to patients with involvement of other extranodal sites.

Costs

As the demand for cardiac replacement has outstripped the available donor supply, the number of patients on waiting lists has grown

significantly over the past decade.[45] The consequent increases in waiting time have resulted in a greater proportion of severely ill patients
awaiting and receiving transplants. While success rates and long-term
survival have not been affected by this trend, remaining relatively stable throughout the past decade, the costs of pre- and post-transplant
medical care have risen substantially.[46] In 1992, we performed a cost
analysis of the cardiac transplantation program at Columbia-Presbyterian,[45] finding that average total hospital and post-discharge charges
had nearly tripled over 4 years, from $45,000 in 1988 to $121,000 in 1992.
These increases were accompanied by nearly two-fold increases in average pre- and post-transplant hospital lengths of stay, and a dramatic
increase in the proportion of transplant recipients who were bound to
intensive care units preoperatively. Despite these shifts toward more
critically ill transplant recipients, 30-day and 1-year survival figures
were no different between ICU-bound and non-ICU-bound, hemodynamically stable patients. Based on these data, we concluded that the
remarkable success of heart transplantation in severely ill patients
would continue to promote the selection of sicker patients from waiting lists, further increasing costs. In a similar analysis of the United Network for Organ Sharing (UNOS) data base,[47] it has been shown that increasing average costs of heart transplantation have been associated
with an increase in the proportion of transplants performed in Status 1
patients, in whom average charges were more than twice the charges in
Status 2 recipients.

Future Directions

While the current success of heart transplantation can be largely attributed to the use of cyclosporine over the past 15 years, continued improvements in immunosuppression regimens, diagnosis and treatment
of rejection, and management of critically ill patients have allowed survival rates to remain favorably high in the face of an increasingly sicker
cohort of transplant recipients. The dramatic progress observed in the
science of clinical cardiac transplantation over the past 2 decades is certain to be matched by further technological developments in the years
to come.

An area of current investigation involves the development of new
immunosuppressive agents, and early success with FK-506 in animal
models[48] and mycophenolate mofetil (MMF) in salvage therapy of refractory acute rejection[49] may herald a new era of multiple agent immunosuppression, with the potential for reduced toxicity. Additionally, an appreciation of the prognostic importance of pretransplant
sensitization to HLA antigens,[50] as well as the recent identification in

our transplant laboratory of anti-HLA antibody subtypes associated with higher rates of vascular (humoral) rejection, have prompted investigations of alternative methods of immunomodulation, including anti-B cell induction therapy with agents such as cyclophosphamide, in combination with peri-transplant plasmapheresis in highly sensitized patients.

Despite the formidable obstacles imposed by the cross-species transplantation barrier, current investigations in our laboratory[51] are beginning to characterize the nature and function of human preformed xenoantibodies in an effort to develop strategies to overcome the pig-to-human immunologic barrier. While the ethical implications of the use of animal organs in human transplantation are understandably complex, economic issues and the success of other cardiac replacement therapies such as mechanical assistance and cardiac gene therapy, will be equally important in determining the eventual role of xenotransplantation in the treatment of human heart disease.

Summary

In the nearly 30 years since the first successful human heart transplant, a variety of developments have allowed this form of cardiac replacement therapy to flourish. These have included improvements in surgical and critical care technology as well as breakthroughs in immunosuppressive pharmacology, the most notable of which was the introduction of cyclosporine in 1980. Subsequently, indications and exclusion criteria for heart transplantation have evolved, guided by the constraints of a limited donor supply and facilitated by an improved understanding of prognostic risk factors.

Current 1- and 5-year survival estimates are encouraging, and despite the frequency of acute rejection, current management strategies have for the most part limited the fatal consequences of this complication. Graft atherosclerosis, however, has continued to complicate the post-transplant course of many patients, and despite therapeutic strategies aimed at a variety of potential pathogenic mechanisms, this entity remains the most common cause of late death after transplantation. In these and other victims of allograft failure, retransplantation remains a viable option. Finally, the recent trend of selecting increasingly critically ill transplant recipients, while not associated with inferior survival, has driven the costs of this form of cardiac replacement therapy to unprecedented levels. These issues, as well as current developments in the fields of mechanical cardiac assistance, xenotransplantation, and cardiac gene therapy will certainly result in a continually evolving role for cardiac transplantation in the treatment of end-stage heart disease.

References

1. Barnard CN. The operation. *S Afr Med J* 1967;41:1271–1274.
2. White DJG. Immunosuppression for heart transplantation. *Br J Biomed Sci* 1993;50:277–283.
3. Caves PK, Stinson EB, Billingham ME, et al. Diagnosis of human cardiac allograft rejection by serial cardiac biopsy. *J Thorac Cardiovasc Surg* 1973;66: 461–466.
4. Bieber CP, Griepp RB, Oyer PE, et al. Relationship of rabbit ATG clearance rate to circulating T cell level rejection and survival in cardiac transplantation. *Transplant Proc* 1977;9:1031.
5. Hosenpud JD. The Registry of the International Society of Heart and Lung Transplantation: Eleventh official report—1994. *J Heart Lung Transplant* 1994;13:561–570.
6. Kaye MP. The Registry of the International Society of Heart and Lung Transplantation: Ninth official report—1992. *J Heart Lung Transplant* 1992; 11:599–606.
7. Michler RE, Chen JM, Mancini DM, et al. Sixteen years of cardiac transplantation: The Columbia-Presbyterian Medical Center Experience 1977 to 1993. In: *Clinical Transplants,* Los Angeles:1993:109–118.
8. Mancini DM, Eisen H, Kussmaul W, et al. Value of peak exercise oxygen consumption for optimal timing of cardiac transplantation in ambulatory patients with heart failure. *Circulation* 1991;83:778–786.
9. Goldstein DJ, Oz MC, Rose EA, et al. Experience with heart transplantation for cardiac tumors. *J Heart Lung Transplant* 1995;14:382–386.
10. Jeevanandam V, Auteri JS, Oz MC, et al. Myocardial revascularization by laser-induced channels. *Surgical Forum* 1990;XLVI:225–227.
11. Sil P, Misono K, Sen S. Myotrophin in human cardiomyopathic heart. *Circ Res* 1993;73:98–108.
12. Sarris GE, Moore KA, Schroeder JS, et al. Cardiac transplantation: The Stanford experience in the cyclosporine era. *J Thorac Cardiovasc Surg* 1994;108: 240–252.
13. Semigran MJ, Cockrill BA, Kacmarek R, et al. Hemodynamic effects of inhaled nitric oxide in heart failure. *J Am Coll Cardiol* 1994;24:982–988.
14. Oz MC, Argenziano M, Catanese KA, et al. Bridge experience with long-term implantable left ventricular assist devices: Are they an alternative to transplantation? *Circulation* 1996 (submitted).
15. Argenziano M, Moazami N, Gardocki M, et al. Infection in patients with heart failure is not a contraindication to LVAD insertion as a bridge to transplantation. *J Heart Lung Transplant* (in press).
16. Catanese KA, Argenziano M, Moazami N, et al. Infections in patients with left ventricular assist devices do not preclude successful tranplantation. *J Heart Lung Transplant* (in press).
17. Adatia I, Perry S, Landzberg M, et al. Inhaled nitric oxide and hemodynamic evaluation of patients with pulmonary hypertension before transplantation. *J Am Coll Cardiol* 1995;25:1656–1664.
18. Rich GF, Murphy GD, Roos CM, Johns RA. Inhaled nitric oxide: Selective pulmonary vasodilatation in cardiac surgical patients. *Anesthesiology* 1993; 78:1028–1035.
19. Rose EA, Goldstein DJ. Wearable long-term mechanical support for patients with end-stage heart disease: A tenable goal. *Ann Thorac Surg* 1996 (in press).

20. Jeevanandam V, Auteri JS, Marboe C, et al. Extending the limits of donor heart preservation: A trial with University of Wisconsin solution. *Transplant Proc* 1991;23(1 Pt 1):697–698.
21. Gao SZ, Schroeder JS, Alderman EL, et al. Prevalence of accelerated coronary artery disease in heart transplant survivors: Comparison of cyclosporine and azathioprine regimens. *Circulation* 1989;80(suppl III):III100–105.
22. Johnson DE, Alderman EL, Schroeder JS, et al. Transplant coronary artery disease: Histopathologic correlations with angiographic morphology. *J Am Coll Cardiol* 1991;17:449–457.
23. Ventura HO, Mehra MR, Smart FW, Stapleton DD. Cardiac allograft vasculopathy: Current concepts. *Am Heart J* 1995;129:791–798.
24. Uretsky BF, Murali S, Reddy PS, et al. Development of coronary artery disease in cardiac transplant recipients receiving immunosuppressive therapy with cyclosporine and prednisone. *Circulation* 1987;76:827–834.
25. Billingham ME. Histopathology of graft coronary disease. *J Heart Lung Transplant* 1992;3:538–544.
26. Young JB, Windsor NT, Kleiman NS, et al.The relationship of soluble interleukin-2 receptor levels in allograft arteriopathy after heart transplantation. *J Heart Lung Transplant* 1992;11:579–582.
27. Ventura HO, Smart FW, Jain SP, et al. Soluble interleukin-2 receptor levels and allograft vasculopathy: An intravascular ultrasound study. *J Am Coll Cardiol* 1994;23(special issue):438A.
28. Olivari MT, Homans DC, Wilson RF, et al. Coronary artery disease in cardiac transplant patients receiving triple-drug immunosuppressive therapy. *Circulation* 1989;80(suppl III):III111–115.
29. Hammond EH, Yowell RL, Price GD, et al. Vascular rejection and its relationship to allograft coronary artert disease. *J Heart Lung Transplant* 1992;11:S111–119.
30. Costanzo-Nordin MR. Cardiac allograft vasculopathy: Relationship with acute cellular rejection and histocompatibility. *J Heart Lung Transplant* 1992;11:S90–104.
31. Johnson MR. Transplant coronary disease: Nonimmunologic risk factors. *J Heart Lung Transplant* 1992;11:S124–132.
32. Gratten MT, Moreno-Cabral CE, Starnes VA, et al. Cytomegalovirus infection is associated with cardiac graft rejection and atherosclerosis. *JAMA* 1989;261:3561–3562.
33. McDonald K, Rector TS, Braunlin EA, et al. Association of coronary artery disease in transplant recipients with cytomegalovirus infection. *Am J Cardiol* 1989;64:359–362.
34. Kendall TJ, Wilson JE, Radio SJ, et al. Cytomegalovirus and other herpes viruses: Do they have a role in the development of accelerated coronary arterial disease in human allografts? *J Heart Lung Transplant* 1992;11:S14–20.
35. Hajjar DP, Pomerantz KB, Flacone DJ, et al. Herpes simplex virus infection in human arterial cells: Implications in arteriosclerosis. *J Clin Invest* 1987;80:1317–1321.
36. Griepp RB, Stinson EB, Bieber CD, et al. Control of graft atherosclerosis in human heart transplant recipients. *Surgery* 1977;81:262–269.
37. Schroeder JS, Gao SZ, Alderman EL, et al. A preliminary study of diltiazem in the prevention of coronary artery disease in heart transplant recipients. *N Engl J Med* 1993;328:164–170.
38. Michler RE, McLauglin MJ, Chen JM, et al. Clinical experience with cardiac retransplantation. *J Thorac Cardiovasc Surg* 1993;106:622–631.

39. Michler RE, Edwards NM, Hsu D, et al. Pediatric retransplantation. *J Heart Lung Transplant* 1993;12:S319–327.
40. Penn I. Cancer is a complication of severe immunosuppression. *Surg Gynecol Obstet* 1986;162:603–610.
41. Chen JM, Barr ML, Chadburn A, et al. Management of lymphoproliferative disorders after cardiac transplantation. *Ann Thorac Surg* 1993;56:527–538.
42. Penn I. The changing pattern of posttransplant malignancies. *Transplant Proc* 1991;23:1101–1103.
43. Hanto DW, Frizzera G, Gajl-Peczalska KJ, et al. Epstein-Barr virus-induced B-cell lymphoma after renal transplantation: Acyclovir therapy and transition from polyclonal to monoclonal B-cell proliferation. *N Engl J Med* 1982;306:913–918.
44. Armitage JM, Kormos RL, Stuart S, et al. Posttransplant lymphoproliferative disease in thoracic organ transplant patients: Ten years of cyclosporine-based immunosuppression. *J Heart Lung Transplant* 1991;10:877–887.
45. Reemtsma K, Berland G, Merrill J, et al. Evaluation of surgical procedures: Changing patterns of patient selection and costs in heart transplantation. *J Thorac Cardiovasc Surg* 1992;104:1308–1313.
46. Evans RW. Organ transplantation costs, insurance coverage and reimbursement. In Terasaki PI ed: *Clinical Transplants*. Los Angeles:1990:343.
47. Votapka TV, Swartz MT, Reedy JE, et al. Heart transplantation charges: Status 1 versus status 2 patients. *J Heart Lung Transplant* 1995;14:366–372.
48. Ochai T, Nkajima K, Susuki T, et al. Effects of a new immunosuppressive agent FK506 on heterotopic cardiac allotransplantation in rats. *Transplant Proc* 1987;19:1284–1287.
49. Kirklin JK, Bourge RC, Naftel DC, et al. Treatment of recurrent heart rejection with mycophenolate mofetil (RS-61443): Initial clinical experience. *J Heart Lung Transplant* 1994;13:444–450.
50. Lavee J, Kormos RL, Duquesnoy RJ, et al. Influence of panel-reactive antibody and lymphocytotoxic crossmatch on survival after heart transplantation. *J Heart Lung Transplant* 1991;10:921–930.
51. Chen JM, Michler RE. Heart xenotransplantation: Lessons learned and future prospects. *J Heart Lung Transplant* 1993;12:869.

Chapter 10

Cardiac Transplantation:
Trends, Techniques, and Bridges

Valluvan Jeevanandam, MD

Introduction

The treatment of heart failure has progressed significantly over the last 2 decades. With the introduction of angiotensin converting enzyme (ACE) inhibitors, there is for the first time a documented decline in mortality and hospitalization for the medical management of heart failure. Newer pharmacological agents such as carvedilol also show promise in improving prognosis of patients with this illness. Furthermore, by understanding the peripheral and circulatory physiology of congestive heart failure (CHF), rehabilitation has improved the patient's overall quality of life.

With improvement in cardiopulmonary bypass equipment, myocardial preservation, and critical care management, it has also been possible to obtain satisfactory outcomes in patients undergoing revascularization, or in other procedures in patients with depressed ejection fractions. At Temple University Hospital, of 53 consecutive revascularization procedures performed in patients with chronic heart failure symptoms of greater than 2 months duration and with a mean ejection fraction of 17.2%, the operative mortality has been zero, with an actuarial 1-year survival of 92%. However, despite improvements in medical and surgical management of these difficult patients, the only acceptable therapy for end-stage heart disease is replacement with allotransplantation.

Historical Perspective

The era of human heart transplantation was started in 1967 by Dr. Christian Barnard, in South Africa. Unfortunately, most patients died

From: Balady GJ, Piña IL (eds). *Exercise and Heart Failure*. Armonk, NY: Futura Publishing Company, Inc.; ©1997.

within the first year after transplantation from rejection or opportunistic infection, and the procedure was abandoned in all but a few centers. Dr. Norman Shumway from Stanford University performed the first heart transplant in the United States in 1968. However, with a 6-month survival of only 29% in the first 13 patients, the results were discouraging. Persistent pioneering work by the Stanford group, with regard to immunosuppression and improved detection and management of rejection, allowed heart transplantation to evolve from a laboratory curiosity into a clinical reality. Finally, with the introduction of the immunosuppressant, cyclosporine A, in the 1980s, the number of cardiac transplants performed increased exponentially. One-year survival steadily improved from 20% to the current 80% to 85%.

Heart transplantation has now entered the mainstream of surgical management of CHF, with approximately 2000 procedures performed annually in the United States and 3000, worldwide. In contrast to the revolutionary progress in the 1980s, the decade of the 1990s has brought an evolution and maturation of the procedure. There have been forces that act to both decrease and to increase supply and demand. There have been subtle changes in the actual technique that may provide for a more physiological approach to myocardial dynamics. There has been a remarkable increase in the use of mechanical circulatory support devices as a method to "bridge" patients to transplantation. And finally, as heart transplantation moves out of the novelty phase into a clinical mainstay, there are socioeconomic pressures to justify and reduce the cost of the procedure.

Need and Demand for Transplantation

Overall, there is a great need for cardiac transplantation. Over 800,000 people die from heart disease annually in the US. Of people with end-stage heart disease, it is estimated that 41,000 are under 65 years of age, and may benefit from transplantation. Considering the possible contraindications related to transplantation, it is expected that between 10,000 and 14,000 patients each year are candidates for circulatory support.[1] Another factor that increases need for transplantation is the wider recognition of heart failure as a clinical entity, as modalities to treat it evolve. Patients are also becoming more accepting of heart transplantation as it steers into the mainstream of medicine and as its costs are covered by an increasing number of insurance companies. Furthermore, with advances in thrombolytic therapy and angioplasty in the acute setting, the immediate mortality form myocardial infarction has decreased; however, some of these patients are left with significant myocardial injury that can progress to heart failure over time.

As the outcome for transplantation improves, criteria for the acceptable recipient also expands. The maximal age limit is rising with some groups, now considering patients in their 70s. Permanent end-organ dysfunction, as long as the other organ can be replaced by transplantation (ie, heart/kidney transplant), is no longer a contraindication. Patients with active systemic infections and in the presence of diabetes are transplanted. There is a clear trend towards expanding the number of patients who could benefit from this procedure. This is manifested as an increasing number of patients waiting for transplant. Evans defines total demand as the number of patients waiting at the end of the year, plus the number dying on the list, and the number transplanted. In 1993, the total demand was 5686, with 2200 transplants and 782 deaths.[2] The "back log" is the number of patients listed per year minus the deaths and the transplants. This is growing by about 500 cases per year. As bridges to transplantation decrease mortality on the waiting list, the demand will grow even larger.

Supply

The only way to keep pace with demand is to increase supply. In 1993, there were 4895 donors with 43% yielding hearts. It is estimated that there will only be 6900 to 10,700 potential donors in the country per year with potentially 70% yielding hearts.[2] An increase in donors will require a long standing change in the attitude of the population towards donation, the education of medical personnel, and increased donor awareness. These efforts are well underway, but will take time to come to fruition. There are other factors that decrease donor supply. New strains of hepatitis are being discovered. Five years ago, hepatitis C could not be detected, and donors with the disease were used frequently. Currently, those donors are eliminated, but unfortunately they represent 15% of all donors. Other factors decreasing donation are improved vehicle safety, and conversely, more violent penetrating trauma where the victims arrive at the hospital without any signs of life.

The average procurement rate for organ procurement organizations (OPO) is currently 18 per 1,000,000 population base. The best OPOs reach 25 per 1,000,000. Approximately half of these donors should yield hearts. The only way to immediately impact on increasing the donor pool is to liberalize criteria for transplantation without sacrificing patient outcome.[3] The use of older donors (>50 years of age) has been described. Since there is a higher incidence of intimal thickening and focal lesions in these organs, and if obstructive lesions are present, some advocate bypass before implantation. Hearts with severe myocardial dysfunction due to causes other than structural damage can be successfully resuscitated with excellent long-term results. At Temple University Hospital, we routinely undersize the hearts by less than 50%. These hearts can grow and provide excellent myocardial function.[4] University of Wisconsin solution can be used to store hearts for up to 8 hours in cold nonperfused fashion. These recipients do not have an increase in morbidity or mortality in our experience. Hearts from infected donors (other than fungus or endocarditis) can also be used with minimal deleterious effects. Using the wider criteria, we were able to increase our donor pool by 50% without effect on patient outcome.[3]

Technique

Standard orthotopic heart transplantation (SOHT) was originally described by Shumway and Lower,[5] and has been used successfully in over 20,000 transplants. This procedure involves anastomoses between the recipient and donor atria, pulmonary artery, and aorta. Dreyfus and Carpentier[6] describe a procedure which left the pulmonary veins intact, with anastomosis directly to the left atrium. The right atrium was left intact and bicaval connections were made. The amount of left atrium left behind for anastomosis depends on whether a lung transplant is simultaneously occurring from the same donor.

We studied the effect of standard and bicaval techniques on postoperative and long-term myocardial function and patient outcome. One hundred eleven transplants between July, 1993 and March, 1994 were studied: 59 patients received SOHT (group A) and 52 consecutive subsequent patients received bicaval orthotopic heart transplantation (BOHT) (group B). All patients received standard triple immunosuppression. The two groups were similar with regard to: (1) recipient and donor demographics; (2) total cardiopulmonary bypass time; (3) postoperative and 12-month hemodynamics; and (4) need for permanent pacemakers. Significant differences at $P<0.05$ include (group A versus group B): time for implantation (40.2 ± 10.6 minutes versus 51.2 ± 13.2 minutes); isoproterenol requirements at postoperative day (POD) 1 (1.5 ± 0.2 μg/min versus 0.2 ± 0.1 μg/min); need for temporary external pacing before POD 7 (67% versus 10%); intrinsic heart rate at 1 week (67.4 ± 10.2 bpm versus 85.4 ± 12.1 bpm); sinus node dysfunction requiring temporary oral terbutaline (37% versus 2%), and 1-year survival (75% versus 85%). Although BOHT adds an anastomosis and requires longer time for completion, the total cardiopulmonary bypass time was similar. In addition, the high incidence of abnormal sinus node recovery time observed with the SOHT was eliminated by the bicaval technique.

Other advantages include maintaining a normal atrial geometry, eliminating the large compliant atrial chamber, and decreasing stasis. There is improved blood transport between the donor atrioventricular valves, which produces faster filling of the ventricle and enhanced performance.[7,8] Thus, BOHT is becoming the standard technique of choice. While it is more technically challenging and requires longer cross clamp time, it can be beneficial to patients.

Heterotopic heart transplantation has also been used as a method to circumvent problems of pulmonary hypertension and to allow use of undersized hearts.[9] The donor heart is connected in parallel to the recipient and acts as a "booster". Although initially appealing, this procedure is now rarely used. Patients require anticoagulation, since there are many potential stasis points. Endomyocardial biopsy is difficult, as the route to the donor right ventricle is circuitous. The recipient heart can atrophy over a period of time and the combination of the two hearts perform worse than comparable orthotopic transplants. Finally, there is pulmonary compromise from the large amount of space required to accommodate the extra organ. It is now recognized that "undersized" organs can be safely used in the orthotopic position and that drugs such as nitric oxide can improve survival in patients with pulmonary hypertension.

Bridges to Transplantation

With an increasing demand for hearts and an unyielding supply, there are a growing number of patients not being transplanted. Some of these patients improve and can be safely taken off the waiting list. However, many patients never receive a transplant (United Network of Organ Sharing (UNOS) 25%) and are taken off this list when they develop contraindications to transplantation. Most of these patients eventually die while waiting for a heart. Mechanical circulatory systems have been sought as a method of heart replacement since the 1960s. Originally developed in conjunction with the space program, the goal was to develop a totally implantable mechanical device as a permanent alternative to transplantation. Thirty years later, this goal is closer but has still not been reached. The Jarvik hearts reminded the medical community that the blending of mechanical and biological forces is not simple. All patients developed significant thromboembolic events despite anticoagulation, were coagulopathic, and had episodes of bleeding, and developed significant infections.

It became apparent that in order to develop any experience with these devices, they had to be initially used on a temporary basis and then progress to permanent replacement. This generated the concept of "bridge to transplantation". In addition, it was recognized that a total heart replacement might not be necessary. Assist devices that support only the left heart could perform adequately with potentially less infectious complications than those that support the total artificial heart. Furthermore, in case of mechanical failure, assist devices had a natural back-up mechanism: the native heart.

The currently available devices can be divided into groups depending on the anticipated duration of support. The short-term devices were primarily developed as postcardiotomy devices, (ie, for patients who cannot be weaned off cardiopulmonary bypass), but have now been extended for use as bridge devices. They can be used as support to allow for cardiac recovery, as a bridge to another longer term device, or as a bridge to transplantation.

The least invasive of these devices is the intra-aortic balloon pump (IABP). The IABP was the most commonly used bridge device before the development of other assist devices. It can significantly augment circulation especially in the face of ischemic cardiomyopathy if the patient has myocardial reserve that responds to increased blood supply. Its effectiveness in idiopathic cardiomyopathy is less dramatic, but has been reported to increase output by 5% to 15%, by essentially decreasing afterload of the native heart.[10] IABP are adequate bridge devices over a short period of time. In the past, this was acceptable, as the wait for status 1 patients was short. As the time periods lengthened, patients began to exhibit problems with immobilization and chronic low cardiac output. They were either dying or receiving heart transplantation in the face of severe physical debilitation (having been immobilized in bed) and with some end-organ damage caused by inadequate circulation. Patients were also subject to a higher incidence of vascular and infectious complications. IABP have been placed in the axillary artery to allow for ambulation, but this can be cumbersome. Another use of the IABP is to stabilize patients in heart failure, help diuresis, and restore adequate hemodynamics. The IABP can then be weaned off and the patient can continue to wait for heart transplantation.

The use of centrifugal pumps as a bridge to transplant was a natural extension of their use in the operating room.[11] Centrifugal pumps use rotating cones or impellers to generate energy in the form of pressure/flow work.[12] They are usually placed in the operating room with cannulation of the left atrium/aorta for left-sided support and the right atrium/pulmonary artery for right-sided support. They can also be placed percutaneously, but this is not common practice. Patients must be anticoagulated to prevent thromboembolic events. Although these devices offer versatility, their use is limited. The devices are extremely traumatic to blood and cause significant hemolysis and inflammatory response. Patients often require large amounts of volume and become anasarcous. The flow generated by the centrifugal pumps is generally nonpulsatile and may result in end-organ dysfunction. With these limitations, these devices are best used for very short periods of time (1 day to 4 days), after which another device can be used or transplantation can be performed. Finally, although the centrifugal pump is a relatively inexpensive device, it requires a perfusion for maintenance. This adds a significant cost, and must be considered when calculating the total expense of the device.

The Abiomed BVS system 5000 is the only FDA-approved device for postcardiotomy support. It is an external pulsatile ventricular assist device with polyurethane valves. It is housed in a rigid shell and is specifically designed for ease of use. It is a gravity-filled device, and is less traumatic to the blood. It is pulsatile and has been shown to allow for recovery of end organs. It is also versatile allowing for use as a left ventricular assist device (LVAD), right ventricular assist device (RVAD), or biventricular assist device (BiVAD). A perfusion is not required for maintenance and hence it is relatively inexpensive to use. However, its best use is as a postcardiotomy pump to allow native heart recovery or to bridge to another more permanent device.

Intermediate-term devices can be thought of as the true bridges to transplant. These were not designed for permanent support, and are intended for explantation during heart transplant. The most widely used of these is the Thoratec Ventricular Assist Device.[13] Patients have been supported for up to 500 days with this device. It is versatile allowing for RVAD, LVAD, or BiVAD configuration. Each ventricle costs approximately $18,000 but can be maintained with minimal personnel. Similar to the Abiomed BVS, the atria are cannulated with outflow grafts sewn into the arteries. The left ventricular apex can also be cannulated, allowing for better drainage. The device can be used as a bridge for transplantation or, if the atria are cannulated, can be used to allow for recovery. There have been many examples of Thoratec use for recovery in patients with viral myocarditis, post partum myocarditis or to allow for recovery of donor hearts in the midst of a rejection. The devices use suction drainage with pulsatile flow, and can be traumatic to the blood, causing hemolysis and need for significant blood transfusions. Heparinization with this device is essential. Because of good pulsatile flow, it allows for recovery of organs. The portable driver permits for some mobility of patients.

Long-term devices were designed in the United States as replacement therapy for patients with heart failure. Work on these artificial hearts began in the late 1960s. It has taken 20 years of rigorous laboratory and clinical evaluation to bring these devices into mainstream use. The two major systems that are available are the ThermoCardio Systems (TCI) HeartMate Device and the Baxter Novacor device.[14] They are paracorporeal systems, in which the blood follows a pathway that is not intrinsically normal. The devices rest below the diaphragm either in the intraperitoneal or the properitoneal position. Although they were designed as replacement therapy, most of the clinical experience has been obtained as bridge to transplantation. This experience will be extrapolated for their use as a transplant alternative. At the current time, in the European market, these devices can be used as transplant alternatives; in the US they can only be used as a bridge to transplantation.

The Novacor device works with a magnetic actuator. The electromagnet activates a pusher plate designed to collapse a bladder, which in the presence of two bio-prosthetic valves, sends blood in one direction from the left ventricular apex to the ascending aorta. As with other left ventricular assist devices, a competent aortic valve is essential for their use. The Novacor device can be placed in the intra or properitoneal position (Figure 1). Warfarin or heparin are essential as the incidence of neurological events approaches 25%, even in the presence of adequate anticoagulation. Redesign of the inlet cannula might eventually allow for a lower incidence of neurological events. The bridge-to-transplant rate is currently 65%. Success with this device is improving with better timing and careful recipient selection. The Novacor device is used extensively in the European market, where it has also been used as an alternative to transplant.[15] Patients have been sent home, some of whom have been supported for up to 18 months.

The TCI HeartMate LVAD[16] currently has a much larger presence in the US market. It is also a paracorporeal device that comes in two versions: a pneumatic version which has obtained FDA approval as a bridge to transplant, and an electric version which is currently under FDA investigation both as a bridge and an alternative to transplant. It is available only in a left ventricular assist device configuration and is connected to the left ventricle by an apical cannula, which allows inflow of blood to the VAD with ejection up to the ascending aorta (Figure 2). There are hemodynamic criteria for device insertion which are outlined in Table 1. It is most important to implant these devices before end-organ damage develops. Although these devices can act as extremely efficient pumps, if there is significant end-organ damage, blood flow alone cannot revive a patient.[17]

The TCI LVAD is unique in that is uses a counter-intuitive approach to surface design. The surface of the device is textured as opposed to smooth. This allows for formation of a protein coat, which over a period of time becomes nonthrombogenic. Hence, anticoagulation with Coumadin is not required for this device and the thromboembolic rate is below 3%. The device has been specifically designed for patients to use in an outpatient setting. The devices are expensive and can cost as much as $70,000 for a fully functional electrical system. The TCI LVAD is designed to allow for rehabilitation, as patients can

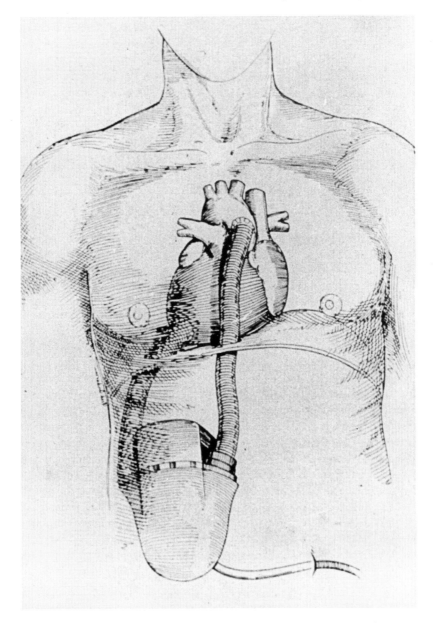

Figure 1: Schematic representation of the Baxter Novacor LVAD.

be off of inotropic support, rebuild their muscle mass, and even leave the hospital. This allows them to return to the hospital and receive their transplant essentially as New York Heart Association (NYHA) Class I patients (Figure 3). In our experience at Temple University Hospital, 27

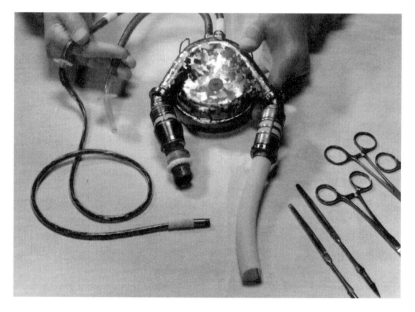

Figure 2: TCI electric Heart Mate LVAD.

of 30 patients supported with the device have been successfully transplanted to date.

It is important to understand the physiology of device implantation. The device is used solely as a left ventricular assist device with an essential pumping efficiency of 100%. Thus, it will pump whatever amount of blood it contains. With the exception of a mechanical problem from a kink in the inflow cannula or with device malfunction, blood flow through the pulmonary and right ventricular circuit will determine how the LVAD can function. Therefore, the primary management goal is to improve right-sided circulatory flow. Right-sided circulatory flow is determined by two factors, right ventricular function and pulmonary vascular resistance. Since left ventricular end-diastolic pressure will drop with the insertion of LVAD, this should reduce the

---

Table 1

Criteria for Assist Device Implantation

- Active heart transplant candidate
- On maximal inotropic support, with or without IABP
- Systolic blood pressure <80 mm Hg with:
    Cardiac index <2.0 L/min/m² or
    Pulmonary capillary wedge pressure >20 mm Hg

IABP = intra-aortic balloon pump.

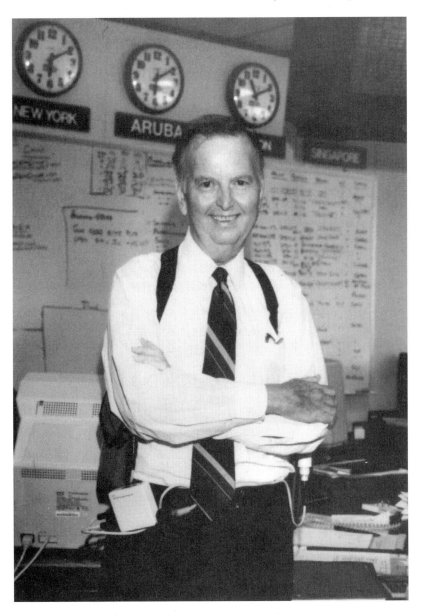

Figure 3: Patient supported on the TCI HeartMate LVAD, who has returned to work as a financial consultant.

afterload of the right ventricle. Therefore, even a poorly functioning right ventricle before LVAD implantation should subsequently improve. However, protection of the right ventricle is essential during LVAD implantation. Patent grafts, essential for right ventricular function, should be preserved and new grafts might be required. Increased pulmonary vascular resistance is an important contributing factor in the development of right-sided circulatory failure. Many patients have underlying pulmonary hypertension as their chronic left ventricular overloaded state causes intraparenchymal edema and increased pulmonary vascular resistance. Increased pulmonary vascular resistance in the immediate perioperative period can occur from an inflammatory reaction elicited by cardiopulmonary bypass. Release of cytokines, neutrophil elastase, and interleukins can cause pulmonary dysfunction. This effect, compounded by perioperative volume resuscitation, can further increase pulmonary vascular resistance. Treatment efforts to reduce pulmonary vascular resistance include hyperventilation, maximal oxygenation, nitric oxide, or use of an RVAD. Insertion of RVAD in the presence of a TCI LVAD is associated with over a 75% mortality.[17] Therefore, it is important to maintain meticulous hemostasis, minimize need for blood products, and maximize pulmonary function during implantation.

Conclusions

Heart transplantation is now a clinical reality, and is the treatment of choice for end-stage heart disease which is refractory to maximal medical management. Goals of research include: preservation, efforts to expand the donor pool, improve immunosuppression, and decrease transplant arteriopathy. Mechanical assistance holds promise in the near future as a potential alternative to transplantation, and may eventually take the forefront of surgical management of end-stage heart disease.

References

1. Evans RW, Manninen DL, Garrison LP, Maier AM. Donor availability as the primary determinant of the future of heart transplantation. *JAMA* 1986;255:1892–1898.
2. Evans RW. Socioeconomic aspects of heart transplantation. *Curr Opin Cardiol* 1995;10:169–1792.
3. Jeevanandam V, Furukawa S, Prendergast TW, et al. Standard criteria for an acceptable donor heart are restricting heart transplantation. *Ann Thor Surg* (in press).
4. Jeevanandam V, Mather P, Furukawa S, et al. Adult orthotopic heart transplantation using undersized pediatric donor hearts technique and postoperative management. *Circulation* 1994;90:II-74–II-77.
5. Lower RR, Stofen RR, Shumway NE. Homovital transplantation of the heart. *J Thorac Cardiovasc Surg* 1961;41:196.
6. Dreyfus G, Jebara V, Mihaileanu S, Carpentier AF. Total orthotopic heart

transplantation: An alternative to the standard technique. *Ann Thorac Surg* 1991;52:1181–1184.

7. Leyh RG, Jahnke AW, Kraatz EG, Sievers HH. Cardiovascular dynamics and dimensions after bicaval and standard cardiac transplantation. *Ann Thorac Surg* 1995;59(6):1495–1500.

8. El-Gamel A, Deiraniya AK, Rahman AN, et al. Orthotopic heart transplantation hemodynamics: Does atrial preservation improve cardiac output after transplantation? *J Heart Lung Transplant* 1996;15:564–571.

9. Barnard CN, Wolpowitz A. Heterotopic versus orthotopic heart transplantation. *Trans Proc* 1979;11:309.

10. Hardesty RL, Griffith BP, Trento A, et al. Mortally ill patients and excellent survival following heart transplantation. *Ann Thorac Surg* 1986;41:126–129.

11. Joyce LD, Emery RW, Eales F, et al. Mechanical circulatory support as a bridge to cardiac transplant. *J Thorac Cardiovasc Surg* 1989;98:935–941.

12. Golding LAR, Stewart RW, Sinkewich M, et al. Nonpulsatile ventricular assist bridging to transplantation. *Trans Am Soc Artif Int Organs* 1988;34:476–479.

13. Farrar DJ, Hill JD. Univentricular and biventricular Thoratec VAD support as bridge to transplantation. *Ann Thorac Surg* 1993;55:276–282.

14. Pennington DG, McBride LR, Swartz MT. Implantation technique for the Novacor left ventricular assist system. *J Thorac Cardiovasc Surg* 1994;108:604–608.

15. Loisance DY, Deleuze PH, Mazzucotelli JP, et al. Clinical implantation of the wearable Baxter Novacor ventricular assist system. *Ann Thorac Surg* 1994;58:551–554.

16. Jeevanandam V, Rose EA. TCI HeartMate LVAD: Results with chronic support. Mechanical Cardiac Assist (State of the Art Reviews). In Ott RA, Gutfinger DE eds: *CARDIAC SURGERY: State of the art reviews* Vol 7/ No.2. Philadelphia: Hanley & Belfus, Inc;1993.

17. Frazier OH, Rose EA, Macmanus Q, et al. Multicenter clinical evaluation of the HeartMate 1000 IP left ventricular assist device. *Ann Thorac Surg* 1992;53:1080–1090.

Chapter 11

Long-Term Implant of Left Ventricular Assist Devices

Brian E. Jaski, MD and Richard S. Maly, MS

Introduction

In response to the increasing number of patients with advanced heart failure who could potentially benefit from cardiac transplantation, cardiologists and cardiac surgeons have explored methods of sustaining patients to surgery as well as possible alternatives to cardiac transplantation, including mechanical cardiac assistance.[1-4] Recently, the FDA approved the use of the Thermo Cardiosystems (TCI) pneumatic HeartMate left ventricular assist device (LVAD) as a bridge to transplantation. The investigational use of the related portable Vented Electric (VE) LVAD in an outpatient setting for over 500 days in humans suggests that in the future, long-term use of the system may serve as an alternative to cardiac transplantation in selected patients.[5,6]

Consideration of these devices for long-term outpatient use, however, requires that patients maintain adequate circulatory function during activities of daily life. We have previously reported results of patients implanted with the pneumatic LVAD during treadmill and supine bicycle testing.[7,8] This review of the use of the LVAD in patients with refractory heart failure will emphasize our experience with the pneumatic HeartMate LVAD, although principles should be similar to other implanted pneumatic and electric LVADs including the Baxter Novacor LVAD.

Supported in part by the Rose Azus Cardiac Research Education Fund, Sharp Hospital Foundation, San Diego, and the San Diego Foundation for Cardiovascular Research and Education, San Diego, CA.

From: Balady GJ, Piña IL (eds). *Exercise and Heart Failure.* Armonk, NY: Futura Publishing Company, Inc.; ©1997.

LVAD Construction and Function

Pneumatic HeartMate LVAD 1000 IP

The TCI pneumatic HeartMate is constructed of a titanium housing, titanium-Dacron cannulae, and a flexible polyurethane diaphragm within the LVAD. Texturized titanium and diaphragmatic surfaces are used within the LVAD to allow the formation of an endogenous cellular coating, thereby reducing required anticoagulation therapy.[9,10] The LVAD is typically implanted in an anterior abdominal wall pocket, with a percutaneous driveline exiting the skin to an external control console, although intraperitoneal approaches are also used.[11,12] Blood arrives at the pump through a cannula placed in the left ventricle and exits via a Dacron graft sutured to the ascending aorta, distal to the coronary ostia. The apical inflow cannula is a moderately flexible, Dacron-titanium conduit with a 1.9 cm internal diameter (cross sectional area=2.8 cm^2). A cylindrical piece of myocardium at the apex is removed for cannula placement into the left ventricle. Unidirectional movement of blood through the LVAD is controlled by two 25 mm porcine heterograft valves in the inflow and outflow cannulae.[13]

The pump is normally operated in an asynchronous, fill-to-empty mode, ejecting approximately 83 cc when full, to a maximal LVAD rate of 140 bpm. As stroke volume remains relatively constant, the pump may achieve a maximal cardiac output of approximately 11 L/min. Deformation of the diaphragm during LVAD ejection results in an up to −20 mm Hg intra-LVAD filling pressure as the diaphragm returns to its baseline shape. After the LVAD reaches its maximal filling volume, pump ejection is actuated pneumatically from the external console to force the pusher plate and polyurethane diaphragm toward the pump housing, displacing blood within the LVAD. The console digitally displays beat-to-beat LVAD rate and stroke volume. A 6-beat moving average of LVAD output calculated from instantaneous LVAD rate and stroke volume is also displayed. Displayed stroke volume may vary with vigorous exercise due to changes in instantaneous afterload, errors due to the internal sensor malfunction, or regurgitation across the valve.

LVAD ejection duration (200 to 450 milliseconds) is selected by the operator by manually increasing from 200 milliseconds, to achieve complete emptying of the LVAD at rest without adversely affecting LVAD filling volume. By design, minimal LVAD filling time is 50% of selected LVAD ejection duration so that maximal possible LVAD rate may be calculated by the equation: Maximum LVAD rate = 60 / [1.5 * ejection duration * 0.001] (Personal communications, Thermo Cardiosystems, Inc.). Thus, maximum possible LVAD rate varies from 89 bpm to the designed limit of 140 bpm.

Vented Electric (VE) or Sealed Electric (SE) HeartMate LVADs

LVAD housing and cannulae, and filling characteristics of the Vented Electric (VE) and Sealed Electric (SE) LVADs are similar to those of the pneumatic pump. The electric LVADs, however, differ in pump actuation, power source, and systolic function. After an assigned time interval of LVAD pump stasis during LVAD filling, pumping is initiated from an external controller. Energy is transferred to a circular copper coil, creating an intra-LVAD electromagnetic field to actuate rotor assembly rotation. Interaction of the rotor bearings and the diaphragm-mounted helical cams push the diaphragm toward the LVAD housing. Blood is subsequently displaced similarly to with the pneumatic LVAD. Power for the VE derives from 6 hour to 8 hour batteries worn on the individual or from an external 12 volt power source.

The VE and SE pumps do not use a Hall sensor for diaphragm displacement measurement. Ejection duration is constant in the VE and SE, with rate varying by automatic changes in LVAD filling time when the rotor assembly is in a static position. With increased venous return and improved LVAD filling, the pump-controller detects a decreased "no load time" before diaphragm cam and rotor interaction. The subsequent time of rotor stasis is then reduced by the LVAD controller. Thus, with a decrease in LVAD filling time, overall LVAD rate and output increase.

Due to the increased ejection power of the electric LVAD, changes in afterload minimally affect pump performance. Overall performance is limited only by LVAD filling and designed maximum LVAD rate of approximately 140 bpm.

Design of the VE includes an LVAD vent line placed subcutaneously to minimize negative pressure build-up within the LVAD during diaphragm ejection. Similarly, the SE uses an implantable compliance chamber, although this is currently under development. In addition, the SE is totally implantable with power transduction occurring through transcutaneous induction coils and no percutaneous lines.

Indications and Contraindications

The U. S. Food and Drug Administration has currently approved the TCI LVAD only as a bridge for patients with profound cardiogenic shock listed for cardiac transplantation (Table 1).[14] Maximal inotropic therapy associated with high left ventricular filling pressures, low cardiac output, refractory or progressive hypotension,

Table 1

Indications for LVAD Implantation

Refractory Heart Failure (Category I)	Cardiac Arrest (Category II)
Approved transplant candidate	Cardiac arrest
On inotropic therapy	Approved transplant candidate
On IABP (not necessary)	On inotropic therapy
PCW or LAP 20 mm Hg with either:	On IABP (not necessary)
a. Systolic blood pressure <80 mm Hg	Systolic blood pressure <60 mm
b. Cardiac index <2.0 L/min/m²	Hg

LVAD = left ventricular assist device; IABP = intra-aortic balloon pump.

and possibly intra-aortic balloon pump (IABP) support indicates LVAD use. However, patients not meeting all criteria, including patients during cardiac arrest, have been implanted with the pneumatic pump. The clinical decision for LVAD implantation should also include the metabolic status of the patient as well as the rate of hemodynamic compromise.

Most relative contraindications to LVAD implantation are similar to those of cardiac transplantation including severe chronic pulmonary disease, irreversible renal or hepatic failure, history of malignancy, or active systemic infection (Table 2). Other possible contraindications affecting pump efficacy include severely depressed right heart function, intractable ventricular tachycardia, or blood dyscrasia. A body surface area <1.5 m² is the only absolute contraindication by the FDA.

Table 2

Contraindications for TCI LVAD Implantation

Body surface area <1.5 m²	Severe hepatic disease
Age >70 years	Cerebral vascular disease
<7 days following AMI with severe LV failure	Active systemic infection
Chronic renal failure	Cardiac arrest
Severe emphysema or COPD	Systolic blood pressure <60 mm Hg
Elevated PVR	Unresolved malignancy
Dysfunctional RV	BUN >100 mg %
Intractible ventricular tachycardia	Creatinine >5.0 mg %

AMI = acute myocardial infarction; BUN = blood urea nitrogen; COPD = chronic obstructive lung disease; LV = left ventricle; PVR = pulmonary vascular resistance; RV = right ventricle; TCI = Thermo Cardiosystems.

LVAD-Supported Hemodynamics at Rest and During Supine Bicycle Exercise

Resting Hemodynamics

Table 3 provides a summary of hemodynamic findings in 10 patients following LVAD implantation, partially presented in a previous report.[7] Native heart rate was higher than LVAD rate at rest (87 ± 12 bpm versus 82 ± 18 bpm). Total Fick cardiac output was 5.0 ± 1.2 L/min at a similar LVAD output of 5.4 ± 0.9 L/min. Operator-set LVAD ejection duration ranged from 280 to 435 milliseconds. Resting oxygen consumption was 3.2 ± 0.6 ccO_2/min/kg, with arterial blood oxygen saturations of $97\pm2\%$ and venous saturations at $66\pm5\%$. Central hemodynamic measurements were within normal range in all but one patient who had elevated right atrial (RA) and pulmonary capillary wedge (PCW) pressures and a high systemic vascular resistance (SVR).

Hemodynamics During Supine Bicycle Exercise

With supine bicycle exercise, LVAD and heart rate increased in parallel (peak LVAD rate = 107 ± 21 bpm versus peak heart rate = 117 ± 14 bpm). Fick cardiac output increased with exercise in all patients and exceeded LVAD output because of parallel ejection through the native aortic valve verified by Doppler echocardiography (Figure 1).[8] This was associated with increased tissue oxygen utilization and reductions in venous oxygen supply to $38\pm10\%$. Maximal oxygen consumption reached 8.2 ± 1.7 ml O_2/min/kg. This was slightly more than half that achieved by the same patients during upright treadmill exercise (13.8 ± 2.7 ccO_2/min/kg).

PCW and RA pressures increased in all patients during supine exercise while SVR and pulmonary vascular resistance (PVR) declined. Abrupt increases in capillary wedge pressures accompanied patients reaching peak LVAD rate and output (Figure 2). Peak power exercise output achieved was between 75 watts and 150 watts.

Echocardiographic Studies

Echocardiographic studies completed at baseline and peak exercise revealed little or no ejection through the aortic valve at rest, however valve opening was observed during exercise. Diastolic left ventricular size increased with activity while diastolic right ventricular dimensions and perimeter calculations surprisingly either did not change or decreased, despite increased right-heart filling pressures.[8] This is consistent with a decrease in functional right ventricular diastolic compliance secondary to left and right ventricular interaction.

Table 3

Hemodynamic and Oxygen Consumption Data During Supine Bicycle and Treadmill Exercise

	Supine Bicycle		Treadmill	
	Baseline	Maximal Exercise	Baseline	Maximal Exercise
Heart rate (beats/min)	87 ± 12	117 ± 14	95 ± 7	147 ± 17*
LVAD rate (beats/min)	82 ± 18	107 ± 21	72 ± 13*	111 ± 21
Systolic BP (mm Hg)	142 ± 32	153 ± 26	122 ± 16*	124 ± 21*
Diastolic BP (mm Hg)	73 ± 8	79 ± 13	75 ± 9	75 ± 18
LVAD output (L/min)	5.4 ± 0.9	7.0 ± 1.4	4.4 ± 0.8*	7.6 ± 1.9
LVAD SV (mL/min)	65 ± 6	66 ± 7	62 ± 8	70 ± 10
VO$_2$/kg (mL O$_2$/min per kg)	3.2 ± 0.6	8.2 ± 1.7	4.8 ± 1.7*	13.8 ± 2.7*
RA (mm Hg)	6 ± 4	12 ± 5		
PA (mm Hg)	17 ± 3	31 ± 7		
PCW (mm Hg)	5 ± 3	13 ± 8		
Fick CO (L/min)	5.0 ± 1.2	7.8 ± 2.5		
PVR (dynes·s per cm^5)	216 ± 83	202 ± 96		
SVR (dynes·s per cm^5)	1478 ± 369	899 ± 357		
% Art SAT	97 ± 2	94 ± 2		
% PA SAT	66 ± 5	38 ± 10		
Ejection duration (ms)	326 ± 63		314 ± 46	

LVAD = left ventricular assist device; BP = blood pressure; RA = mean right atrial pressure; PA (mean) = mean pulmonary artery pressure; PCW = mean pulmonary capillary wedge pressure; CO = cardiac output; SV = stroke volume; PVR = pulmonary vascular resistance; SVR = systemic vascular resistance; Art SAT = arterial oxygen saturation; PA SAT = pulmonary artery saturation; VO$_2$/kg = oxygen consumption; Ejection Duration = LVAD systolic ejection duration; Hgb = blood hemoglobin content; PO = post operative. Data reported as mean ± SD.

* = P<.05 treadmill vs. supine bicycle.

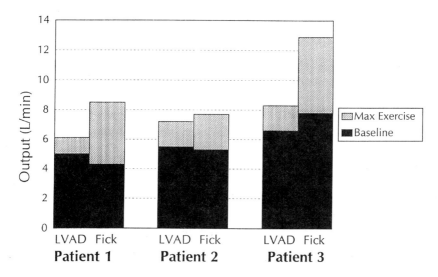

Figure 1: Comparison of left ventricular assist device (LVAD) output and calculated Fick cardiac output during baseline study (solid bars) and maximal (Max) supine bicycle exercise (hatched bars). L = liters.

LVAD-Supported Hemodynamics During Upright Treadmill Exercise

Patients performed upright treadmill exercise testing 50 ± 22 days after being implanted with a LVAD. Heart rate increased from 95 ± 7 bpm at rest to 147 ± 17 bpm at peak exercise ($P<.001$). LVAD rate increased from a baseline value of 72 ± 13 bpm to a peak exercise value of 111 ± 21 bpm ($P<.001$). There was no change in systolic or diastolic blood pressure during treadmill exercise. Pump output also increased with exercise from 4.4 ± 0.8 L/min to 8.0 ± 1.9 L/min ($P<.001$), with minimal change in LVAD stroke volume. Oxygen consumption increased from 4.8 ± 1.7 to 14.1 ± 2.7 with treadmill exercise ($P<.001$). (Relative workload, 4.0 ± 0.8 METS, ranging from 2.8 METS to 5.3 METS). Heart rate and LVAD rate increased in parallel throughout exercise (Table 1).

Comparative Hemodynamic and Oxygen Consumption Measurements During Supine Bike and Upright Treadmill Exercise

Although baseline heart rates were not significantly different between bike and treadmill exercise, at peak exercise mean treadmill

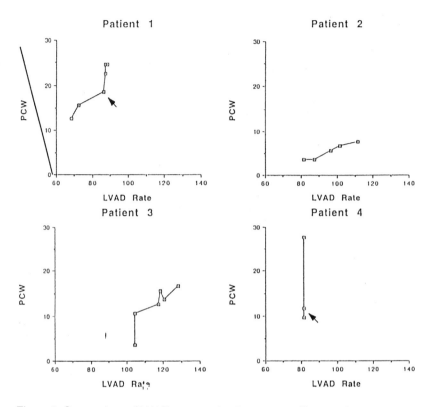

Figure 2: Comparison of LVAD rates and pulmonary capillary wedge pressures during supine bicycle exercise. LVAD rate reached a plateau after 3 minutes for Patient 1 and did not increase for Patient 4 throughout exercise *(arrows).*

heart rate was significantly greater than supine bike heart rate (147±17 bpm and 117±17 bpm, respectively, *P*<.01). Systolic blood pressure (SBP) was greater at rest and at maximal exercise, however, during supine bike exercise (*P*<.01). Assist device output was lower during baseline treadmill evaluation than supine bike evaluation (4.4±0.8 versus 5.4±0.9 mL/kg/min, *P*<.01), but was similar at maximal exercise. Oxygen consumption was observed to be significantly greater during treadmill testing at rest (*P*<.01) and at maximal exertion (*P*<.01). There was a trend for higher R values during baseline treadmill evaluation than during baseline bicycle evaluation (*P*=.06), with a significant difference at peak exercise (1.33±0.23 versus 1.10±0.12, *P*<.01).

Determinants of "LV-LVAD Complex" Function

Figure 3 summarizes the factors affecting the performance of the LV-LVAD complex with activity. As stroke volume is designed to be

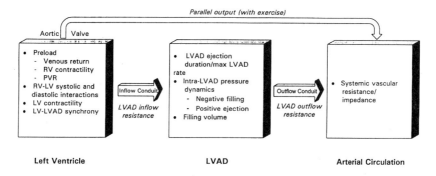

Figure 3: Model of the determinants affecting the left ventricular (LV)-LVAD complex performance at rest and during activity. Significant parallel ejection through the native aortic valve is common with exerercise.

constant when operating in a fill-to-empty mode, the rate of LVAD filling is the primary determinant of total LVAD output until peak LVAD rate is reached. In patients with little or no residual left ventricular systolic function, peak LVAD rate may be blunted due to poor LVAD filling, and result in elevated left- and right-heart filling pressures. Finally, right ventricular delivery of venous return to the left ventricle will be affected by total vascular volume as related to oral intake and diuretic use, right ventricular contractility, and pulmonary vascular resistance. Thus, limitations to LV-LVAD peak performance may be related to left ventricular preload and residual contractility, relative timing of the LV-LVAD complex, LVAD inflow resistance, or total LVAD active suction.

Left ventricular systolic function can contribute to active filling of the LVAD through a ventricular "kick". As the LVAD works on a fill-to-empty mode, this may assist in overcoming inflow cannula impedance, shorten LVAD diastolic filling time, and increase potential output per unit time.[8] With the increase in LV preload during exercise, systolic left ventricular pressure can exceed aortic pressure, allowing additional contributions to total cardiac output flow through the native aortic valve. In patients with irreversible and profoundly depressed LV function, cardiac reserve may be blunted due to extended filling times and little parallel contribution to total cardiac output.

By design, ejection duration, which determines maximum possible LVAD rate, is manually set to achieve a balance between complete LVAD emptying and filling. Therefore, observed peak LVAD rate, if not limited by LV-assisted filling, is ultimately confined by approaching this LVAD frequency limit. Furthermore, ejection duration required to achieve complete ejection, correlates with systemic vascular resistance.[8] Whether vasodilator therapy can allow a decrease in ejection duration and increase in peak LVAD rate during long-term implantation is unknown. Patients supported with the VE LVAD, however, presumably would not have this limitation, but elevated systemic vascular resistance could increase rate of power consumption and mechanical wear.

Complications During Left Ventricular Assist Device Support

Table 4 lists potential problems in three phases based on the time postimplant: (1) immediately postoperative (<2 days), (2) early implantation (<30 days), and (3) late implantation (>30 days). Previous reports have generally considered acute postoperative complications, including right ventricular failure, surgical complications, infections, and thromboembolism.[15-18] Long-term LVAD support, however, may be complicated by infection, LVAD pump component deterioration and malfunction, and progressive cardiac problems such as the development of arrhythmias, alterations in pulmonary vascular resistance, or advancement of coronary artery disease.[19] These categories are arbitrary but can serve as guidelines when diagnosing clinical problems associated with LVAD implantation.

Conclusions

As the number of patients awaiting cardiac transplant increases without concomitant increases in donor heart availability, mechanical bridging or other alternatives to transplant will become more common in the future. Long-term outpatient LVAD implantation requires the ability of the LVAD patient to function during activities of daily life. Although the right ventricle is important in the acute postoperative phase, residual left ventricular function may contribute to active filling of the LVAD, overcoming LVAD inflow impedance, and parallel flow out of the aortic valve. Patients with adequate reserve of LV-LVAD complex may be ideal candidates for long-term, outpatient LVAD implantation. Additional investigation into optimal anticoagulation therapies, improvement in diagnostic procedures for cardiac and LVAD malfunction, and other issues involved in implantation will be important for long-term care of the LVAD patient.

Table 4

Postoperative, Early, and Late Complications with LVAD Support

Time Period:	Postoperative (<48 hours):	Early (<30 days):	Late (>30 days):
LVAD-related complications:	Mechanical malfunction	Mechanical malfunction	Mechanical malfunction
	In/outflow cannula obstruction	In/outflow cannula obstruction	In/outflow cannula obstruction
	Thromboembolism	Thromboembolism	Thromboembolism
	Hemolysis	Hemolysis	—
	Excessive Bleeding	—	LVAD valve failure/calcification
	—	—	Worn cams/rollers in LVAD
Cardiac-related complications:	Left ventricular dysfunction	Left ventricular dysfunction	Left ventricular dysfunction
	RV failure	—	—
	—	—	Valvular insufficiency
	—	—	Myocardial ischemia (CAD)
Systemic-related complications:	Multi-organ failure	Infection	Infection
	Pulmonary hypertension	Multi-organ failure	—
	—	—	—

References

1. Adamson RM, Dembitsky WP, Reichman RT, et al. Mechanical support: Assist or nemesis. *J Thorac Cardiovasc Surg* 1989;98:915–921.
2. Hill DJ. Bridging to cardiac transplantation. *Ann Thorac Surg* 1989;47: 167–71.
3. Birovljev S, Radovancevic B, Burnett CM, et al. Heart transplantation after mechanical circulatory support: Four years' experience. *J Heart Lung Transplant* 1992;11:240–245.
4. McCarthy PM, James KB, Savage RM, et al. Implantable left ventricular assist device: Approaching an alternative for end-stage heart failure. *Circulation* 1994;90(Part 2):83–86.
5. Frazier OH. First use of an untethered, vented electric left ventricular assist device for long-term support. *Circulation* 1994;89:2908–2914.
6. Myers TJ, Dasse KA, Macris MP, et al. Use of a left ventricular assist device in an outpatient setting. *ASAIO Journal* 1994;40:M471–M475.
7. Jaski BE, Branch KR, Gordon JB, et al. Exercise hemodynamics in patients awaiting heart transplant with a left ventricular assist device. *J Am Coll Cardiol* 1993;22:1574–1580.
8. Branch KR, Dembitsky WP, Peterson KL, et al. Physiology of the native heart and the left ventricular assist device complex at rest and during exercise: Implications for chronic support. *J Heart Lung Transplant* 1994;13: 641–651.
9. Graham TR, Salih V, Coumbe A, et al. Evaluation of biological linings forming on texturized biomaterial surfaces during clinical use of an implantable left ventricular assist device [Abstr]. *J Heart Lung Transplant* 1992;11:196.
10. Rose EA, Levin HR, Oz MC, et al. Artificial circulatory support with texturized interior surfaces: A counterintuitive approach to minimizing thromboembolism. *Circulation* 1994;90(Part 2):87–91.
11. McCarthy PM, Wang N, Vargo R. Preperitoneal insertion of the HeartMate 1000 IP implantable left ventricular assist device. *Ann Thorac Surg* 1994; 57:634–637.
12. Parnis SM, McGee MG, Igo SR, et al. Anatomic considerations for abdominally placed permanent left ventricular assist devices. *ASAIO Transactions* 1989;35:728–730.
13. Frazier OH, Rose EA, Macmanus Q, et al. Multicenter clinical evaluation of the HeartMate 1000 IP left ventricular assist device. *Ann Thorac Surg* 1992; 53:1080–1090.
14. HeartMate IP LVAS: Directions for Use. Woburn, MA.: Thermo Cardiosystems, Inc., 1994.
15. Jaski BE, Branch KR, Dasse KA. Diagnosis and treatment of complications in patients implanted with a TCI left ventricular assist device. *J Interventional Cardiol* 1995;8:275–282.
16. Mandarino WA, Morita S, Kormos RL, et al. Quantitation of right ventricular shape changes after left ventricular assist device implantation. *ASAIO Journal* 1992;38:M228–M231.
17. Sato N, Mohri H, Miura M, et al. Right ventricular failure during the use of a left ventricular assist device. *ASAIO Transactions* 1989;35:550–552.
18. Hobson KS. Physiologic aspects of the TCI HeartMate mechanical left ventricular assist device. *J Cardiovasc Nurs* 1994;8:16–35.
19. Phillips WS, Burton NA, MacManus Q, Lefrak EA. Surgical complications in bridging to transplantation: The Thermo Cardiosystems LVAD. *Ann Thorac Surg* 1992;53:482–486.

Exercise Testing and Expired Gas Analysis

Chapter 12

Exercise Testing Protocols for Use in Heart Failure

Ileana L. Piña, MD

Exercise testing of heart failure patients had not been the standard of practice among clinical cardiologists until recent years, when it was shown to be safe and to provide the health care team with useful information. Early exercise studies of patients with heart failure used the Modified Naughton protocol in 2-minute stages with measurements of gas exchange.[1] Thus, the Modified Naughton became the rule rather than the exception when choosing exercise protocols. In fact, most randomized trials that have studied the effects of a particular drug on exercise function in heart failure patients have also chosen this protocol. Exercise testing, however, can be performed using a variety of published protocols. The protocol chosen often depends on the experience of the testing physician and on the norms of any specific testing facility.

Treadmill Versus Bicycle Ergometry

Testing of heart failure patients can be performed either on a treadmill or on a bicycle ergometer. The bicycle ergometer offers the convenience of a stable sitting position, which allows more accurate measurements of blood pressure and particularly of concomitant hemodynamic measurements. Walking is more familiar to the average U.S. population and patients may be capable of performing at a higher level. The exercise testing results, however, will vary with the testing mode. More specifically, peak VO_2, the anaerobic threshold, and the minute ventilation will be higher with treadmill testing than with bicycle ergometry. On the other hand, heart rate, systolic blood pressure, respiratory exchange ratio (RER), and RPE can be identical with both testing modali-

From: Balady GJ, Piña IL (eds). *Exercise and Heart Failure*. Armonk, NY: Futura Publishing Company, Inc.; ©1997.

ties.[2] These differences must be kept in mind when applying the results of published studies to the general population. It is interesting to note that key multicenter trials in heart failure (V-Heft I and V-Heft II) that have underscored the relevance of exercise testing and have used bicycle ergometry as the testing modality[3] have found similar $\dot{V}O_2$ values for predicting mortality, as have other notable studies that have used treadmill testing instead.[4]

Treadmill Protocols: Fast or Slow?

The selection of protocols for testing heart failure patients should, however, follow the same criteria as when choosing protocols for other testing purposes, eg, ischemia. An exercise protocol should yield the maximum amount of information and truly assess a patient's maximal or near-maximal function with a high degree of confidence and reproducibility. Patients with heart failure stop performing activity usually due to one of two reasons: feelings of breathlessness or feelings of fatigue. Breathlessness may be the salient symptom when exercise is of sudden onset, whereas fatigue predominates at slow but longer-lasting activity. To examine this observation more closely, Lipkin and colleagues exercised heart failure patients on a fast and a slow protocol.[5] The slow protocol consisted of 6-minute stages with gradual increases in workload from 1.0 mph and 0% grade to 2.5 mph and a 12.5% elevation. The fast protocol consisted of a sudden increase in workload to the level at which the patient had stopped exercising on the slow test. That particular workload was then maintained for 3 minutes and incremented every 2 minutes. Although there was no difference in pulmonary capillary pressure achieved with either protocol, the fast protocol yielded a higher $\dot{V}O_{2max}$, higher cardiac output, and a greater degree of breathlessness. In contrast, the slower protocol provoked fatigue at a lower $\dot{V}O_{2max}$ and cardiac output. The authors speculate that a longer protocol may lead to a higher production of lactic acid in skeletal muscle, leading to fatigue. In addition, longer protocols may also be associated with boredom and lack of motivation on the part of the patient. Therefore, although steady state may not be reached with shorter stages, longer protocols may not yield an accurate assessment of $\dot{V}O_{2max}$.

Pollock and co-workers studied a group of normal individuals with various levels of physical conditioning using four separate treadmill protocols: The Balke, Bruce, Ellestad, and Modified Astrand Protocols.[6] As seen in Figure 1, the protocols differ in the work rate and degree of difficulty. The speed of the Modified Astrand, after warm up, was determined by the subject's ability to run on the Balke protocol. In the sedentary group of subjects tested, the $\dot{V}O_{2max}$ was highest on the Astrand protocol, and the longest duration was on the Balke. The great-

TREADMILL PROTOCOLS

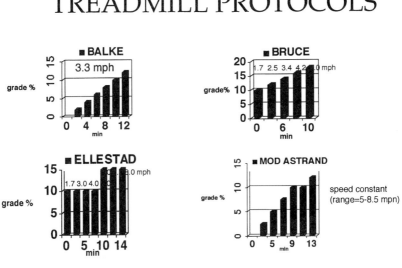

adapted from Pollock et al., 1976

Figure 1: Comparison of four treadmill protocols used primarily in testing normals. See text for dicussion. Adapted from Reference 6.

est degree of effort was noted on the Bruce and the Ellestad and was mirrored by the highest minute ventilation, indicative of a greater effort. These observations notwithstanding, the differences in all measured parameters were of no clinical relevance, and therefore in the more deconditioned patient (more compatible with heart failure patients), the choice of protocols may not be as important as in fit individuals. It is more crucial that the patient be able to perform a certain workload comfortably in order to determine a true level of functional capacity for that individual. Subsequently, the Balke, Ellestead and Modified Astrand protocols apply speeds that may be too difficult for a patient with heart failure to achieve. Similarly, the Bruce protocol may be too challenging and difficult because of its large increments in workload per stage, and although heart failure patients can perform this protocol, the duration of exercise may be short-lived.[7] Table 1 lists the work rates and stages of commonly used protocols for testing heart failure patients. The ramp protocol shown in Table 1 can be modified in accordance with the patient's capabilities

Ramp protocols provide an interesting alternative to the standard 2- and 3-minute per stage protocols. In addition, ramp protocols can be created across various levels of difficulty, thus ensuring the patient's ability to perform in accordance with individual capabilities. Most ramp protocols are in stages lasting ≤1 minute, with speed and elevation changes

Table 1

Treadmill Protocols Per Stage

	I	II	III	IV	V	VI	VII	VII	IX	X
	1.7	*2.5*	*3.4*	*4.2*	*5.0*	*5.5*				
Bruce	10%	12%	14%	16%	18%	20%				
	1.0	*1.5*	*2.0*	*2.0*	*2.0*	*3.0*	*3.0*	*3.0*	*3.0*	*3.0*
Naughton	0%	0%	0%	3.5%	7%	5%	7.5%	10%	12.5%	15%
	2.0	*2.0*	*2.0*	*2.0*	*2.0*					
Ramp	3.5%	7.0%	10.5%	14%	17.5%					

NOTE: The Naughton and Bruce protocols have 3 min/stage. The Naughton can be modified to 2 min/stage. The Ramp protocol uses 1 min/stage but can be modified as well to the patient's capacity. Numbers in italics represent speed (mph); numbers followed by % represent grade.

allowing a desirable time of completion of <10 minutes. An additional benefit to ramp protocols lies in the linear increase in $\dot{V}O_2$ versus time, allowing a better visualization of a maximum $\dot{V}O_2$ or "plateau", if attained.

Since most heart failure centers use gas exchange in addition to ECG monitoring, it is more important to achieve, at the very least, an anaerobic threshold and, preferably, as close to a true maximum $\dot{V}O_2$ as possible, than to use the same protocol routinely. Exercise that is sufficient to reach an anaerobic threshold demonstrates a significant level of effort expended. Furthermore, as shown in Figure 2, the anaerobic threshold is effort- and protocol-independent and should be a minimal target in testing.[7] If properly measured, the anaerobic threshold is also reproducible in repeated testing and can be used as a clinical and prognostic tool as well[8] (Figure 2). Several investigators have provided the means to extrapolate maximum $\dot{V}O_2$, provided the respiratory exchange ratio (RER) exceeds 1.0.[9]

6-Minute Walk Test

Among exercise testing potocols, the 6-minute walk is worthy of noting. This testing modality has become more popular in recent years due to its ease of administration and its approximation to daily tasks. In addition, the 6-minute walk can be used to supplement clinical information. The test uses a 20 meter long, level, enclosed corridor. Instructions are given to the patient to cover as much ground as possible in 6 minutes by walking continuously, if possible. The 6-minute walk test is less likely to discriminate between New York Heart Association (NYHA) Class II and Class III than an $\dot{V}O_{2max}$ test, and may be better suited for the patients with moderate to severe heart failure in whom repeated testing is used for serial monitoring.[10] Of interest, a substudy of the SOLVD (Studies of Left Ventricular Dysfunction) registry has reported that the 6-minute

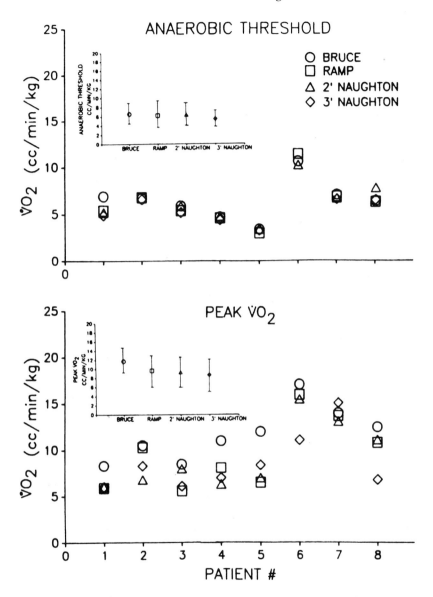

Figure 2: Comparison of four treadmill protocols for oxygen uptake and anaerobic threshold in eight heart failure patients. The protocols were administered randomly. The anaerobic threshold is more reproducible across all protocols than the peak oxygen uptake. The means and standard deviation are shown in the inset. From Reference 7.

walk test is safe and simple to perform, as well as an independent, strong predictor of mortality and morbidity. Among 898 patients, those with the higher performance level had the lowest chance of death and hospitalization during the follow-up period.[11]

The 9-Minute Self-Powered Treadmill Test

The 9-minute self-powered treadmill test has also been used in the assessment of functional exercise capacity in patients with heart failure. The patient is asked to walk on a self-powered treadmill for a total of 9 minutes. The treadmill is usually placed on a small incline. When compared to a standard maximum treadmill test, the 9-minute self-powered treadmill yields a lower peak $\dot{V}O_2$, and a shorter distance covered. The 9-minute treadmill test has been shown to be as reproducible as standard treadmill testing.[12] In two separate recently-conducted multi-center trials comparing a β-blocking agent to placebo, the 9-minute self-powered treadmill test was used to assess functional capacity along with the 6-minute walk.[13,14] Whether this test will ever take the place of a 6-minute walk or a standard assessment of functional capacity with gas exchange is yet to be determined. At this time, the 9-minute self-powered test does not appear to offer any significant advantage over the two.

Summary

Ideally, a protocol should be tailored to the physical capabilities of the patient and should be challenging enough and of sufficient duration to achieve target endpoints within 8 to 10 minutes. Protocols lasting longer than 10 minutes may ultimately become boring to both patient and supervising staff, and not necessarily render any more pertinent information.

References

1. Weber KT, Kinasewitz GT, Janicki JS, Fishman AP. Oxygen utilization and ventilation during exercise in patients with chronic cardiac failure. *Circulation* 1982;65:1213–1223.
2. Page E, Cohen-Solal A, Jondeau G, et al. Comparison of treadmill and bicycle exercise in patients with chronic heart failure. *Chest* 1994;106:1002–1006.
3. Cohn JN, Johnson GR, Shabetai R, et al. Ejection fraction, peak exercise oxygen consumption, cardiothoracic ratio, ventricular arrhythmias, and plasma norepinephrine as determinants of prognosis in heart failure. *Circulation* 1993;87(suppl VI):VI-5–VI-16.
4. Mancini D, Eisen HE, Kussmaul W, et al. Value of peak exercise oxygen cardiac transplantation in ambulatory patients with heart failure. *Circulation* 1991;83:778–786.
5. Lipkin DP, Canepa-Anson R, Stephens MR, Poole-Wilson PA. Factors determining symptoms in heart failure: Comparison of fast and slow exercise tests. *Br Heart J* 1986;55:439–445.
6. Pollock ML, Bohannon RL, Cooper KH, et al. A comparative analysis of four protocols for maximal treadmill stress testing. *Am Heart J* 1976;92:39–46.

7. Piña IL, Karalis DG. Comparison of four exercise protocols using anaerobic threshold measurement of functional capacity in congestive heart failure. *Am J Cardiol* 1990;65:1269–1271.

8. Weber KT, Janicki JS. Lactate production during maximal and submaximal exercise in patients with chronic heart failure. *J Am Coll Cardiol* 1985;6:717–724.

9. Clark AL, Poole-Wilson PA, Coats AJ. Effects of motivation of the patients on indices of exercise capacity in chronic failure. *Br Heart J* 1994;71:162–165.

10. Lipkin DP, Scriven AJ, Crake T, Poole-Wilson PA. Six minute walking test for assessing exercise capacity in chronic heart failure. *Br Heart J* 1986;292: 653–655.

11. Bittner V, Weiner DH, Yusuf S, et al. Prediction of mortality and morbidity with a 6-minute walk test in patients with left ventricular dysfunction. SOLVD Investigators. *JAMA* 1993;270:1702–1707.

12. Yamani MF, Wells L, Massie BM, et al. Relation of the nine-minute self-powered treadmill test to maximal exercise capacity and skeletal muscle function in patients with congestive heart failure. *Am J Cardiol* 1995;76: 788–792.

13. Packer M, Colucci WS, Sackner-Bernstein J, et al. and the PRECISE Study Group. Prospective randomized evaluation of carvedilol on symptoms and exercise tolerance in chronic heart failure: Results of the PRECISE trial. *Circulation* 1995;92: I-143.

14. Bristow M, Gilbert EM, Abraham WT, et al. for the MOCHA Investigators. Multicenter oral carvedilol heart failure assessment (MOCHA): A six-month dose-response evaluation in class II-IV patients. *Circulation* 1995;92: I-142.

Chapter 13

Ventilatory Gas Exchange in Heart Failure:
Techniques, Problems, and Pitfalls

Jonathan Myers, PhD

Ventilatory gas exchange data obtained during exercise testing provide a more precise and reproducible measure of total body work and substantially increase the yield of information on cardiopulmonary function when compared to exercise time.[1-3] These techniques are particularly useful in patients with chronic heart failure whose hallmark symptoms include exercise intolerance and exertional dyspnea due in part to a mismatching of ventilation to perfusion in the lung.[4-6] Proper application of gas data analysis requires an understanding of basic exercise physiology, the mechanics of the technique, and a degree of expertise by the technician involved, since attention to calibration, validation, and quality control are essential. Likewise, proper application of the results by the clinician requires an understanding of the principles of ventilatory gas exchange. The purpose of this chapter is to outline techniques of measuring ventilatory gas exchange during exercise testing and to discuss common problems and pitfalls of the technology.

Instrumentation

In its simplest terms, the determination of oxygen uptake requires the ability to measure three variables: (1) the fraction of oxygen in the expired air; (2) the fraction of carbon dioxide in the expired air; and (3) the volume of the inspired or expired air. Oxygen uptake can be roughly described as simply the product of ventilation (VE) in a given

From: Balady GJ, Piña IL (eds). *Exercise and Heart Failure.* Armonk, NY: Futura Publishing Company, Inc.;©1997.

interval and the fraction of oxygen in that ventilation which has been consumed by the working muscle:

$$\dot{V}O_2 \text{ mL/min (STPD)} = VE \times (FiO_2 - FeO_2)$$

where FiO_2 is the fraction of inspired oxygen and FeO_2 is the fraction of expired oxygen. FiO_2 is equal to 20.93% at sea level and 0% humidity, and ventilation is converted to standard temperature and pressure, dry (STPD). $FiO_2 - FeO_2$ represents the amount of oxygen consumed by the working muscle for a given sample, sometimes called "true O_2". This process is illustrated in Figure 1.

For the sake of explanation, the above equation is oversimplified, as it assumes that expired air is dry and that the inspired and expired volumes are not different. Because this is generally not the case (inspired and expired volumes are similar only when the respiratory exchange ratio equals one), several additional calculations are necessary to accurately determine oxygen uptake. First, FiO_2 is affected by the ambient temperature, barometric pressure, and humidity; all three of these variables must be measured and FiO_2 must be adjusted accordingly (Figure 2). Second, because oxygen uptake is defined by the difference between the fraction of oxygen in the inspired and expired ventilation, both in-

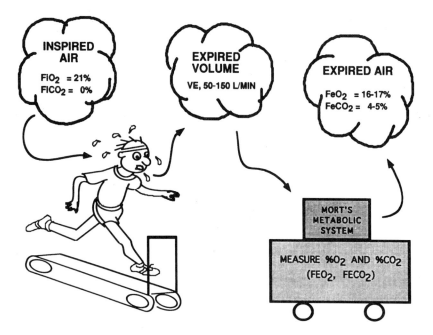

Figure 1: Method of obtaining oxygen uptake by measuring the volume and concentration of exhaled air.

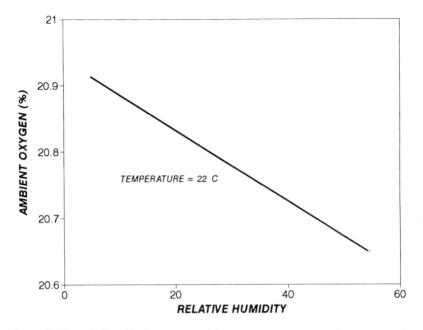

Figure 2: The relationship between ambient oxygen, expressed as a percentage, and relative humidity, at a temperature of 22°C. The slope of this relationship steepens slightly as temperature increases, and flattens as temperature decreases.

spired and expired ventilation must be known precisely. Ventilatory volume is frequently measured only from the expired air. Inspired volume however, can be determined from the expired volume and the fractions of oxygen and carbon dioxide. This is possible because nitrogen (N_2) and other inert gasses do not affect the body's gas exchange processes. In other words, the amount of N_2 inspired is equal to the amount of N_2 expired. One needs only to be concerned with differences in the concentrations of O_2 and CO_2 between the inspired and expired air. The concentrations of N_2, CO_2, and O_2 in the inspired air are known to approximate 0.7904, 0, and 0.2093, respectively (when dry). The fraction of inert gasses in the expired air (FeN2) is:

$$FeN_2 = 1 - FeO_2 - FeCO_2$$

Thus, inspiratory volume (VI) can be expressed as the difference between the fraction of inert gasses in the expired air and the fraction of inert gasses in the atmosphere:

$$VI = \frac{[VE \times (1 - FeO_2 - FeCO_2]}{0.7904}$$

And the equation for oxygen uptake becomes:

$$VO_2 \text{ L/min STPD} = \frac{(1 - FeO_2 - FeCO_2)}{0.7904} \times (FiO_2 - FeO_2)$$
$$\times VE \text{ L/min STPD}$$

Collection of Expired Ventilation

The measurement of ventilation during exercise requires that the patient have a mouthpiece in place that seals tightly and the nose sealed with a clip, or have a face mask that covers the mouth and nose securely. All breathing valves have a "dead space"— a volume of air that fills the valve apparatus and does not participate in gas exchange. A balance exists between the dead space volume and the valve's resistance; the smaller the dead space, the higher the resistance. Both high dead space and high resistance are undesirable, and most exercise testing is performed using a valve with a dead space somewhat less than 100 mL. Extreme care must be taken so that leaking does not occur at high ventilation rates. Newer face masks are designed so that they are less prone to leaking, have a small dead space (40 mL), and are more comfortable, since they permit the subject to swallow or speak. Speaking should be discouraged however, because it can interfere with the metabolic system's ability to define breaths.

Unlike past years during which ventilation was gathered in collection bags or mixing chambers, today ventilation is commonly obtained "online"; various types of flow meters are used, including mass transducers, Fleisch pneumotachometers, hot wire devices, or small propellers and turbines. These rapidly responding systems permit the measurement of gas exchange data on a breath-by-breath basis. With these systems, the patient's responses are available immediately, and with the help of a computer, rapid computations can be made and displayed continuously during the test. Pneumotachometers are the most common types of flow meters today. They measure changes in pressure caused by airflow through a tube or a series of wire screens. The relationship between flow and a drop in pressure is stated by Bernoulli's Law (flow is proportional to the square root of the pressure difference), and ventilation is determined.

A recent advance has been the development of small, lightweight, disposable pneumotachometers, which measure the volume of flow at the mouth (Figure 3). These clever devices obviate the need for headgear, the valve apparatus, and collection tubes, which can often be cumbersome. As relatively low-cost disposable devices, these systems also reduce the risk of contamination. Flow is determined as a difference in

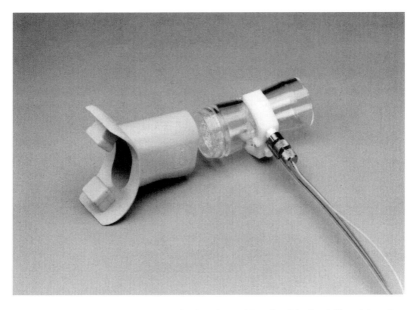

Figure 3: Disposable pneumotach developed by the Medical Graphics Corporation. Ventilatory volume is measured as a difference in pressure between the front and back of a strut positioned in the center.

pressure between the front and back of a strut or a series of screens positioned in the center of the pneumotachometer.

Gas Analyzers

The development of rapidly-responding computer-assisted gas analyzers is relatively recent. Early gas analysis systems consisted mainly of Haldane and Scholander methods, which were so cumbersome as to make them impractical in the exercise laboratory. The two types of oxygen analyzers that are commonly used today are the paramagnetic and electrochemical oxygen analyzers. These oxygen analyzers actually measure partial pressures; the gas is expressed as a percentage by taking the ratio of the partial pressure of oxygen to the barometric pressure.

Electrochemical analyzers are most commonly used by the currently available automated systems. These analyzers frequently use a zirconium oxide cell that is heated to extreme temperatures. Differences in the partial pressure of oxygen on either side of the cell's semipermeable membrane (ie, room air versus the air inside the sensor) generate a magnetic field current caused by changes in the concentration of oxygen.

Carbon dioxide is generally measured with an infrared analyzer. This is based on the concept that carbon dioxide absorbs energy from a specific portion of the infrared spectrum. Infrared light passes through a cell containing a given amount of carbon dioxide, and the volume of light transmitted is compared to a known constant value. The difference is proportional to the partial pressure of carbon dioxide in the sample. Infrared carbon dioxide analyzers have been well-validated, have very fast response times, and are used in virtually all of the commercially available metabolic systems.

Correction of Gas Volumes to Standard Conditions

Generally, metabolic systems measure ventilatory volume under conditions of *atmospheric temperature* and *pressure, saturated* with water vapor (ATPS). That is, the system receives air from the patient that is saturated with water vapor under variable (ambient) conditions of temperature and pressure. An important distinction that must be made is that between a gas volume designated ATPS, and those designated body temperature and pressure saturated (BTPS), or standard temperature and pressure, dry (STPD). $\dot{V}O_2$ and $\dot{V}CO_2$ measurements must be expressed under STPD conditions to make them proportional to gas exchanged in moles (an expression which incorporates both the absolute and molecular weight of a gas). "Standard" conditions are defined as those with a temperature of 0°C, a pressure of 760 mm Hg, and a completely dry gas. As a general rule, gas exchange variables pertaining to volumes within the lung are expressed as BTPS, while those involving the exchange of gas between the lung and the bloodstream are expressed STPD. Therefore, VE is usually expressed in BTPS, whereas $\dot{V}O_2$ and $\dot{V}CO_2$ are usually expressed in STPD.

These differences are critical, since water vapor can greatly influence the data. The concentration of water molecules in a gas sample also varies with both the temperature and the barometric pressure. Thus, it is important that the system take into account each of these variables, and that the data be expressed under the appropriate conditions. One expression of ventilatory volume can be converted to another through some simple equations. Ventilation expressed as BTPS can be converted to ATPS by the following:

$$VE \text{ (BTPS)} = VE \text{ (ATPS)} \times \frac{Pb - Pa \text{ (H}_2\text{0)}}{Pb - 47 \text{ mm Hg}} \times \frac{310}{273 + Ta}$$

Where Pb is the barometric pressure, Ta is ambient temperature, and Pa (H_2O) is the water vapor pressure.

When the system uses VI rather than VE to measure volume,

VI is an atmospheric condition (ATPS), and this conversion applies similarly.

Ventilation expressed as STPD can be converted to ATPS by the following:

$$\text{VE (STPD)} = \text{VE (ATPS)} \times \frac{Pb - Pa\ (H_2O)}{760\ mm\ Hg} \times \frac{273}{273 + Ta}$$

Conversion factors to change volumes measured under ATPS conditions to BTPS and STPD conditions at given temperature and water vapor pressures are available in tabular form.

Data Validation and Quality Control

Gas exchange analysis is an imperfect science—considerable errors can occur if specific procedures are not followed to minimize them. To ensure that the data obtained are valid, the technician must possess some basic skills in gas exchange analysis, maintain quality control, and have the wherewithal to identify errors and the reasons underlying them. It is important to be able to identify errors in the calibration prior to the test, as well as errors which may occur during the test and while interpreting the results. The reliability and accuracy of an analyzer is only as good as the calibration techniques used. Moreover, the calibration procedure is meaningless if the calibration gas is unreliable. Studies have documented inconsistencies in gas exchange data among laboratories in both Britain and Canada.[7,8] These studies suggest that variations between laboratories as high as 25% can occur, which are more than likely attributable to a lack of attention paid to quality control.

Gas analyzers and flow meters are prone to drift, which can occur from day to day and even from test to test. It is therefore essential that the system be calibrated immediately prior to each test performed. Because ambient conditions can affect the concentration of oxygen in the inspired air, it is necessary to have a thermometer, a barometer, and a hygrometer in the laboratory. A fan is useful when the laboratory is small or when flow is measured with a pneumotach or turbine system at the mouth. This ensures an appropriate fraction of inspired oxygen. A record of the calibration results should accompany each test; valid interpretation of test results is possible only in the presence of appropriate calibration values. Modern gas-exchange systems, which are commercially available have convenient calibration procedures controlled by a microprocessor. The calibration procedure should include documentation of the ambient environment and the accuracy of airflow and of both the oxygen and carbon dioxide analyzers (Table 1).

Table 1

Information that Calibration Report Should Contain

Ambient Environment
- Temperature
- Barometric pressure
- Relative humidity
- O_2 concentration (%)
- CO_2 concentration (%)

Equipment Specifications
- O_2 concentration in calibration tank
- CO_2 concentration in calibration tank
- Valve dead space
- Syringe size for volume calibration

System Performance
- Volume:
  Flow meter measured volume
  Calibration factor
  Deviation (% error)
- O_2 analyzer
  % O_2 measured from calibration gas
  Deviation (% error)
  System response time or "phase delay"
  Ambient O_2 during calibration test or response test
- CO_2 analyzer:
  % CO_2 measured from calibration gas
  Deviation (% error)
  System response time or "phase delay"
  Ambient O_2 during calibration test or response test

System Validation

In addition to pretest calibration procedures, other methods can be used to validate the system on a routine basis. Gas exchange variables are highly reproducible within a given subject. One commonly used validation method is outlined by Jones,[17] in which laboratory staff members are tested at submaximal steady-state workloads on a periodic basis. It is recommended that several staff members participate in this process, each using a somewhat different steady-state workload, and that these procedures be performed on a monthly basis. Oxygen uptake, ventilation, and CO_2 production should be reproducible and the data should approximate the predicted oxygen cost of a given steady-state workload (Table 2).

A clever calibration device that has recently become available is a gas exchange validator developed by Huszczuk and coworkers,[9] and distributed by the Medical Graphics Corporation (St. Paul, MN). This

Table 2

Limits of Variation in Values Obtained by Repeated Study of the Same Subject at a Given Power Output in a Steady State ($\pm$ 1 SD)

Variable	Limit ($\pm$)
Oxygen intake	5.1%
Carbon dioxide output	6.2
Ventilation	5.0
Heart rate	4.7
Mixed venous PCO_2	2.7
Cardiac output	8.9

From Jones NL. *Clinical Exercise Testing*. Philadelphia: W.B. Saunders; 1988.

system simulates a wide range of respiratory gas exchange rates for on-line calibration of metabolic systems. It uses a pump, which intakes a mixture of room air and a known volume of calibration gas. It then expels a gas mixture at a concentration and volume that resemble those of normal human respiration. The mixture of "inspired" air and flow rate can be set to simulate any given metabolic rate. Routine use of such a system would greatly facilitate the validation process and increase confidence in gas exchange responses considerably. While its use is somewhat limited at the moment, it seems imminent that this, or devices similar to it, will become the norm for validation and calibration of metabolic systems.

Other Sources of Error

Aside from the flow meter or gas analyzers, other common sources of error include leaking of the valves, mouthpiece, or face mask, or a blockage in the sample line due to a kink or collection of dust. Many of these sources of error can be identified while collecting resting data from the patient prior to the test. A resting period of 1 to 5 minutes not only identifies most errors before starting, but also provides the opportunity to ascertain that the test begins with the patient in a relaxed, basal state. Inappropriate gas exchange responses may also be observed when the treadmill or cycle ergometer are not calibrated properly.

Problems, Pitfalls, and Gray Areas

Several areas in gas exchange analysis have generated a significant amount of disagreement, and are therefore applied inconsistently among laboratories. These areas include gas exchange data sampling, the ventilatory or anaerobic threshold, plateau in oxygen uptake, normal reference values for exercise capacity, and the application of algorithms. Each will now be discussed briefly.

Gas Exchange Data Sampling

Not long ago, gas exchange analysis was an awkward process, which required the user to fill and empty ventilation bags at precise intervals. Sampling was limited to each minute, and the process was subject to a great deal of error. The recent availability of rapidly responding gas analyzers has provided the user with choices as to how to sample the data online. This technology has certainly facilitated precision and convenience, but it has led to confusion regarding data sampling. For example, differences in sampling (ie, breath by breath, 30 seconds, 60 seconds, or "running" breath averaging) has a profound effect on both the precision and variability of oxygen uptake. Figure 4 illustrates the standard deviations of various oxygen uptake samples during steady state exercise in 10 subjects.[10] Not surprisingly, the variability in oxygen uptake is considerably greater as the sampling interval shortens (ie, 4.5 mL/kg/min for breath-by-breath versus 0.8 mL/kg/min for 60-second samples). Thus, a given value for oxygen uptake carries an inherent variability, and this variability depends on the sampling interval. Shorter sampling intervals increase resolution, making it possible to assess precise periods for certain applications, but also increase the variability.

Data derived from small sampling intervals should be interpreted with caution, and one should resist the tendency to use breath-by-breath data simply because the technology is available. Breath-by-breath sampling can be invaluable for certain research applications such as when measuring oxygen kinetics or when end-tidal pressures are needed, but it is inappropriate for general clinical applications. Breath averaging would appear to represent a reasonable balance between precision (when high precision is needed) and variability. For most clinical uses, the variability associated with samples <30 seconds is unacceptably high. It is useful to configure the system to report the test results using 30-second samples printed every 10 seconds. This smoothes the data, yet permits adequate resolution for choosing test endpoints, the ventilatory threshold, and other relevant analysis points. Regardless of the sample chosen, investigators should report the sampling interval used, and the intervals should be consistent throughout a given trial when studying an intervention.

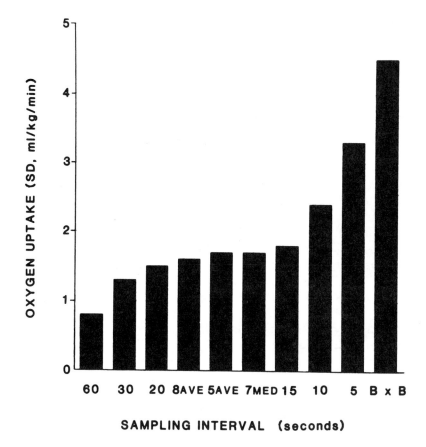

Figure 4: Variability in oxygen uptake expressed as the standard deviation for different sampling intervals during steady state exercise. 8 AVE and 5 AVE are "moving" breath averages, 7 MED is the median of seven breaths, and B x B is breath by breath.

Ventilatory Threshold

Few areas of the exercise sciences have generated as much debate as the ventilatory or "anaerobic" threshold, and a great deal of confusion exists in terms of how to apply this point clinically. A physiological link between exercise capacity, lactate accumulation in the blood, and respiratory gas exchange was made by researchers in the United States and Europe in the early part of this century.[11,12] A sudden rise in the blood lactate level during exercise has long been associated with muscle anaerobiosis and has therefore been termed the "anaerobic threshold."[13] Historically, the anaerobic threshold has been defined as the highest oxygen uptake during exercise, above which a sustained lactic acidosis occurs. When this level of exercise is reached, excess H^+ ions of lactate must be buffered to maintain physiological pH. Because bicarbonate buffering of lactate yields an additional source of CO_2 in the blood, ventilation is further simulated. This point of nonlinear increase in ventilation has been used to detect the anaerobic threshold noninvasively and is often called the gas exchange anaerobic threshold (ATge), or the ventilatory threshold (VT). Much confusion exists concerning the mechanism underlying this point and how it might be determined and applied clinically.[14–16]

Changes in oxygen uptake at the VT have been used during pharmacological and other investigations to imply that a change in oxygen supply to the working muscle has occurred. The anaerobic threshold has recently come under scrutiny, however, on both theoretical[14,15] and pragmatic[17–19] grounds. For example, Connett et al[20] studied dog gracilis muscle, which is a pure red fiber containing only type I and type IIA fibers, and observed lactate accumulation in those fibers under fully aerobic, mild (10% $\dot{V}O_{2max}$) conditions. These investigators also observed that lactate accumulation occurred, even though no anoxic areas were present in the muscle. This suggests that lactate production and muscle hypoxia are unrelated. Additionally, the advent of isotopic tracer technology has raised strong questions about the cause-and-effect relationship between oxygen availability to the muscle and the anaerobic threshold. Many studies now suggest that lactate production occurs at all times, even in resting conditions.[14,20] Further, the turnover rate of lactate (the ratio appearance and disappearance) is linearly related to oxygen uptake during exercise.[15,21,22] This relationship is possible because recent studies have shown that lactate is "shuttled" from fibers where it is produced (presumably fast-twitch muscle) to those where it is used as an energy source (such as the heart and slow-twitch fibers). The "lactate shuttle" hypothesis has engendered the concept that production, transport, and use of lactate represents an important source of energy from carbohydrates during exercise.[14,15]

Recent arguments have also been raised as to whether lactate in fact increases in a pattern that is mathematically "continuous" during exercise, rather than as a threshold.[23,26] The cumulative effect of these studies has led many to conclude that the "anaerobic" threshold is not related to muscle anaerobiosis but instead reflects simply an imbalance between lactate appearance and disappearance.[14,15] When using gas exchange techniques, the term "ventilatory threshold" has been suggested as preferable to "anaerobic," as it does not imply the onset of anaerobiosis. Lactate production and appearance in the blood during exercise appear to be related to several factors, including the rate of glycolytic flux, the isozyme form of lactate dehydrogenase (which catalyzes the conversion of pyruvate to lactate), as well as the availability of oxygen.[27] The precise mechanism underlying the VT will continue to be argued. Irrespective of whether the VT is directly related to anaerobiosis, lactate does accumulate in the blood during exercise and ventilation must respond to maintain physiological pH; a breakpoint in ventilation appears to occur reproducibly,[1] and this point is related to various measures of cardiopulmonary performance in normals[28–30] and patients with heart disease.[16,31–35]

From the many studies in this area, the following might be concluded: (1) regardless of the mechanism, ventilatory changes are correlated with lactate accumulation in the blood; (2) an alteration in the VT reflects a change in the balance between lactate production and removal; (3) references to muscle anaerobiosis should be avoided; (4) lactate accumulation in the blood, and thus the VT, is associated with: a) metabolic acidosis; b) hyperventilation; c) slowed oxygen uptake kinetics; d) accelerated glucose turnover; e) muscle fatigue; and f) a reduced capacity to perform work. Therefore, a change in the lactate response to exercise that can be attributed to an intervention may add important information concerning the intervention. In this context, the VT during exercise testing remains an interesting and applicable index for use during exercise studies. However, the commonly used application of a given boundary (such as 40% or 50% $\dot{V}O_{2max}$) separating cardiovascular from pulmonary disorders requires further study.

An additional concern has been the method of choosing the VT. Our laboratory,[19] along with others,[17,18,36] has observed that the VT can vary markedly depending on the presence or absence of disease, the method of determination, the evaluator, and the exercise protocol. Although several methods of determination have been proposed, Caiozzo et al[37] report that the use of the ventilatory equivalents for oxygen uptake ($VE/\dot{V}O_2$) and carbon dioxide ($VE/\dot{V}CO_2$) most closely reflect a lactate inflection point. Many laboratories have therefore defined the VT as the beginning of a systematic increase in $VE/\dot{V}O_2$ without a concomitant increase in $VE/\dot{V}CO_2$. However, methods which rely on minute ventilation (such as the $VE/\dot{V}O_2$ method) may not be reliable under certain conditions (ie, obesity, airflow obstruction, chemoreceptor insensitivity), in which ventilation may lag behind metabolic events. Beaver et al[38] therefore regresses $\dot{V}CO_2$ versus $\dot{V}O_2$ (the V-slope), since carbon dioxide production more directly addresses lactate accumulation and is less influenced by noise or oscillatory changes in ventilation often noted in certain patients. These investigators report that the detection of the ATge was less difficult with the V-slope method.

In regard to interobserver agreement, we have successfully used a method outlined by Sullivan et al[1] and modified by Shimuzu[19] in which two or more experienced, blinded (to patient name and test purpose such as whether the test represents a drug or placebo phase) observers independently choose the VT for each exercise test. When a discrepancy exists, an additional observer is also blinded and chooses the VT independently. The VT is determined as the minute sample in which two of the three observers agree. The VT is not included in the analysis for that particular patient when all observers differ. Using 1-minute samples of the ventilatory equivalents, we have found that out of three independent observers, two observers agree on 100% of exercise tests, and all three observers agree on 71% of the tests.[1] In a more recent study, 7% of tests were excluded because all three observers disagreed.[19] This technique avoids interobserver bias and provides a means by which the VT can be determined objectively. Methods, problems, and advantages and disadvantages of various methods of choosing the VT or lactate inflection points have been the subjects of numerous reports.[14–19,23–26,36–41]

Plateau in Oxygen Uptake

A question frequently raised is "what exactly defines 'maximal' oxygen uptake?" From early studies using interrupted protocols, a test was only considered maximal when there was no further increase in oxygen uptake, despite further increases in workload (ie, a plateau). Conversely, oxygen uptake has been considered "peak" when the subject reaches a point of fatigue while no plateau in oxygen uptake was observed. Unfortunately, the many problems associated with the determination and criteria for the plateau in oxygen uptake make these definitions more semantic than physiological.

In 1955, Taylor and associates[42] established the criteria of plateauing as a failure to increase oxygen uptake more than 150 mL/kg/min with an increase in workload. This original research was performed using interrupted, progressive treadmill protocols. With interrupted protocols, stages of exercise could be separated by rest periods ranging from minutes to days. Taylor and coworkers found that 75% of their subjects fulfilled these criteria. Using continuous treadmill protocols, Pollock et al[43] found that 69%, 69%, 59%, and 80% of subjects plateaued when tested using the Balke, Bruce, Ellestad, and Astrand protocols, respectively. Froelicher et al[44] found that only 33%, 17%, and 7% of healthy air crewmen met these criteria during testing with the Taylor, Balke, and Bruce protocols, respectively, although there were no significant differences between the protocols in maximal heart rate, maximal blood pressure, or maximal oxygen uptake. Taylor et al later reported that plateauing generally did not occur when they used continuous treadmill protocols. More recent studies using a variety of empirical criteria, report the occurrence of a plateau ranging from 7% to 90% of tests.

The plateau concept is long-ingrained in exercise physiology. Intuitively, the body's respiratory and metabolic systems must reach some finite limit, beyond which oxygen uptake can no longer increase, and some subjects who are highly motivated may exhibit a plateau. However, the plateau has been subjected to many interpretations and criteria. The newer, automated gas exchange systems that allow breath-by-breath or any specified sampling interval have raised new questions in regard to interpreting a plateau.[45,46] Although the definitions of plateauing vary considerably, all focus on the concept that oxygen uptake at some point will fail to continue to rise as work increases. Recent studies have pointed out that the occurrence of a plateau depends as much on the criteria applied, the sampling interval, and the methodology as on the subject's health, fitness, and motivation. The demonstration of a plateau is unlikely to be crucial to clinical decision-making. These studies suggest that the plateau concept has limitations for general application during standard exercise testing.[45–48]

Normal Reference Values for Exercise Capacity

Normal reference values are fundamental to cardiopulmonary exercise testing. However, the decision as to what constitutes "normal" can be complex. Although numerous studies have been performed in this area, few of the population samples have been large enough to firmly establish "normal standards," and all are specific to the population from which they were drawn. In addition, the data are rather sparse in terms of normal standards for variables other than maximal oxygen uptake, such as maximal ventilation, Vd/Vt, breathing frequency, and end-tidal pressures.

Many clever attempts have been made to improve the prediction of what represents a normal exercise capacity, by including height, weight, body composition, activity status, exercise mode, and such clinical and demographic factors as smoking history, heart disease, and medications. It is important to note that a "normal" value is only a number that has been inferred from some population. A predicted normal value usually refers to age and gender, but many other factors affect one's exercise capacity. These include some that are not so easily measured, such as genetics and the type and extent of disease, in addition to those mentioned above. In the classic studies of Bruce and associates,[49] gender and age were the most important factors influencing exercise capacity (compared with activity status, weight, height, or smoking). This has since been confirmed by our laboratory[50] and others.[51]

However, the relation between age and exercise capacity is highly imprecise. Figure 5 illustrates the relationship between maximal oxygen uptake and age for a group of male subjects, with different levels of current physical activity considered. The wide scatter and relatively poor correlation coefficient underscores the common observation that a great deal of variability exists when exercise capacity is predicted from age, even when considering other factors such as gender or activity level. Choosing the most appropriate reference equation is therefore critical. Table 3 outlines the various factors to consider when applying reference formulae.

Application of Algorithms

Gas exchange algorithms are used by some laboratories as "decision tree" aids in classifying patients by disease. These approaches can provide useful guidelines for using cardiopulmonary responses to help stratify patients when the cause of exercise intolerance is unclear, but they have several pitfalls. First, mathematically, studies have shown that the highest proportion of data that is useful for classifying patients is contained in the pretest information, which algorithms do not con-

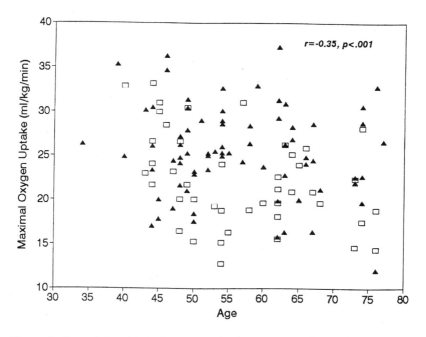

Figure 5: The relationship between maximal oxygen uptake and age among active ▲ and sedentary ☐ healthy males referred for exercise testing.

Table 3

Factors to Consider in Reference Population When Applying Formulae for Exercise Capacity

- Population tested:
  - Age
  - Gender
  - Anthropometric characteristics
  - Health and fitness
  - Heart disease
  - Pulmonary disease
- Exercise mode and protocol
- Reason tested:
  - Clinical referral
  - Screening apparently healthy volunteers
- Exercise capacity estimated versus measured directly
- Units of measurement
- Variability of measurements (usually 10% to 30%)

sider. Second, the use of cutpoints for normal/abnormal at each branching point is required. This raises some ambiguity, since substantial overlap exists in terms of what represents "normal." Third, many patients referred to exercise testing for clinical reasons, although having one major complaint, have a mixture of disease processes that underlie their exercise intolerance. Finally, a given response to any diagnostic test only changes the balance between pre- and post-test probability of disease, and it is unknown what these probabilities are in this context. When applying the cardiopulmonary exercise test to classify disease, stratify risk, or quantify exercise capacity, it is most useful to consider all clinical and exercise test information, including symptoms, hemodynamic and electrocardiographic responses, pretest characteristics, and gas exchange information.

Summary

The value of ventilatory gas exchange techniques during exercise testing, including improved precision and greater yield of clinically useful information, is underscored by a growing body of literature. However, proper application of cardiopulmonary exercise testing requires an understanding of the theory and instrumentation involved. The incorporation of microprocessors into the exercise laboratory has greatly facilitated precision and convenience, but advances in technology have raised new questions with regard to application. The greater automation often leaves the user "blinded" as to appropriate validation procedures and how the data are expressed.

Several caveats were discussed in this chapter in regard to interpretation and application of gas exchange responses to exercise. Strict attention to quality control is essential to ensure that valid data are obtained. Common sources of error in cardiopulmonary exercise testing include an oxygen or carbon dioxide analyzer that is out of calibration, a flow meter with an unstable baseline, a treadmill or cycle ergometer that is out of calibration, or a leaking valve, face mask, or mouthpiece. Performing system analyzer calibration procedures outlined by the manufacturer before each test can alleviate most problems encountered using a metabolic system.

Despite significant disagreement over the mechanisms leading to lactate accumulation in the blood and how to define its ventilatory consequences, the ventilatory threshold maintains widespread application as a marker for cardiopulmonary performance both in the sport sciences and in clinical medicine. Although a plateau in oxygen uptake has historically been considered a marker for maximal effort, it is often not observed clinically, and its use has been limited by the many ways it has been defined and the differences in how gas exchange data are sampled. Reference standards for maximal oxygen uptake and other gas exchange variables depend greatly on the populations from which they are derived. All normal standards are population-specific, and considerable variability exists (10% to 30%) even among homogenous populations. The consideration of other variables in addition to age and gender, such as activity status, exercise mode, medications, and other clinical and demographic factors has been shown to reduce this variation only modestly and only in some studies. Although algorithms are popular for stratifying patients based on gas-exchange responses, they have several shortcomings, including substantial overlap in terms of what constitutes abnormal at several branching points. Test accuracy is highest and the information yield is greatest when all clinical and exercise test information is considered, including symptoms, hemodynamic and electrocardiographic responses, pretest characteristics, and ventilatory gas exchange information.

References

1. Sullivan M, Genter F, Savvides M, et al. The reproducibility of hemodynamic, electrocardiographic, and gas exchange data during treadmill exercise in patients with stable angina pectoris. Chest 1984;86:375–382.
2. Elborn JS, Stanford CF, Nichols DP. Reproducibility of cardiopulmonary parameters during exercise in patients with chronic cardiac failure: The need for a preliminary test. Eur Heart J 1990;11:75–81.

3. Myers J, Froelicher VF. Optimizing the exercise test for pharmacological investigations in angina pectoris. In Ardissino D, Savonitto S, Opie LH eds: *Drug Evaluation in Angina Pectoris.* Norwell, MA: Klewer Academic Publishers.

4. Myers J, Salleh A, Buchanan N, et al. Ventilatory mechanisms of exercise intolerance in chronic heart failure. *Am Heart J* 1992;124:710–719.

5. Clark AL, Chua TP, Coats AJ. Anatomical dead space, ventilatory pattern, and exercise capacity in chronic heart failure. *Br Heart J* 1995;74:377–380.

6. Sullivan MJ, Higginbotham MB, Cobb FR. Increased exercise ventilation in patients with chronic heart failure: Intact ventilatory control despite hemodynamic and pulmonary abnormalities. *Circulation* 1988;77:552–559.

7. Contes JE, Woolmer RE. A comparison between 27 laboratories of the results of analysis of an expired gas sample. *J Physiol* 1962;163:36P–37P.

8. Jones NL, Kane JW. Quality control of exercise test measurements. *Med Sci Sports* 1979;11:368–372.

9. Huszczuk A, Whipp BJ, Wasserman K. A respiratory gas exchange simulator for routine calibration in metabolic studies. *Eur Resp J* 1990;3:465–468.

10. Myers J, Walsh D, Sullivan M, Froelicher VF. Effect of sampling on variability and plateau in oxygen uptake. *J Appl Physiol* 1990;68:404–410.

11. Hill AV, Lupton H. Muscular exercise, lactic acid, and the supply and utilization of oxygen. *Q J Med* 1923;16:135–171.

12. Hollman W. Historical remarks on the development of the aerobic-anaerobic threshold up to 1966. *Int J Sports Med* 1985;6:109–116.

13. Wasserman K, McElroy MB. Detecting the threshold of anaerobic metabolism in cardiac patients during exercise. *Am J Cardiol* 1964;14:844–852.

14. Brooks GA. Lactate production under fully aerobic conditions: The lactate shuttle during rest and exercise. *Fed Proc* 1986;45:2924–2929.

15. Brooks GA. Anaerobic threshold: Review of the concept and directions for future research. *Med Sci Sports Exerc* 1985;17:22–31.

16. Davis JA. Anaerobic threshold: Review of the concept and directions for future research. *Med Sci Sports Exerc* 1985;17:6–18.

17. Gladden LB, Yates JW, Stremel RW, Stamford BA. Gas exchange and lactate anaerobic thresholds: Inter- and intra-evaluator agreement. *J Appl Physiol* 1985;58:2082–2089.

18. Yeh MP, Gardner RM, Adams TD, et al. Anaerobic threshold: Problems of determination and validation. *J Applied Physiol* 1983;55:1178–1186.

19. Shimizu M, Myers J, Buchanan N, et al. The ventilatory threshold: Method, protocol, and evaluator agreement. *Am Heart J* 1991;122:509–516.

20. Connett RJ, Gayeski TEJ, Honig GR. Lactate accumulation in fully aerobic working dog gracilis muscle. *Am J Physiol* 1984;246:H120–H128.

21. Issekutz B, Shaw WAS, Issekutz AC. Lactate metabolism in resting and exercising dogs. *J Appl Physiol* 1976;40:312–319.

22. Stanley WC, Neese RA, Wisneski JA, Gertz EW. Lactate kinetics during submaximal exercise in humans: Studies with isotoipc tracers. *J Cardiopulmonary Rehabil* 1988;9:331–340.

23. Beaver WL, Wasserman K, Whipp BJ. Improving detection of lactate threshold during exercise using a log-log transformation. *J Appl Physiol* 1985;59:1936–1940.

24. Hughson RL, Weisiger KH, Swanson GD. Blood lactate concentration increases as a continuous function during progressive exercise. *J Appl Physiol* 1987;62:1975–1981.

25. Myers J, Walsh D, Buchanan N, et al. Increase in blood lactate during ramp

exercise: Comparison of continuous versus threshold models. *Med Sci Sports Exer* 1994;26:1413–1419.

26. Dennis SC, Noakes TD, Bosch AN. Ventilation and blood lactate increase exponentially during incremental exercise. *J Sports Sci* 1992;10:437–449.

27. Graham T. Mechanisms of blood lactate increase during exercise. *Physiologist* 1984;27:299.

28. Davis JA, Frank MH, Whipp BJ, Wasserman K. Anaerobic threshold alterations caused by endurance training in middle-aged men. *J Appl Physiol* 1979;46:1039–1046.

29. Ready AE, Quinney HA, Alterations in anaerobic threshold as the result of endurance training and detraining. *Med Sci Sports Exerc* 1982;14:292–296.

30. Tanaka K, Matsura Y, Matsuzaka A, Hirakoba K. A longitudinal assessment of anaerobic threshold and distance running performance. *Med Sci Sports Exerc* 1986;16:278–282.

31. Sullivan MJ, Cobb FR. The anaerobic threshold in chronic heart failure: Relationship to blood lactate, ventilatory basis, reproducibility, and response to exercise training. *Circulation* 1990;81:1147–1158.

32. Matsumura N, Nishijima H, Kojima S, et al. Determination of anaerobic threshold for assessment of functional state in patients with chronic heart failure. *Circulation* 1983;68:360–367.

33. Weber KT, Kinasewitz GT, Janicki JS, Fishman AP. Oxygen utilization and ventilation during exercise in patients with chronic cardiac failure. *Circulation* 1982;65:1213–1223.

34. Myers J, Atwood JE, Sullivan M, et al. Perceived exertion and gas exchange after calcium and beta-blockade in atrial fibrillation. *J Appl Physiol* 1987;63:97–104.

35. Sullivan M, Atwood AE, Myers J, et al. Increased exercise capacity after digoxin administration in patients with heart failure. *J Am Coll Cardiol* 1989;13:1138–1143.

36. Dickstein K, Barvik S, Aarsland T, et al. A comparison of methodologies in detection of the anaerobic threshold. *Circulation* 1990;81(suppl II):II-38–II-46.

37. Caiozzo VJ, Davis JA, Ellis JF, et al. A comparison of gas exchange indices used to detect the anaerobic threshold. *J Appl Physiol* 1982;53:1184–1189.

38. Beaver WL, Wasserman K, Whipp BJ. A new method for detecting anaerobic threshold by gas exchange. *J Appl Physiol* 1986;60:2020–2027.

39. Hughes EF, Turner SC, Brooks GA. Effects of glycogen depletion and pedaling speed on "anaerobic threshold." *J Appl Physiol* 1982;52:1598–1607.

40. Whipp BJ, Ward SA, Wasserman K. Respiratory markers of the anaerobic threshold. *Adv Cardiol* 1986;35:47–64.

41. Gaesser GA, Poole DC. Lactate and ventilatory threshold: Disparity in time course of adaptations to training. *J Appl Physiol* 1986;61:999–1004.

42. Taylor HL, Buskirk E, Heuschel A. Maximal oxygen intake as an objective measurement of cardiorespiratory performance. *J Appl Physiol* 1955;8:73–80.

43. Pollack ML, Bohannon RL, Cooper KH, et al. A comparative analysis of four protocols for maximal treadmill stress testing. *Am Heart J* 1976;92:39–46.

44. Froelicher VF, Brammel H, Davis G, et al. A comparison of the reproducibility and physiologic response to three maximal treadmill exercise protocols. *Chest* 1974;65:512–517.

45. Myers J, Walsh D, Buchanan N, Froelicher VF. Can maximal cardiopul-

monary capacity be recognized by a plateau in oxygen uptake? *Chest* 1989;96:1312–1316.

46. Myers J, Walsh D, Sullivan M, Froelicher VF. Effect of sampling on variability and plateau in oxygen uptake. *J Appl Physiol* 1990;68:404–410.
47. Katch VL, Sady SS, Freedson P. Biological variability in maximum aerobic power. *Med Sci Sports Exerc* 1982;14:21–25.
48. Noakes TD. Implication of exercise testing for prediction of athletic performance: A contemporary perspective. *Med Sci Sports Exerc* 1988;20:319–330.
49. Bruce RA, Kusumi F, Hosmer D. Maximal oxygen uptake and nomographic assessment of functional aerobic impairment in cardiovascular disease. *Am Heart J* 1973;85:546–562.
50. Myers J, Do D, Herbert W, et al. A nomogram to predict exercise capacity from a specific questionnaire and clinical data. *Am J Cardiol* 1994;73:591–596.
51. Kline GM, Porcari JP, Hintermeister R, et al. Estimation of $VO_{2\,max}$ from a one-mile track walk, gender, age, and body weight. *Med Sci Sports Exerc* 1987;19:253–259.

Chapter 14

Clinical Utility of Cardiopulmonary Exercise Testing Data in Heart Failure

Rebecca J. Quigg, MD

Introduction

Cardiopulmonary exercise stress testing has become an important clinical tool to assess severity of illness and guide therapy in patients with heart failure due to left ventricular systolic dysfunction. Important clinical information can be obtained by the measurement of inspired and expired gases and assessment of anaerobic threshold. A determination of the etiology of exercise limitation and measurement of both peak exercise workload and peak exercise oxygen consumption (peak VO_2) for objective functional classification can be made. This information may be used to guide therapy to improve functional class and survival and to identify patients with the greatest need for cardiac transplantation.

Etiologies of Exercise Limitation in Systolic Heart Failure

Patients with heart failure due to left ventricular systolic dysfunction may have cardiac, noncardiac, or a combination of both etiologies for their exercise limitation and exertional dyspnea (Table 1). Potential cardiovascular abnormalities contributing to exercise intolerance include: poor cardiac output response to exercise; rest or exercise pulmonary congestion; peripheral blood flow abnormalities; exercise chronotropic in-

From: Balady GJ, Piña IL (eds). *Exercise and Heart Failure*. Armonk, NY: Futura Publishing Company, Inc.; ©1997.

Table 1

Reasons for Exercise Limitation in Patients
with Systolic Heart Failure

Cardiovascular Causes	Noncardiac Causes
Poor cardiac output response to exercise	Skeletal muscle deconditioning
Pulmonary congestion	Chronic obstructive pulmonary disease
Decreased leg blood flow	Age and gender
Exercise chronotropic incompetence	Reduced muscle mass
Atrial fibrillation with rapid ventricular response	Poor motivation
Cardiac ischemia	

competence; atrial fibrillation with uncontrolled ventricular response; and cardiac ischemia in patients with coronary artery disease. Noncardiac etiologies that may contribute to exercise intolerance include skeletal muscle deconditioning and underlying pulmonary disease. Exercise tolerance is also related to age, gender, muscle mass, and patient motivation. The performance of an initial cardiopulmonary exercise test in a patient who presents with systolic heart failure may elucidate one or more contributing factors that limit exercise capacity. Clarifying the factors that contribute to exercise limitation may dramatically alter therapy.

The syndrome of heart failure is defined as an inability to adequately increase cardiac output to supply blood flow to exercising muscles, or in its severest form, to muscles at rest. The inability of the heart to increase forward cardiac output may also result in pulmonary congestion due to elevated pulmonary filling pressures, which may worsen during exercise. In addition, peripheral vasoconstriction, which occurs due to high sympathetic tone, may further limit blood flow to the periphery during exercise. Therapies that have been shown to improve these physiological abnormalities that contribute to heart failure symptoms such as positive inotropes and vasodilator therapy, result in an improvement in exercise tolerance.[1-10]

Exercise chronotropic incompetence may be another identifiable etiology of exercise intolerance in this patient population. Patients with systolic heart failure develop cardiac β-receptor downregulation due to elevated plasma norepinephrine levels.[11] Elevated norepinephrine levels may result in a high resting heart rate, while β-receptor downregulation leads to a blunted and delayed heart rate response during exercise.[12] Some patients develop a severe degree of chronotropic incompetence during exercise, which significantly limits their peak exercise capacity.[12]

In addition, β-adrenergic blockers[13] and amiodarone,[14] which have been increasingly used in this patient population, may exacerbate this problem. When exercise chronotropic incompetence is determined to be a major contributing factor to exercise intolerance, medications that contribute to this problem should be discontinued, if feasible, and/or placement of a rate-responsive pacemaker should be considered. Therapy aimed at improving the heart failure syndrome may result also in upregulation of β-receptors over time[15] with a resultant improvement in exercise heart rate response.

Atrial fibrillation is a common problem in patients with systolic heart failure as a result of chronic volume overload, elevation of atrial filling pressures and atrial enlargement. Although the ventricular response rate to atrial fibrillation may be well controlled at rest, ventricular rate may increase dramatically with exercise, resulting in decreased ventricular filling and exercise cardiac output. Whenever possible, chemical or electric cardioversion to normal sinus rhythm should be attempted, to improve cardiac function. If atrial fibrillation remains refractory to all therapies, alternatively, tight control of the ventricular rate during exercise should be attempted with digoxin. If the ventricular response rate continues to remain poorly controlled during exercise, calcium channel blockers with minimal negative inotropic activity may be added to digoxin for their atrial-ventricular nodal blocking effects. Repeat exercise testing should be performed to confirm rate control and reassess exercise performance.

Approximately 50% to 70% of patients with systolic heart failure have coronary artery disease as the underlying etiology of their cardiomyopathy (Table 2).[16-23] Ongoing cardiac ischemia may be identified as an important component of exercise intolerance in patients with or without previous myocardial infarction. The addition of cardiac nuclear perfusion imaging techniques during cardiopulmonary exercise testing may assist in assessing the extent and severity of ischemia. If ischemia is present and myocardial viability can be demonstrated, coronary revascularization should be considered, if possible. When revascularization is not possible, medical therapy with anti-ischemic drugs should be used with nitrates and/or calcium channel blocker therapy. Calcium channel blockers with minimal negative inotropic effect, that have been shown to be safe in systolic heart failure, such as amlodipine or felodipine, should be used.[24,25] Effective treatment of ischemia may result in a dramatic improvement in exercise capacity and peak $\dot{V}O_2$.

Patients with severe heart failure may develop significant musculoskeletal deconditioning due to frequent decompensations and hospitalizations. Often heart failure patients are inappropriately told by their physicians or family members to limit their activity, which may result in worsening-of-deconditioning. Musculoskeletal abnormalities that are

Table 2

Studies Demonstrating the Relationship Between Peak Exercise Oxygen Consumption and Survival in Patients with Heart Failure

Investigator	Number Patients n/(m/f)	NYHA Class n (%)	Heart Failure Etiology Type (%)	Oral Medical Therapy Drug (%)*	Peak VO$_2$ (mL/kg/min)	p Value Univariate Analysis	1 Year Survival (%)**	Follow-up Survival %/time
Szlachcic 1985[16]	27 (27/0)	II (22%) III (59%) IV (19%)	ISCM (70%) DCM (30%)	No Vasodilators (100%)	≤10.0 >10.0 to <18	<0.001	23% 79%	23% 2 yr 64% 2 yr
V-HeFt I 1986[17]	642 (642/0)	I–IV (N/A)	ISCM (44%) DCM (56%)	Hydralzine/Nitrates (29%) Prazosin (28%) No vasodilators (43%)	≤14.5 >14.5	<0.0001	46% 67%	56% x̄ 2.3 yr (overall)
Likoff 1987[18]	201 (150/51)	I (01%) II (23%) III (43%) IV (33%)	ISCM (60%) DCM (34%) HTN (03%)	Digoxin (92%) ACEI (60%) Antiarrhythmics (39%)	≤13.0 >13.0	<0.001	64% 90%	55% x̄ 1.5 yr 75% x̄ 1.5 yr
Mancini 1991[19]	122 (103/19)	II (13%) III (70%) IV (17%)	ISCM (46%) DCM (54%)	ACEI (96%) Vasodilators (98%)	≤14.0 listed for TX ≤14.0 not TX candidate >14.0	<0.005	70% 47% 94%	NA 32% 2 yr 84% 2 yr
van der Brock 1992[20]	90 (74/16)	II–IV NA	ISCM (80%) DCM (20%)	Diuretics (93%) Digitalis (56%) ACEI (93%) Vasodilators (33%) Antiarrythmics (14%)	≤14.0 >14.0 to <20.0	<0.05	70% 93%	2 yr 3 yr 57% 52% 93% 78%

Parameshwar 1992[21]	127 (113/14)	NA	ISCM (67%) DCM (33%)	NA	≤13.7 >13.7	<0.01	70% 80%	45% 2 yr 55% 2 yr
V-HeFt II 1991[22]	804 (804/0)	I (6%) II (51%) III (43%) IV (<1%)	ISCM (53%) DCM (47%)	Enalapril (50%) Hydralazine/Nitrates (50%)	≤14.5 >14.5	<0.00005	59% 94%	65% x̄ 2.5 yr (overall)
Roul 1994[23]	75 (1)	II (43%) III (57%)	ISCM (55%) DCM (45%)	ACEI (96%) Nitrates (97%) β-blocker (20%) Amiodarone (15%)	≤14.0 >14.0	<0.01	61% 100%	NA

n = number of patients; m = males; f = females; NYHA = New York Heart Association; NA = not available; peak VO_2 = peak exercise oxygen consumption; V-HeFT = Veterans' heart failure trial; ISCM = ischemic cardiomyopathy; DCM = dilated cardiomyopathy; HTN = hypertensive cardiomyopathy; ACEI = angiotensin converting enzyme inhibitor; x̄ = mean; yr = year.

*All patients on digoxin unless otherwise noted; **data may be extrapolated from survival curves.

similar to those seen in other forms of deconditioning have been well-documented in patients with heart failure.[26] Cardiac rehabilitation in this patient population has been shown to reverse musculoskeletal deconditioning, improve peak $\dot{V}O_2$, and to be both safe and efficacious.[26-30]

Patients with systolic heart failure due to coronary artery disease or hypertension may also have a long-standing history of tobacco use, which may be associated with chronic obstructive pulmonary disease. If obstructive pulmonary disease is present, it may be an important component to exercise limitation. Pulmonary function tests should be performed prior to exercise testing and an assessment of oxygen saturation during exercise with a pulse oximeter or indwelling arterial catheter should be made. If significant obstructive lung disease is present, treatment should be initiated with inhaled bronchodilator therapy, especially prior to exercise. Exercise testing should be repeated following therapy to assess improvement.

Therapies For Systolic Heart Failure Known to Improve Exercise Capacity

Once the etiologies contributing to exercise intolerance have been identified, therapy can be initiated in an attempt to improve these parameters. Several effective oral medical therapies for the treatment of systolic heart failure, that result in both improved symptoms and survival, have been developed over the past 2 decades. Standard oral therapy for symptomatic heart failure now includes a triple-drug regimen including digoxin, diuretics, and vasodilator therapy with angiotensin converting enzyme (ACE) inhibitors and/or hydralazine/nitrate combination.[17,31] Treatment with digoxin in addition to diuretics has been shown to improve both exercise time[1,2] and peak $\dot{V}O_2$ an average of 2.6 mL/kg/min.[1] Conversely, when digoxin is withdrawn, exercise time has been demonstrated to worsen.[32,33] Treatment with the ACE enzyme inhibitor, captopril, has been shown in several studies to result in an increase in exercise time[4] and peak $\dot{V}O_2$.[5] Exercise capacity has also been shown to improve with enalapril,[6-9] with the maximum effect on exercise capacity occurring within 3 months after the initiation of therapy.[9] The newer, long-acting ACE inhibitors quinapril,[34] fosinipril[35] and benazapril[36] have also been shown to result in improved exercise duration. Lisinopril has been demonstrated to improve both exercise duration and peak $\dot{V}O_2$.[37,38] The second Veterans' Heart Failure (V-HeFT) trial demonstrated that although enalapril had a more marked effect in improving survival,[31] the combination of hydralazine and nitrates was superior to enalapril in improving peak exercise $\dot{V}O_2$.[10]

If musculoskeletal deconditioning is a major contributing factor to exercise limitation, a formal cardiac rehabilitation program should be prescribed. Sullivan,[39] Coats[28] and Belardinelli[26] have demonstrated average improvements in peak $\dot{V}O_2$ values of 3.6, 2.4 and 2.8 mL/kg/min respectively, with cardiac rehabilitation in patients with systolic heart failure. This improvement may be a result of improved peripheral skeletal muscle oxidative capacity.[29]

Although cardiac transplantation has been shown to improve survival in patients with end-stage cardiomyopathy, the effect on maximal exercise capacity has been disappointing, with peak $\dot{V}O_2$ values remaining at an average of 20.0 mL/kg/min following transplantation.[40] Potential explanations for poor peak $\dot{V}O_2$ after cardiac transplantation include parasympathetic and sympathetic denervation causing chronotropic incompetence during exercise, ischemic injury, diastolic dysfunction, and transplant coronary artery disease. Implantable assist devices have been increasingly studied as a bridge to transplantation and hold promise as a potential alternative to transplantation. Peak $\dot{V}O_2$ has been measured in patients on assist devices and has been demonstrated to improve an average of 5 mL/kg/min.[41,42] These topics will be discussed in more detail in Section V of this book.

Association of Exercise Capacity And Survival in Left Ventricular Systolic Dysfunction

Patients with systolic heart failure due to left ventricular dysfunction have a 1-year survival of between 55% and 65% and a 5-year survival of 25% to 35%.[43] Survival in this patient population has been shown to correlate with New York Heart Association (NYHA) functional class,[44] left ventricular ejection fraction,[18,22,44,45] right ventricular ejection fraction,[46] severity of ventricular arrhythmias,[44,47] degree of neurohormonal aberration,[44,48] and objective exercise capacity as measured by peak $\dot{V}O_2$ (Table 2).[16-23]

It has long been known that peak workload achieved during exercise testing, as measured by metabolic equivalents, correlates with survival in patients with known coronary disease with or without left ventricular dysfunction.[49] As cardiopulmonary exercise testing has been increasingly used in the heart failure population, it has been repeatedly demonstrated that peak exercise $\dot{V}O_2$ is an important predictor of survival in patients with systolic dysfunction (Table 2). However, there is a poor association between peak $\dot{V}O_2$ and NYHA functional class[50] and left ventricular ejection fraction,[51] making peak $\dot{V}O_2$ an important independent prognostic indicator.

In 1985 Szlachcic, et al[16] were the first to demonstrate a poor survival in 27 patients with NYHA Class II to Class IV heart failure on digoxin and diuretics, who had peak $\dot{V}_2$ values ≤ 10.0 mL/kg/min. In 1986, the V-HeFT I trial[31] demonstrated that 642 male patients with Class I to Class IV heart failure randomized to treatment with hydralazine/nitrate combination had an improvement in survival when compared to those patients receiving prazosin or placebo in addition to digoxin and diuretics. However, patients in all study arms who had peak $\dot{V}O_2$ values ≤ 14.5 mL/kg/min had a worse survival.[17] In 1987, Likoff et al[18] reported data further supporting these results in a series of 201 patients with NYHA Class I to Class IV heart failure. A striking difference in survival was demonstrated in patients who had peak $\dot{V}O_2$ values ≤ 13.0 mL/kg/min. In this study, exercise peak $\dot{V}O_2$ was a better predictor of survival then the subjective assessment of NYHA functional class.

This series of studies began to elucidate the important association of objectively-measured exercise capacity and peak $\dot{V}O_2$ with survival in patients with systolic heart failure. In the late 1980s most major academic heart failure and cardiac transplantation centers began to use peak exercise $\dot{V}O_2$ as an important predictor of survival to guide therapy and determine the need for cardiac transplantation. In 1991, Mancini, et al[19] reported a landmark study where they triaged ambulatory patients for cardiac transplantation listing based solely on a peak $\dot{V}O_2$ value ≤ 14.0 mL/kg/min alone. She observed that patients who had peak $\dot{V}O_2$ values >14.0 mL/kg/min initially or after optimization of therapy had a 1- and 2-year survival with medical therapy of 94% and 84%, respectively, which was similar to patients who had undergone transplantation at their center.

In 1992 van den Brock, et al[20] again confirmed that a peak $\dot{V}O_2$ ≤ 14.0 mL/kg/min was associated with a poor survival in 90 patients with NYHA Class II to Class IV heart failure. Of note was that patients with peak $\dot{V}O_2$ values >14.0 mL/kg/min died more often from sudden cardiac death than from the progression of heart failure. Also in 1992, Parameshwar et al[21] reported 127 patients with chronic heart failure, who had a worsened survival if their peak $\dot{V}O_2$ was <13.7 mL/kg/min. Report of the second V-HeFT trial (V-HeFT II)[52] in 1993 again confirmed the clear association of peak $\dot{V}O_2$ values and survival in 804 patients treated with either enalapril or hydralazine/nitrate combination in addition to digoxin and diuretics. When the results of the two V-HeFT trials were combined in a substudy analysis,[22] the data showed a consistent association of peak $\dot{V}O_2$ and survival irrespective of treatment arm. This appeared to be a continuous relationship, with survival worsening as peak $\dot{V}O_2$ decreased progressively below 14.5 mL/kg/min. Data from the combined V-HeFT trials also demonstrated that patients with peak $\dot{V}O_2$ values >14.5 mL/kg/min tended to die more often from sudden cardiac death than from progressive pump failure,[53] confirming the previous report by van den Brock.[20]

Recently, Wilson, et al[54,55] show that poor peak exercise $\dot{V}O_2$ values do not correlate with resting or exercise hemodynamics. In a follow-up preliminary study, Wilson, et al[56] demonstrate that patients with a peak exercise $\dot{V}O_2$ <15 mL/kg/min, but who have a preserved cardiac output response to exercise have a 1-year survival of 92%. They suggest that patients with low peak $\dot{V}O_2$ values despite a preserved cardiac output response to exercise are limited by deconditioning and may improve with cardiac rehabilitation.[57] Alternatively, patients with peak $\dot{V}O_2$ values <15 mL/kg/min and a reduced cardiac output response to exercise have a poor survival with medical therapy alone and should be considered for cardiac transplantation. This interesting observation, if confirmed by other investigators, may dramatically alter treatment options in this subset of patients with low peak $\dot{V}O_2$ values.

It has been well established that predicted exercise $\dot{V}O_2$ is dependent on patient age and gender, with peak $\dot{V}O_2$ values expected to be lower in females and older individuals. Several investigators have attempted to determine whether risk-stratifying patients by their percentage of predicted peak $\dot{V}O_2$ adds additional prognostic benefit in patients with severe heart failure. In 1995, DiSalvo et al[46] demonstrated that peak $\dot{V}O_2$ values <30% of predicted were associated with a poor survival and were a better predictor of outcome than was absolute peak $\dot{V}O_2$. Also in 1995 Aaronson, et al[58] reported that patients with peak $\dot{V}O_2$ values below 50% of predicted had a worse survival. However they concluded that there was little additive prognostic value in assessing peak $\dot{V}O_2$ as a percentage of predicted when compared to absolute values. In 1996 Stelken et al[59] also confirmed that patients with less than 50% of age- and sex-predicted $\dot{V}O_2$ values had a worse survival. However, their data suggest that percentage of predicted peak $\dot{V}O_2$ was a more important predictor of cardiac death or need for urgent transplantation than absolute $\dot{V}O_2$ measurements. Based on these studies, it appears that a peak $\dot{V}O_2$ of less than 50% of predicted is an indicator of poor prognosis.

Exercise Oxygen Consumption as a Criteria for Cardiac Transplantation

In the late 1980s and early 1990s, a large body of data was accumulated independently by several groups of investigators who reported that peak exercise $\dot{V}O_2$ values <14 to <15 mL/kg/min were associated with a poor survival with continued medical therapy (Table 2). In the early 1990s, peak $\dot{V}O_2$ values as a criteria for cardiac transplantation listing began to be incorporated into recipient criteria guidelines (Table 3).[60,61] However, as pointed out by Piña[62] in a recent editorial entitled,

---

Table 3

Published Guidelines for Peak Exercise Oxygen Consumption
as a Criteria for Cardiac Transplantation

Bethesda Conference on Cardiac Transplantation
Task Force 3: Recipient Guidelines/Prioritization 1993[61]

Category for transplant	Peak VO_2 value (mL/kg/min)
Accepted indications	<10
Probable indications	<14
Inadequate indications	>15

Consensus Conference on Candidate Selection
for Heart Transplantation—1993[62]

Category for transplant	Peak VO_2 value (mL/kg/min)
Definite indications	<10
Probable indications	≤14
Inadequate indications	>14

"Optimal Candidates for Heart Transplantation: Is 14 The Magic Number?", peak exercise $VO_2 \leq 14.0$ mL/kg/min should not be used as the sole indication for cardiac transplantation. When peak VO_2 was evaluated as a prognostic indicator in the combined analysis of the two V-HeFT trials,[22] survival progressively worsened as peak VO_2 decreased, indicating that an absolute cutoff value to indicate poor survival is not appropriate. A recent preliminary study by Aaronson et al[63] also demonstrates in a large number of patients referred for cardiac transplant that the relationship between peak VO_2 and survival is a continuous relationship without an abrupt cutoff at 14.0 mL/kg/min.

Most cardiac transplant centers evaluate a variety of prognostic indicators to assess patients with advanced heart failure and determine an individual patient's expected prognosis. The expected prognosis with continued medical therapy for heart failure is usually compared to projected outcome with cardiac transplantation[64] to assess the potential survival benefit with transplantation. In addition to the well-described prognostic indicators in the general heart failure population, several transplant centers have identified additional factors that may have equal or greater prognostic value in individual patients. These include persistent elevation of pulmonary filling pressures despite intensive therapy,[19,65] severity of reduction of left ventricular ejection fraction below 20%,[18,19,22] degree of left ventricular dilatation,[66] and untreatable ischemia.[67] Therefore, the decision whether to list a patient for transplantation should be individualized based on the overall clinical parameters including peak VO_2, along with an understanding of the expected waiting time for a donor organ due to the patient's blood type and body size.

Improvement of Peak Exercise Oxygen Consumption with Therapy for Heart Failure

Although an individual patient may have a low peak $\dot{V}O_2$ on initial exercise testing, this value may improve as therapy for heart failure is optimized. A variety of noninvasive or invasive techniques may be used by a heart failure/cardiac transplant specialist to optimize medical therapy. Since measurement of pulmonary pressures and pulmonary vascular resistance are required for evaluation for cardiac transplantation, maximization of therapy may be most expediently performed by use of a right heart catheter to measure baseline hemodynamics and to monitor the response to intravenous and/or oral therapy for heart failure. Positive inotropic drugs such as dobutamine or the phosphodiesterase inhibitor, milrinone, which also has peripheral and central vasodilator activity, may be used to improve resting hemodynamics. "Tailored Therapy" with the use of intravenous vasodilator therapy alone with nitroprusside is also described extensively by Stevenson, et al[65] to facilitate the optimization of oral vasodilator therapy. Initiating or increasing the dose of ACE inhibitors or hydralazine by this or other techniques may result in short- and long-term improvements in exercise capacity and peak $\dot{V}O_2$.[5]

Use of Serial Exercise Testing to Guide Therapy in Patients with Systolic Heart Failure

Cardiopulmonary exercise testing should be repeated approximately 3 months after adjustments in heart failure therapy have been made, to assess improvement in exercise duration and peak $\dot{V}O_2$.[9] In a preliminary study,[68] we have demonstrated that peak $\dot{V}O_2$ improves in a subset of patients referred for transplantation, which prevented the need to be listed or allowed them to be removed from the transplant list. Mancini et al[19] observe that 6% of patients listed for transplant improved their peak $\dot{V}O_2$ values to above 14 mL/kg/min with optimization of medical therapy. Stevenson, et al[69] demonstrate that as many as 29% of ambulatory transplant candidates could be removed from the transplant list due to improvement in peak $\dot{V}O_2$ after optimization of therapy.

As additional therapies for heart failure that may have a beneficial effect on survival and/or exercise capacity are developed, they may be added to standard triple-drug therapy for heart failure. New drugs which have shown promise in the treatment of systolic heart failure include the β-blockers metoprolol,[13] carvedilol[70] and bucindolol,[71] and in patients with nonischemic cardiomyopathy, amlodipine[24] and amiodarone.[14] Although β-blockers have been shown to increase left ventricular ejection fraction, there is little data on the effect of these drugs on exercise $\dot{V}O_2$.

Conclusions

In conclusion, cardiopulmonary exercise testing with measurement of peak exercise $\dot{V}O_2$ provides crucial information in the assessment of patients with systolic heart failure. Determination of the contributing factors to exercise intolerance and measurement of objective functional class will assist in the management of these patients and guide decisions regarding medical and surgical therapy for systolic heart failure.

References

1. Sullivan M, Atwood JE, Myers J, et al. Increased exercise capacity after digoxin administration in patients with heart failure. *J Am Coll Cardiol* 1989;13:1138–1143.
2. Fleg JL, Rothfeld B, Gottlieb SH, et al. Effect of maintenance digoxin therapy on aerobic performance and exercise left ventricular function in mild to moderate heart failure due to coronary artery disease: A randomized, placebo-controlled, crossover trial. *J Am Coll Cardiol* 1991;17:743–751.
3. The Captopril Multicenter Research Group. Comparative effects of therapy with captopril and digoxin in patients with mild to moderate heart failure. *JAMA* 1988;259:539–544.
4. Creager MA, Faxon DP, Halperin JL, et al. Determinants of clinical response and survival in patients with congestive heart failure treated with captopril. *Am Heart J* 1982;104:1147–1154.
5. Mancini DM, Davis L, Wexler JP, et al. Dependence of enhanced maximal exercise performance on increased peak skeletal muscle perfusion during long-term captopril therapy in heart failure. *J Am Coll Cardiol* 1987;10:845–850.
6. Sharpe DN, Murphy J, Coxon R, et al. Enalapril in patients with chronic heart failure: A placebo-controlled, randomized, double-blind study. *Circulation* 1984;70:271–278.
7. Cleland JCF, Dargie HJ, Ball SG, et al. Effects of enalapril in heart failure: A double blind study of effects on exercise performance, renal function, hormones, and metabolic state. *Br Heart J* 1985;54:305–312.
8. Athanassiadis DI, Bay G, Balestrini A, et al. Long-term effects of enalapril in patients with congestive heart failure: A multicenter, placebo-controlled trial. *HF* 1987;102–107.
9. Davies RF, Beanlands D, Nadeau C, et al. Enalapril versus digoxin in patients with congestive heart failure: A multicenter study. *J Am Coll Cardiol* 1991;18:1602–1609.
10. Ziesche S, Cobb FR, Cohn JN, et al. Hydralazine and isosorbide dinitrate combination improves exercise tolerance in heart failure. *Circulation* 1993;87:VI-56–VI-64.
11. Denniss AR, Marsh JD, Quigg RJ, et al. B-Adrenergic receptor number and

adenylate cyclase function in denervated transplanted and cardiomyopathic human hearts. *Circulation* 1989;79:1028–1034.

12. Colucci WS, Ribeiro JP, Rocco MB, et al. Impaired chronotropic response to exercise in patients with congestive heart failure. Role of postsynaptic β-adrenergic desensitization. *Circulation* 1989;80:314–323.

13. Waagstein F, Bristow MR, Swedberg K, et al. Beneficial effects of metoprolol in idiopathic dilated cardiomyopathy. *Lancet* 1993;342:1441–1446.

14. Singh SN, Fletcher RD, Fisher SG, et al. Amiodarone in patients with congestive heart failure and asymptomatic ventricular arrhythmia. *N Engl J Med* 1995;333:77–82.

15. Heilbrunn SM, Shah P, Bristow MR, et al. Increased B-receptor density and improved hemodynamic response to catecholamine stimulation during long-term metoprolol therapy in heart failure from dilated cardiomyopathy. *Circulation* 1989;79:483–490.

16. Szlachcic J, Massie BM, Kramer BL, et al. Correlates and prognostic implication of exercise capacity in chronic congestive heart failure. *Am J Cardiol* 1985;55:1037–1042.

17. Cohn JN, Archibald DG, Ziesche S, et al. Effect of vasodilator therapy on mortality in chronic congestive heart failure. *N Engl J Med* 1986;314:1547.

18. Likoff MJ, Chandler SL, Kay HR. Clinical determinants of mortality in chronic congestive heart failure secondary to idiopathic dilated or to ischemic cardiomyopathy. *Am J Cardiol* 1987;59:634–638.

19. Mancini DM, Eisen H, Kussmaul W, et al. Value of peak exercise oxygen consumption for optimal timing of cardiac transplantation in ambulatory patients with heart failure. *Circulation* 1991;83:778–786.

20. van den Brock SAJ, Van Veldhuisen DJ, De Graeff PA, et al. Mode of death in patients with congestive heart failure: Comparison between possible candidates for heart transplantation and patients with less advanced disease. *J Heart Lung Transplant* 1993;12:367–371.

21. Parameshwar J, Keegan J, Sparrow J, et al. Predictors of prognosis in severe chronic heart failure. *Am Heart J* 1992;123:421–426.

22. Cohn JN, Johnson GR, Shabetai R, et al. Ejection fraction, peak exercise oxygen consumption, cardiothoracic ratio, ventricular arrhythmias, and plasma norepinephrine as determinants of prognosis in heart failure. *Circulation* 1993;87[suppl VI]:VI-5–VI-16.

23. Roul G, Moulichon ME, Bareiss P, et al. Exercise peak VO_2 determination in chronic heart failure: Is it still of value? *Eur Heart J* 1994;15:495–502.

24. O'Connor CM, Belkin RN, Carson PE, et al. Effect of amlodipine on mode of death in severe chronic heart failure: The PRAISE trial. *Circulation* 1995; 92, No.8.

25. Cohn JN, Ziesche SM, Loss LE, et al. Effect of Felodipine on short-term exercise and neurohormone and long-term mortality in heart failure: Results of V-HeFT VIII. *Circulation* 1995;92,No.8:I-143

26. Hambrecht R, Neibauer J, Fiehn E, et al. Physical training in patients with stable chronic heart failure: Effects on cardiorespiratory fitness and ultrastructural abnormalities of leg muscles. *J Am Coll Cardiol* 1995;25:1239–1249.

27. Sullivan MJ, Higginbotham MB, Cobb FR. Exercise training in patients with chronic heart failure delays ventilatory anaerobic threshold and improves submaximal exercise performance. *Circulation* 1989;79:324–329.

28. Coats AJS, Adamopoulos S, Radaelli A, et al. Controlled trial of physical training in chronic heart failure: Exercise performance, hemodynamics, ventilation, and autonomic function. *Circulation* 1992;85:2119–2131.

29. Adamopoulos S, Coats AJS, Brunotte F, et al. Physical training improves skeletal muscle metabolism in patients with chronic heart failure. *J Am Coll Cardiol* 1993;21:1101–1106.
30. Belardinelli R, Georgiou D, Scocco V, et al. Low intensity exercise training in patients with chronic heart failure. *J Am Coll Cardiol* 1995;26: 975–982.
31. Cohn JN, Johnson G, Ziesche S, et al. A comparison of enalapril with hydralazine-isosorbide dinitrate in the treatment of chronic congestive heart failure. *N Engl J Med* 1991;325:303–310.
32. Uretsky BF, Young JB, Eden Shahidi F, et al. Randomized study assessing the effect of digoxin withdrawal in patients with mild to moderate chronic congestive heart failure: Results of the PROVED trial. *J Am Coll Cardiol* 1993;22:955–962.
33. Packer M, Gheorghiade M, Young JB, et al. Withdrawal of digoxin from patients with chronic heart failure treated with angiotensin-converting-enzyme inhibitors. *N Engl J Med* 1993;329:1–7.
34. Riegger GAJ. The effects of ACE inhibitors on exercise capacity in the treatment of congestive heart failure. *J Cardiovasc Pharmacol* 1990;15:S41–S46.
35. Brown EJ, Chew PH, MacLean A, et al. Effects of fosinopril on exercise tolerance and clinical deterioration in patients with chronic congestive heart failure not taking digitalis. *Am J Cardiol* 1995;75:596–600.
36. Colfer HT, Ribner HS, Gradman A, et al. Effects of once-daily benazepril therapy on exercise tolerance and manifestations of chronic congestive heart failure. *Am J Cardiol* 1992;70:354–358.
37. Zannad F, van den Brock SAJ, Bory M, et al. Comparison of treatment with lisinopril versus enalapril for congestive heart failure. *Am J Cardiol* 1992; 70:78C–83C.
38. Jessup M, Spielman S, Hare T, et al. Lisinopril in the treatment of chronic cardiac failure: A controlled trial. *HF* 1987;114–127.
39. Sullivan MJ, Higginbotham MB, Cobb FR. Exercise training in patients with severe left ventricular dysfunction: Hemodynamic and metabolic effects. *Circulation* 1988;78:506–515.
40. Quigg RJ, Rocco MB, Gauthier DF, et al. Mechanisms of the attenuated peak heart rate response to exercise after orthotopic cardiac transplantation. *J Am Coll Cardiol* 1989;14:338–344.
41. Kormos RL, Murali S, Dew MA, et al. Chronic mechanical circulatory support: Rehabilitation, low morbidity, and superior survival. *Ann Thorac Surg* 1994;57:51–58.
42. Jaski BE, Branch KR, Adamson R, et al. Exercise hemodynamics during long-term implantation of a left ventricular assist device in patients awaiting heart transplantation. *J Am Coll Cardiol* 1993;22:1574–1580.
43. Ho KKL, Anderson KM, Kannel WB, et al. Survival after the onset of congestive heart failure in Framingham Heart Study subjects. *Circulation* 1993; 88:107–115.
44. Keogh AM, Baron DW, Hickie JB. Prognostic guidelines in patients with idiopathic or ischemic dilated cardiomyopathy assessed for cardiac transplantation. *Am J Cardiol* 1990;65:903–908.
45. Cohn JN, Archibald DG, Francis GS, et al. Veterans Administration Cooperative Study on Vasodilator therapy of heart failure: Influence of prerandomization variables on the reduction of mortality by treatment with hydralazine and isosorbide dinitrate. *Circulation* 1987;75:IV-49–IV-54.
46. DiSalvo TG, Mathier M, Semigran MJ, et al. Preserved right ventricular

ejection fraction predicts exercise capacity and survival in advanced heart failure. *J Am Coll Cardiol* 1995;25:1143–1153.

47. Reese DB, Silverman ME, Gold MR, et al. Prognostic importance of the length of ventricular tachycardia in patients with nonischemic congestive heart failure. *Am Heart J* 1995;130:489–493.

48. Francis GS, Cohn JN, Johnson G, et al. Plasma norepinephrine, plasma renin activity, and congestive heart failure: Relations to survival and the effects of therapy in V-HeFT II. *Circulation* 1993;87(suppl VI):VI40–VI48.

49. Morris CK, Ueshima K, Kawaguchi T, et al. The prognostic value of exercise capacity: A review of the literature. *Am Heart J* 1991;122:1423–1431.

50. van den Brock SAJ, Van Veldhuisen DJ, De Graeff PA, et al. Comparison between New York Heart Association classification and peak oxygen consumption in the assessment of functional status and prognosis in patients with mild to moderate chronic congestive heart failure secondary to either ischemic or idiopathic dilated cardiomyopathy. *Am J Cardiol* 1992;70: 359–363.

51. Smith RF, Johnson G, Ziesche S, et al. Functional capacity in heart failure: Comparison of methods for assessment and their relation to other indexes of heart failure. *Circulation* 1993;87(suppl VI):VI88–VI93.

52. Johnson G, Carson P, Francis GS, et al. Influence of prerandomization (baseline) variables on mortality and on the reduction of mortality by enalapril: Veterans Affairs Cooperative Study on Vasodilator Therapy of Heart Failure (V-HeFT II). *Circulation* 1993;87(suppl VI):VI32–VI39.

53. Goldman S, Johnson G, Cohn JN, et al. Mechanism of death in heart failure: The Vasodilator-Heart Failure Trials. *Circulation* 1993;87(suppl VI):VI24–VI31.

54. Wilson JR, Rayos G, Yeoh T, et al. Dissociation between peak exercise oxygen consumption and hemodynamic dysfunction in potential heart transplant candidates. *J Am Coll Cardiol* 1995;26:429–435.

55. Wilson JR, Rayos G, Yeoh TK, et al. Dissociation between exertional symptoms and circulatory function in patients with heart failure. *Circulation* 1995;92:47–53.

56. Wilson JR, Rayos G, Yeoh TK, et al. Identification of patients with heart failure and severe exercise intolerance who are at low risk for mortality. *Circulation* 1995;92, No 8:I-541.

57. Wilson JR, Groves J, Rayos GH, et al. Cardiac output response to exercise identifies patients with heart failure who will benefit from cardiac rehabilitation. *Circulation* 1995;92, No. 8:I-402–I-403.

58. Aaronson KD, Mancini DM. Is percentage of predicted maximal exercise oxygen consumption a better predictor of survival than peak exercise oxygen consumption for patients with severe heart failure? *J Heart Lung Transplant* 1995;14:981–989.

59. Stelken AM, Younis LT, Jennison SH, et al. Prognostic value of cardiopulmonary exercise testing using percent achieved of predicted peak oxygen uptake for patients with ischemic and dilated cardiomyopathy. *J Am Coll Cardiol* 1996;27:345–352.

60. Mudge GH, Goldstein S, Addonizio LJ, et al. Task Force 3: Recipient guidelines/prioritization. *J Am Coll Cardiol* 1993;22:1–64.

61. Miller LW, Kubo SH, Young JB, et al. Medical management of heart and lung failure and candidate selection report of the consensus conference on candidate selection for heart transplantation-1993. *J Heart Lung Transplant* 1995;14:562–571.

62. Piña IL. Optimal candidates for heart transplantation: Is 14 the magic number? *J Am Coll Cardiol* 1995;26:436–437.
63. Aaronson KD, Chen T, Mancini DM. Demonstration of the continuous nature of peak VO_2 for predicting survival in ambulatory patients evaluated for transplant. *J Heart Lung Transplant* 1996;15:S66.
64. Hosenpud JD. The registry of the International Society for Heart and Lung Transplantation: Eleventh official report. *J Heart Lung Transplant* 1994;14: 561–570.
65. Stevenson LW, Dracup KA, Tillisch JH. Efficacy of medical therapy tailored for severe congestive heart failure in patients transferred for urgent cardiac transplantation. *Am J Cardiol* 1989;63:461–464.
66. Wong M, Johnson G, Shabetai R, et al. Echocardiographic variables as prognostic indicators and therapeutic monitors in chronic congestive heart failure: Veterans Affairs Cooperative Studies V-HeFT I and II. *Circulation* 1993;87(suppl VI):VI65–VI70.
67. DiCarli MF, Davidson M, Little R, et al. Value of Metabolic imaging with positron emission tomography for evaluating prognosis in patients with coronary artery disease and left ventricular dysfunction. *Am J Cardiol* 1994;73, No.8:527–533.
68. Quigg R, Roberge P, Sica D, et al. Monitored titration of medical therapy improves prognostic indicators in patients referred for cardiac transplantation. *J Am Coll Cardiol* 1994;356A:941–944.
69. Stevenson LW, Steimle AE, Fonarow G, et al. Improvement in exercise capacity of candidates awaiting heart transplantation. *J Am Coll Cardiol* 1995; 25:163–170.
70. Krum H, Sackner-Bernstein JD, Goldsmith RL, et al. Double-blind, placebo-controlled study of the long-term efficacy of carvedilol in patients with severe chronic heart failure. *Circulation* 1995;92:1499–1506.
71. Anderson JL, Gilbert EM, O'Connell JB, et al. Long-term (2 year) beneficial effects of β-adrenergic blockade with bucindolol in patients with idiopathic dilated cardiomyopathy. *J Am Coll Cardiol* 1991;17:1373–1381.

Physiological Responses to Exercise Training

Chapter 15

Cardiovascular Adaptations to Exercise Training in Left Ventricular Dysfunction

Martin J. Sullivan, MD and Brian D. Duscha, MS

Introduction

The past 20 years have seen the incidence of myocardial infarction decline along with improvements in interventional and medical treatment strategies for coronary artery disease (CAD). It is somewhat of a paradox that this has been accompanied by an increase in the prevalence of chronic heart failure (CHF) due to left ventricular dysfunction (LVD). Although this is due in part to an aging population, it is possible that the improved CAD survival rates, along with better pharmacological management of systemic hypertension, has been responsible for the increased incidence of CHF due to LVD. Chronic heart failure due to LVD is a clinical syndrome characterized by increased intracardiac filling pressures and a decreased cardiac output. In addition to these central hemodynamic abnormalities, it is now clear that peripheral vascular and skeletal muscle factors contribute to the decreased aerobic capacity (peak $\dot{V}O_2$) that is accompanied by the symptoms of dyspnea and fatigue in patients with CHF. Traditionally, CHF patients with LVD have been treated with rest and medical therapy, including loop diuretics, digoxin, and vasodilators. Recent studies now show that

Research from this review was supported by Grant HL-17670 from the National Heart, Lung, and Blood Institute, Bethesda, Maryland, by General Medical Research Funds from the Veterans Administration Medical Center, Durham, North Carolina, and by Grant RR-30 Division of Research Resources, General Clinic Research Centers Program, NIH. Dr. Sullivan was supported by an Established Investigators award from the American Heart Association.

From: Balady GJ, Piña IL (eds). *Exercise and Heart Failure*. Armonk, NY: Futura Publishing Company, Inc.; ©1997.

exercise training may be an important adjunctive form of therapy by improving peak $\dot{V}O_2$ and symptoms of exercise intolerance. Exercise training both effects central hemodynamics, and leads to peripheral adaptations. This chapter will focus on the central hemodynamic abnormalities in CHF due to left ventricular systolic dysfunction, and will outline alterations in cardiac function with exercise training.

Training Effects on Normal Left Ventricular Function

Long-term aerobic conditioning is associated with a number of important physiological adaptations in normal persons that may be beneficial to patients with LVD.[1-3] Exercise training leads to an improvement in both submaximal and maximal exercise performance in normal persons. The improvements seen in exercise tolerance are acquired through both central hemodynamic changes (including increased stroke volume) and peripheral adaptations (including skeletal muscle and vascular alterations). During submaximal exercise after training, cardiac output is unchanged although stroke volume is increased. At peak exercise in normal persons some,[2,3] but not all,[1] studies report an increase in cardiac output mediated through an increase in stroke volume without a change in peak heart rate. This increase in stroke volume is caused by an increase in LV end-diastolic volume (EDV), as indices of LV systolic performance such as ejection fraction do not increase in most training studies. Although strenuous exercise in elite athletes may lead to hypertrophy,[4] it appears that many of the effects on LV volumes after training reflect the use of the Frank-Starling mechanism. It is likely that most of the increase in stroke volume after training is caused by an increased plasma volume and total body hemoglobin coupled with a more efficient "muscle pump," to facilitate venous return during intense exercise. This concept is supported by the rapid decrease in stroke volume that is noted after deconditioning in normal persons, that is not accompanied by changes in cardiac wall thickness.[5]

Exercise Intolerance and Central Hemodynamics at Rest, Submaximal, and Maximal Exercise in Patients with Left Ventricular Dysfunction

Peak oxygen consumption (peak $\dot{V}O_2$) by expired gas analysis is widely used and remains a good indicator of exercise tolerance and functional capacity in CHF due to LVD. Although a number of limitations exist with this technique, this form of testing yields a quantitative and reproducible measurement that may be used for evaluation of disease severity, exercise prescription, or interventional decision making. Assessment of functional capacity also provides important prognostic information on survival outcomes, as illustrated in Figure 1.[6] In addition, peak $\dot{V}O_2$ correlates closely with maximum cardiac output and serves as an indirect measure of stroke volume.[7-9]

One of the most common causes of disability in CHF is exercise intolerance due to dyspnea or fatigue. It is now well established that the degree of LVD, as measured by ejection fraction or pulmonary capillary wedge pressure,[10] is an important measurement for assessing severity of myocardial damage and prognosis, but does not correlate with exercise tolerance, peak $\dot{V}O_2$, or symptom status in CHF patients.[7-9,11-14] Although these findings indicate that systolic function is not a primary determinant of peak $\dot{V}O_2$, they should not necessarily be interpreted to mean that cardiac function does not play a role in determining exercise capacity. It is likely that ejection fraction plays a small role in determining the variability in cardiac output in groups of patients preselected with a low left ventricular ejection fraction (LVEF). Cardiac output (Q), which is the product of heart rate (HR) and stroke volume (SV), is determined not only by LV contractility, but by several other factors, including changes in LVEDV and mitral regurgitation fraction (MRF)

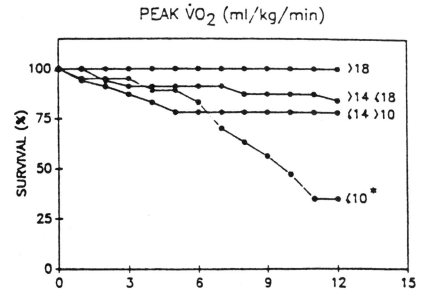

Figure 1: Survival curves of patients with CHF referred for cardiac transplantation, categorized by peak $\dot{V}O_2$. (Reprinted, with permission, from Reference 6).

as follows: $Q = HR \times SV$ or $Q = HR \times [LVEDV \times LVEF \times (1 - MRF)]$. It is clear from this equation that LVEF is only one of several determinants of cardiac output in patients with CHF. The two most powerful predictors of peak oxygen consumption ($\dot{V}O_{2\,max}$) are peak cardiac output and peak leg blood flow, as illustrated in Figure 2.[15–17] The linear relationship between peak cardiac output and peak $\dot{V}O_2$ in patients with LVD has been shown in several studies.[7–9,17,19] Massie et al[18] show high correlations between exercise cardiac index (r = 0.82; p<0.001) and $\dot{V}O_{2max}$ in patients with New York Heart Association (NYHA) Class II to Class IV CHF. This finding supports the view that exercise is dependent on the heart's ability to supply the working muscles with adequate oxygen and fuel to meet demands of increased workloads.

The close relationship of peak $\dot{V}O_2$ and peak cardiac output might be expected from the Fick equation, $Q = \dot{V}O_2 / A - \dot{V}O_2$. Our laboratory at Duke University Medical Center and others have additional evidence to support the important role of cardiac output in determining exercise tolerance. This comes from the finding that at a given submaximal workload, cardiac output is closely related to peak $\dot{V}O_2$.[20] This finding suggests that the cardiac output during submaximal exercise is an important determinant of peak exercise tolerance in patients with LVD. Although this relationship is not clearly understood, it is likely that a decrease in exercise cardiac output reduces the perfusion to the working skeletal muscles, thereby causing early anaerobic metabolism and symptoms of fatigue.

As a result of a decreased cardiac output, the arteriovenous oxy-

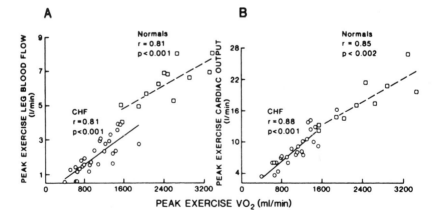

Figure 2: Plots of relations of peak exercise $\dot{V}O_2$ to single leg blood flow (panel A) and cardiac output (panel B) in patients with CHF due to systolic LVD (open circles, solid predicted regression lines) and normal subjects (open box, dashed predicted regression lines); r = correlation coefficient. (Reprinted, with permission, from Reference 15).

gen difference (A − V̇O$_2$ difference)(Figure 3D)[15] is increased at rest and during exercise in patients with CHF compared to normals. Other hemodynamic changes that occur in the periphery, which may have an important effect on symptoms include an increase in systemic vascular resistance and a decrease in blood flow to working muscles.[21] Our laboratory has recently found cardiac output to be normal at submaximal workloads in a subset of CHF patients, while leg blood flow was reduced and leg vascular resistance was elevated.[22] This finding suggests that abnormal peripheral vasoregulation can limit exercise tolerance independent of central hemodynamic abnormalities in CHF patients, and suggests that the relationship of cardiac output and leg blood flow appear to be variable in this disorder. This is supported by Wilson et al[23] who demonstrate that some patients have decreased cardiac output and normal leg blood flow.

Although the relationship between cardiac output and leg blood flow is not yet clearly understood, stroke volume appears to be highly correlated with cardiac output (r = 0.72, P<.01). Stroke volume is re-

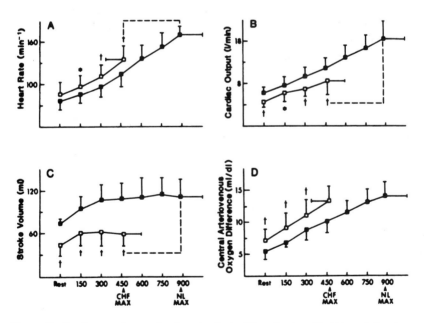

Figure 3: Resting and exercise heart rate in 30 patients with LV systolic dysfunction and 12 normal subjects, and resting and exercise cardiac output, stroke volume, and central arteriovenous oxygen difference in patients with chronic heart failure (n = 25) (open boxes) and normal subjects (n = 10) (closed boxes); * =P<0.05; †=P<0.01, patients versus normal subjects. Dashed lines indicate intergroup comparison of maximal data. (Reproduced, with permission, from Reference 15).

lated to disease severity, and therefore appears to be a primary factor determining the cardiac output response during exercise. Studies have shown[24,25] that even though stroke volume is decreased at rest and at exercise, patients with LV systolic dysfunction actually increase stroke volume from rest to peak exercise similar to normals, 42% versus 48%, without increasing ejection fraction. This is accomplished by the use of the Frank-Starling mechanism. Higginbotham et al[24] explain this accomplishment by demonstrating a three-fold increase in LV end-diastolic volume compared to normals. This increase in LVEDV augmented cardiac output despite impaired contractile reserve. These findings, coupled with the concept that exercise cardiac output is related to exercise leg blood flow, suggest that the reduced cardiac output response to exercise is an important factor limiting exercise in LVD, and that this is partly compensated for by increasing LVEDV.

In comparison to normals, CHF patients exhibit elevations in heart rate and ventilation at matched submaximal workloads, but have depressed peak values. Oxygen consumption is decreased or unchanged both at submaximal and peak exercise. Due to a decreased oxygen consumption and a number of intrinsic peripheral factors, the anaerobic threshold is decreased with a concomitant elevation in blood lactate at submaximal exercise in CHF patients. In an attempt to compensate for these detrimental effects on aerobic capacity and increased anaerobic metabolism, $A - \dot{V}O_2$ difference is enhanced during submaximal exercise. This increase in $A - \dot{V}O_2$ indicates a more efficient oxygen extraction capacity during submaximal exercise, which can be attributed to a preferential redistribution of cardiac output toward the active muscles. An increased anaerobic metabolism in the periphery results in acidosis in the exercising muscles, which contributes to the limited exercise capacity.

Central Hemodynamic Responses to Exercise Training in Patients with Left Ventricular Dysfunction

Significant advances have been made in the last 10 years in understanding exercise physiology and exercise training in CAD and CHF. Exercise training, once thought of as contraindicated for LVD patients, is now being successfully used as an important adjunctive therapy for this population. Lee et al[26] and Conn et al[27] were the first to demonstrate an improved exercise capacity, by implementing aerobic training as part of cardiac rehabilitation for patients with LVD in the late 1970s and early 1980s. These studies, however, failed to show a relationship between the improved exercise capacity and left ventricular function.

Although these studies and most other studies have failed to identify measurable improvements in central hemodynamics,[28–30] a growing number of exercise training studies now confirm that patients with LVD and CHF can improve exercise performance and reduce exertional symptoms[26–28,31–42] without eliciting adverse effects. In addition to these physiological improvements, other researchers have shown improvements in the patient's quality of life.[37]

Our laboratory has demonstrated similar benefits for CHF patients.[31,32] These studies examined the effects of exercise training 4 hours per week at 75% of peak oxygen consumption for 16 to 24 weeks on hemodynamics in CHF patients. Our results show no change in ejection fraction at rest or during exercise following the training program (Figure 4), confirming that LV function is an important criterion for diagnosing the disease, but is not necessarily related to exercise tolerance or symptom status. Stroke volume was unchanged at rest, but tended to increase during exercise, although this increase did not reach statistical significance at submaximal or peak exercise ($P = 0.12$). LV end-systolic and end-diastolic volumes were not altered by exercise training. Although ejection fraction was unchanged, patients showed improvements in peak oxygen consumption (increased by 23%), duration of exercise time, peak workload, and peak A − $\dot{V}O_2$ (Figure 5). The increases in

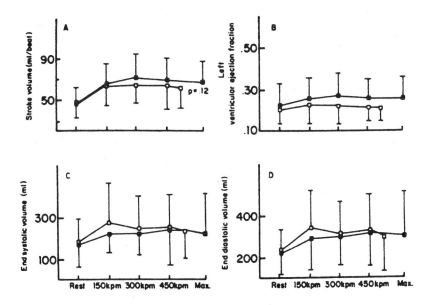

Figure 4: Plots of resting and exercise stroke volume, left ventricular ejection fraction, left ventricular end-systolic and end-diastolic volumes before (□) and after (■) training. No comparison was $P<0.05$ by Wilcoxon signed rank test. (Reproduced with permission from Reference 31).

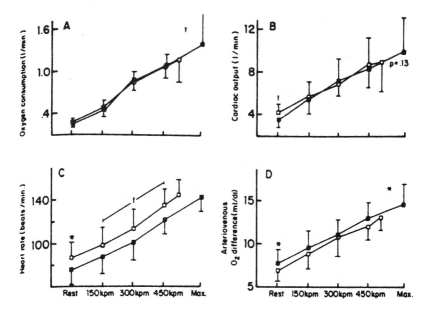

Figure 5: Plots of resting and exercise oxygen consumption, cardiac output, heart rate, and systemic arteriovenous oxygen difference in patients before (□) and after (■) training *$P<0.05$; †$P<0.01$ by Wilcoxon signed rank test. (Reproduced with permission from Reference 31).

maximal oxygen consumption and exercise time seen in CHF patients after training are comparable to those seen in normals and CAD patients without CHF.[43,44] Finally, at submaximal workloads, heart rates were reduced.

Jette et al[39] report an absence of left ventricular hypertrophy, as assessed by end-diastolic diameter following training. This randomized study examined 39 patients with anterior myocardial infarcts less than 10 weeks old. Patients were randomized into one of the following groups based on resting ejection fraction (EF): (1) Training, EF<30%; (2) Training, EF = 31% to 50%; (3) Control, EF<30%; and (4) Control EF = 31% to 50%. Pre- and postexercise tests included a right-heart catheterization, radionuclide ventriculography, echocardiography, and work capacity. The training groups participated in an intense 4-week program of in-hospital exercise. Exercise was performed in the morning (jogging, calisthenics, relaxation training, and cycle ergometry for 15 minutes at a HR of 70% to 80% of $\dot{V}O_{2max}$) and an afternoon session of walking 30 to 60 minutes. Work capacity and $\dot{V}O_{2max}$ improved significantly in patients with an EF<30%, who trained. Resting EF improved in both the trained and control group with EFs of <30%, but were not correlated with work capacity. There was no significant change in cardiac output at rest, submaximal, or peak exercise for any of the four groups. Mean maximal pulmonary wedge pressure increased significantly in the trained patients, with ejection fractions <30%. It was concluded that exercise training could improve exercise tolerance without causing additional ventricular damage or changes in function. This study also suggested that patients with more severe LVD (EF<30%) after a recent anterior myocardial infarction (MI) (10 weeks) have greater improvements in exercise tolerance when compared to both control patients with similar EFs and patients with EFs between 30% and 50%, who participated in a training program. Control patients with EFs <30% actually demonstrated a slight decrease in exercise tolerance. Jette concluded that because resting EF improved in both groups with an EF <30%, the training effect observed was probably the result of improved oxygen use and not necessarily improved cardiac function.

Other studies have found similar improvements in peak $\dot{V}O_2$ without changes in submaximal cardiac output following exercise training.[34,37,41] Hambrecht et al[30] report similar central hemodynamic findings using a thermodilution catheter interfaced with a cardiac output computer, except for an increased peak cardiac output after exercise training (Figure 6). This improvement was significantly correlated with $\dot{V}O_{2max}$. However, like normals, exercise training does not appear to improve cardiac output during submaximal exercise workloads in patients with LVD.

Training intensity also appears to be an important factor in determining exercise training-induced benefits. Previous studies in our laboratory, using higher training intensities (75% of $\dot{V}O_2$ max), have shown an increase in peak leg blood flow without a concomitant increase in leg blood flow during submaximal work, and a decrease in vascular resistance.[31] Belardinelli et al[45] recently show that an exercise regimen using a lower training intensity (40% of peak $\dot{V}O_2$) can elicit peripheral adaptations to the skeletal muscle's oxidative capacity without an increase in limb blood flow. Lactate production has been shown to be independent of leg blood flow, implying that a reduction in lactate production after exercise training is a peripheral adaptation independent of hemodynamic changes.[31] In addition, training resulted in a tendency for peak cardiac output to increase as well, but no change was detected at rest or at submaximal workloads. Belardinelli concluded that low intensity training improves exercise capacity as well as lactate threshold and peak oxygen uptake in patients with mild CHF, similar to those improvements found in studies using higher training intensities (22% to 25% peak $\dot{V}O_2$ improvements). Previous studies in our laboratory[32] and others[34] have shown that the ventilatory anaerobic threshold of CHF patients occurs at a higher $\dot{V}O_2$ after an exercise training program.

The results of at least a dozen studies now demonstrate an in-

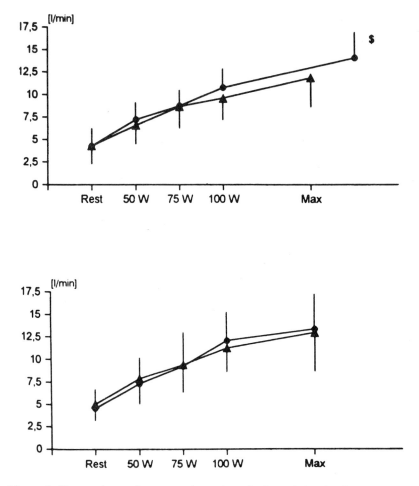

Figure 6: Change in cardiac output in patients in the training (top) and control (bottom) groups at baseline (▲) and at 6-month follow-up (●). Max = maximal exercise. $P<0.05 versus baseline. (Reproduced with permission from Reference 39.)

creased exercise tolerance, as measured by improvements of 15% to 25% in peak $\dot{V}O_2$ and exercise duration, after exercise training in LVD patients. It appears that these improvements are due primarily to peripheral factors, although improved resting ejection fraction and cardiac output is seen in some patients after training. These studies also indicate that cardiac output shows no change, or tends to increase insignificantly, at peak exercise following an exercise training program. Stroke volume appears to also improve slightly, but this change fails to reach significance during both submaximal and peak exercise after training. Other consistencies that have been found between studies include a decreased heart rate at submaximal workloads and improved peak leg blood flow. It appears that in most patients, improved exercise tolerance occurs primarily through more efficient peripheral oxygen extraction and changes in skeletal muscle.

The Effects of Exercise Training on Left Ventricular Geometry

Following myocardial infarction, approximately 8 to 10 weeks are required for early ventricular remodeling and complete scar tissue healing to occur.[46,47] It has been long held that exercise training before that time could be detrimental to the healing process by enhancing ventricular distortion and delaying improvements in resting ventricular function. Patients with decreased LV systolic dysfunction demonstrate large end-diastolic volumes and have little contractile reserve. It has been suggested that training in these patients may induce further increases in LVEDV that would increase wall tension and may be detrimental to LV function. To date, only one study, by Jugdutt et al,[48] report an unfavorable left ventricular remodeling response to exercise training 6 weeks after MI. This study had major limitations, including a very small sample size, a nonrandomized design, and an inadequate exercise stimulus. Larger randomized trials have failed to reproduce these findings. Because of limited long-term clinical trials in patients with LVD, and a lack of a clear understanding of how exercise effects LV geometry following myocardial infarction over time, increased attention has been recently given to how long-term exercise training effects LV geometry. Giannuzzi et al[49,50] have conducted two multicenter studies designed to investigate how exercise influences LV remodeling: (1) Exercise in Anterior Myocardial Infarction (EAMI Trial)[49] and; (2) Exercise and Left Ventricular Dysfunction (ELVD Trial).[50] The EAMI Trial was designed to investigate whether exercise training influenced LV remodeling after an anterior myocardial infarction. Ninety-five patients were studied 4 to 8 weeks after anterior Q wave myocardial infarction and followed up after 6 months of exercise training, with exercise testing and 2-D ECHO. Patients with LVEF <25% were excluded. The training intervention consisted of an initial 2-month supervised period of three exercise sessions per week. Each training session was composed of 30 minutes of continuous bicycle exercise at 80% of heart rate achieved during peak exercise. Following this initial 2-month period, patients were instructed to maintain the prescribed exercise regimen at home and perform a brisk daily walk of ≥30 minutes, returning once every 2 weeks for testing and new training heart rate zones. The results demonstrate an increase in work capacity for the training group. Neither the training group nor the control group demonstrated changes in global ventricular size, regional dilation, or shape distortion by 2-D ECHO. This study concluded that postinfarct patients without clinical complications may benefit from exercise training without causing further ventricular dilation. The authors hypothesized that a decrease in submaximal rate pressure product had a favorable effect on wall stress, and therefore decreased the chance of a negative remodeling response.

The ELVD Trial extended the results of the EAMI trial with a similar study design, using a 6-month exercise training program on patients who had LVD following a first Q wave myocardial infarction. Seventy-five patients with ejection fractions ≤40% were studied 3 to 5 weeks after a first Q wave MI, randomized into either an exercise or control group, and followed up 6 months later by a rest and bicycle stress 2-D ECHO. The exercise training group improved work capacity (from 4462 ± 1095 kpm to 5752 ± 1749 kpm, $P<0.01$), ejection fraction ($34 \pm 5\%$ to $38 \pm 6\%$, $P<0.01$), and showed a decrease in percent wall-motion abnormalities ($49 \pm 8\%$ to $44 \pm 10\%$, $P<0.01$); while the control group had an increase in both end-diastolic (92 ± 24 to 98 ± 26 mL/m^2, $P<0.01$) and end-systolic volumes (61 ± 19 to 67 ± 23 mL/m^2, $P<0.01$) when compared to the exercise group (EDV: 93 ± 28 to 92 ± 28 mL/m^2 and ESV: 61 ± 22 to 57 ± 23 mL/m^2). Not only does this study show no increased dilation with training, but it suggests that exercise training may reduce the unfavorable remodeling response and possibly improve global and regional function. In a similar study by Cannistra et al,[51] it is also found that exercise training does not adversely effect LV remodeling between patients with large MIs and small MIs. These results are consistent with Bellardinelli et al,[52] who recently conclude that 8 weeks of moderate intensity exercise improves myocardial viability in patients with ischemic cardiomyopathy. Based on these studies, it appears that left ventricular dilation occurs as a natural course of the postinfarct period, that exercise training does not adversely effect LV geometry in patients with significant LVD, and that exercise training is beneficial in improving work capacity. One limitation to these studies, and most training studies, is that LVD patients with ejection fractions of <25% have not been well tested or documented. Further research on this subset of patients is needed.

Summary

Although pharmacological therapy is the cornerstone of treatment in patients with left ventricular dysfunction, a growing number of studies now indicate that patients with stable LVD and CHF can safely participate in exercise training to improve exercise performance, reduce exertional symptoms, and improve quality of life. A combination of cardiac, peripheral, and central hemodynamic adaptations probably contributes to the increased functional capacity. It is unlikely that one specific central hemodynamic or peripheral change accounts for all of the increased aerobic capacity. Although stroke volume may improve in selected patients, most studies have not demonstrated an improvement in stroke volume, ejection fraction, or intracardiac filling pressures after training. Important recent studies demonstrate that exercise training does not adversely effect LV remodeling, even after Q wave infarction. Future studies should address the effects exercise training has on morbidity and mortality in patients with LVD. Efforts should be made to determine optimal training intensities that are associated with the least amount of risk. In addition, long-term follow-up data on those patients with LVD who continue to exercise should be gathered.

References

1. Seals DR, Hagberg JM, Hurley BF, et al. Endurance training in older men and women I: Cardiovascular responses to exercise. *J Appl Physiol* 1984;57: 1024–1029.
2. Blomqvist CG Saltin B. Cardiovascular adaptations to physical training. *Annu Rev Physiol* 1983;45:169–189.
3. Scheuer J, Tipton CM. Cardiovascular adaptations to physical training. *Annu Rev Physiol* 1977;39:221–251.
4. Fagard R, Aubert A, Lysens R, et al. Noninvasive assessments of seasonal variations in cardiac structure and function in cyclists. *Circulation* 1983;67 (4):896–901.
5. Sullivan MJ, Binkley PF, Unverferth DV, et al. Prevention of bedrest-induced physical deconditioning by daily dobutamine infusions: Implications for drug-induced physical deconditioning. *J Clin Invest* 1985;76: 1632–1642.
6. Mancini DM, Eisen H, Kussmal W, et al. Value of peak oxygen consumption for optimal timing of cardiac transplantation in ambulatory patients with heart failure. *Circulation* 1991;83:778–786.
7. Weber KT, Kinasewitz GT, Janicki JS, et al. Oxygen utilization and ventilation during exercise in patients with chronic cardiac failure. *Circulation* 1982;65(6):1213–1223.
8. Higginbotham MB, Morris KG, Conn EH, et al. Determinants of variable exercise performance among patients with severe left ventricular dysfunction. *Am J Cardiol* 1983;51:52–60.
9. Franciosa JA, Park M, Levine TB. Lack of correlation between exercise capacity and indexes of resting left ventricular performance in heart failure. *Am J Cardiol* 1981;47:33–39.
10. Sullivan MJ, Higginbotham MB, Cobb FR. Increased exercise ventilation in patients with chronic heart failure: Intact ventilatory control despite hemodynamic and pulmonary abnormalities. *Circulation* 1988;77: 552–559.

11. Benge W, Litchfield RL, Marcus ML. Exercise capacity in patients with severe left ventricular dysfunction. *Circulation* 1980;61:955–959.
12. Szlachcic J, Massie BM, Kramer Bl, et al. Correlates and prognostic implication of exercise capacity in chronic congestive heart failure. *Am J Cardiol* 1985;55:1037–1042.
13. Metra M, Raddino R, Dei Cas L, et al. Assessment of peak oxygen consumption, lactate and ventilatory thresholds and correlation with resting and exercise hemodynamic data in chronic congestive heart failure. *Am J Cardiol* 1990;65:1127–1133.
14. Marantz PR, Tobin JN, Wassertheil-Smoller S, et al. The relationship between left ventricular systolic function and congestive heart failure diagnosed by clinical criteria. *Circulation* 1988;77(3):607–612.
15. Sullivan MJ, Cobb FR. Central hemodynamic response to exercise in patients with chronic heart failure. *Chest* 1992;101(suppl):340S–346S.
16. Sullivan MJ, Knight JD, Higginbotham MB, et al. Relation between central and peripheral hemodynamics during exercise in patients with chronic heart failure: Muscle blood flow is reduced with maintenance of arterial perfusion pressure. *Circulation* 1989;80:769–781.
17. Wilson JR, Ferraro N. Exercise intolerance in patients with chronic heart failure: Relation to oxygen transport and ventilatory abnormalities. *Am J Cardiol* 1983;51:1358–1363.
18. Massie BM. Exercise tolerance in congestive heart failure: Role of cardiac function, peripheral blood flow, and muscle metabolism and effect of treatment. *Am J Med* 1988;84(suppl 3A):75–82.
19. Weber K, Janicki JS. Cardiopulmonary exercise testing for evaluation of chronic heart failure. *Am J Cardiol* 1985;55:22A–31A.
20. Sullivan MJ, Knight JD, Higginbotham MB, Cobb FR. Submaximal exercise cardiac output predicts peak VO_2 in patients with heart failure but not in normal subjects. *Circulation* 1989;80(suppl 2):427.
21. Roubin GS, Anderson SG, Shen WF, et al. Hemodynamic and metabolic basis of impaired exercise tolerance in patients with severe left ventricular dysfunction. *J Amer Coll Cardiol* 1990;15(5):986–994.
22. Jobin J, Cobb FR, Kitzman DW, et al. Peripheral vasoregulatory mechanisms limit exercise heart failure patients with near normal exercise cardiac output (abstract). *Circulation* 1995;992(8):2588.
23. Wilson JR, Mancini DH, Dunkman WB. Exertional fatigue due to skeletal muscle dysfunction in patients with heart failure. *Circulation* 1993;87:470–475.
24. Higginbotham MB, Sullivan MJ, Coleman RE, Cobb FR. Regulation of stroke volume during exercise in patients with severe left ventricular dysfunction: Importance of the Starling mechanism. *J Am Coll Cardiol* 1987;9:58A.
25. Shen WF, Roubin GS, Hirasawa K, et al. Leftventricular volume and ejection fraction response to exercise in chronic congestive heart failure: Difference between dilated cardiomyopathy and previous myocardial infarction. *Am J Cardiol* 1985;55:1027–1031.
26. Lee AP, Ice R, Blessey R, et al. Long term effects of physical training on coronary patients with impaired ventricular function. *Circulation* 1979;60:1519–1526.
27. Conn EH, Williams RS, Wallace AJ. Exercise responses before and after physical conditioning in patients with severly depressed left ventricular function. *Am J Cardiol* 1982;49:296–300.

28. Arvan S. Exercise performance of the high risk acute myocardial infarction patients after cardiac rehabilitation. *Am J Cardiol* 1988;62:197–201.
29. Musch TL, Hilty MR. Effects of dynamic exercise training on the metabolic and cardiocirculatory responses to exercise in the rat model of myocardial infarction and heart failure. *Am J Cardiol* 1988;62:20E–24E.
30. Hambrecht R, Niebauer J, Fiehn E, et al. Physical training in patients with stable chronic heart failure: Effects on cardiorespiratory fitness and ultrastructural abnormalities of leg muscles. *J Am Coll Cardiol* 1995;25(6):1239–1249.
31. Sullivan MJ, Higginbotham MB, Cobb FR. Exercise training in patients with severe left ventricular dysfunction: Hemodynamic and metabolic effects. *Circulation* 1988;78:506–515.
32. Sullivan MJ, Higginbotham MB, Cobb FR. Exercise training in patients with chronic heart failure delays ventilatory anaerobic threshold and improves submaximal exercise performance. *Circulation* 1989;79:324–329.
33. Hagberg JM, Ehsani AA, Halloszy JO. Effect of 12 months of intense exercise training on stroke volume in patients with coronary artery disease. *Circulation* 1983;67:1194.
34. Coats AJS, Adamopoulos S, Radaelli A, et al. Controlled trial of physical training in chronic heart failure: Exercise performance, hemodynamics, ventilation, and autonomic function. *Circulation* 1992;85:2119–2131.
35. Cobb FR, Williams RS, McEwan P, et al. Effects of exercise training on ventricular function in patients with recent myocardial infarction. *Circulation* 1982;60:100.
36. Douard H, Patel P, Broustet JP. Exercise training in patients with chronic heart failure. *Heart Failure* 1994;10(2):80–87.
37. Coats AJS, Adamopoulos S, Meyer T, et al. Effects of physical training in chronic heart failure. *Lancet* 1990;335:63–66.
38. Uren NG, Lipkin DP. Exercise training as therapy for chronic heart failure. *Br Heart J* 1992;67:430–433.
39. Jette M, Heller R, Landry F, et al. Randomized 4-week exercise program in patients with impaired left ventricular function. *Circulation* 1991;84:1561–1567.
40. Kavanagh T, Myers MG, Baigrie RS, et al. Cardiac respiratory training responses to a one-year walking program in patients with chronic heart failure. *Eur Heart J* 1993;14(suppl):415 (Abstract).
41. Minotti JR, Massie BM. Exercise training in heart failure patients: Does reversing the peripheral abnormalities protect the heart? *Circulation* 1992;85:2323–2325.
42. Minotti JR, Johnson EC, Hudson TL, et al. Skeletal muscle response to training exercise in congestive heart failure. *J Clin Invest* 1990;86:751–758.
43. Clausen JP. Circulatory adjustments to dynamic exercise and effect of physical training in normal subjects and in patients with coronary artery disease. *Prog Cardiovasc Dis* 1976;18:459–495.
44. Hambrecht R, Niebauer J, Marburger CH, et al. Various intensities of leisure time physical activity in patients with coronary artery disease: Effects on cardiorespiratory fitness and progression of atherosclerotic lesions. *J Am Coll Cardiol* 1993;22:468–477.
45. Belardinelli R, Georgiou D, Scocco V, et al. Low intensity exercise training in patients with chronic heart failure. *J Am Coll Cardiol* 1995;26(4):975–982.
46. Froelicher V, Jenson D, Genter F, et al. A randomized trial of exercise training in patients with corornary heart disease. *JAMA* 1984;252:1291–1297.
47. Tavazzi L, Ignone G, Giordano, A et al. Cardiac rehabilitation in patients

with recent myocardial infarction and left ventricular dysfunction. *Adv Cardiol* 1986;34:156–169.

48. Jugdutt BI, Michorowski BL, Kappagoda CT. Exercise training after anterior Q wave myocardial infarction: Importance of regional left ventricular wall function topography. *J Am Coll Cardiol* 1988;12:362–372.

49. Giannuzzi P, Tavazzi L, Temporelli UC, et al. Long-term physical training and left ventricular remodeling after anterior myocardial infarction: Results of Exercise in Anterior Myocardial Infarction (EAMI) trial. *J Am Coll Cardiol* 1993;22:1821–1829.

50. Giannuzzi P, Pier L, Temporelli UC, et al. Attenuation of unfavorable remodeling by exercise training in postinfarction patients with left ventricular dysfunction: Results of the Exercise in Left Ventricular Dysfunction (ELVD) trial. *Circulation* 1995;92(8):1899I (Abstract).

51. Cannistra LB, Davidoff R, Picard MH, et al. Effect of exercise training after myocardial infarction on left ventricular remodeling relative to infarct size. *Circulation* 1995;92(8):1900I (Abstract).

52. Bellardinelli R, Georgiou D, Ginzton L. et al. Exercise training improves myocardial viability in patients with chronic coronary artery disease and left ventricular systolic dysfunction. *Circulation* 1995;92(8):1901I (Abstract).

Chapter 16

Skeletal Muscle and The Role of Exercise Training in Chronic Heart Failure

John R. Wilson, MD and Don B. Chomsky, MD

Exercise intolerance remains a major problem for patients with heart failure.[1-3] During normal daily activities, patients frequently report exertional dyspnea and fatigue. During formal exercise testing, the maximal exercise capacity of symptomatic patients is typically less than 50% of normal.[1-3] Even in apparently asymptomatic patients, maximal exercise capacity is usually reduced by 30% to 40%.[4]

The precise reason that patients with heart failure are limited during exertion is not entirely clear, particularly during submaximal exercise. Both skeletal muscle dysfunction and lung dysfunction have been implicated, however, most evidence now suggests that the maximal exercise ability of such patients is limited primarily by skeletal muscle fatigue. During exercise testing, patients typically report progressive leg fatigue, and at peak exercise, patients often identify fatigue as their primary limiting factor.[5] Patients usually exhibit earlier-than-normal increases in blood lactate concentration during exercise, an objective marker of skeletal muscle dysfunction.[1,2]

There is also evidence that skeletal muscle dysfunction is a major factor responsible for lung and ventilatory abnormalities in heart failure. Several groups have documented reduced respiratory muscle strength in patients with heart failure.[6,7] Coats and coinvestigators propose that a link exists between skeletal muscle dysfunction and abnormal ventilatory responses in heart failure, mediated by metabolic receptors in skeletal muscle.[8]

From the Cardiology Division of the Vanderbilt University Medical Center.

Supported by a Grant-in-Aid from the National American Heart Association and by RO-53059 from the NHLBI.

From: Balady GJ, Piña IL (eds). *Exercise and Heart Failure*. Armonk, NY: Futura Publishing Company, Inc.; ©1997.

Mechanism of Skeletal Muscle Dysfunction

Skeletal muscle fatigue in heart failure has traditionally been attributed to inadequate skeletal muscle blood flow. This conclusion was based on the finding that when the cardiac output and leg blood flow response to exercise are evaluated in groups of patients with heart failure, flow responses are, on average, decreased.[1,5] A number of recent observations, however, suggest that muscle fatigue in heart failure may be triggered more by intrinsic muscle abnormalities than by muscle underperfusion.

We have noted that almost half of patients with reduced peak exercise VO2 have cardiac output responses to exercise that are within the normal limits.[9] Leg blood flow in these patients also appears to be normal.[10] Even when leg blood flow is reduced, augmentation of leg flow with hydralazine, dobutamine, or dopamine has minimal effects on exercise performance.[11–13] During exercise, there is little evidence that skeletal muscle myoglobin is deoxygenated, implying that muscle is not ischemic or hypoxic.[14] In contrast, there is now extensive evidence that patients with heart failure can develop intrinsic skeletal muscle changes.

The first evidence that heart failure is associated with intrinsic muscle changes came from 31 phosphorus magnetic resonance spectroscopy studies. We and others used magnetic resonance spectroscopy to noninvasively monitor inorganic phosphate, phosphocreatine, and pH changes in the forearm and calf muscles of patients with heart failure.[15–18] These studies demonstrated that patients with heart failure develop greater-than-normal phosphocreatine depletion and muscle acidification (Figure 1). These changes were noted despite normal limb flow responses to exercise, suggesting that the changes were caused by intrinsic muscle abnormalities.[16] Further supporting intrinsic muscle changes, forearm metabolic abnormalities persisted even when flow to the forearm was removed by cuff-occlusion of the upper arm.[18]

These observations triggered a series of muscle biopsy studies that provided direct evidence of intrinsic abnormalities. Some studies were performed using gastrocnemius muscle biopsies and others using biopsies of the quadriceps muscle; results were similar in both muscle groups. Fiber atrophy, particularly of type II fibers, was noted to be associated with an increase in the proportion of type II fibers.[19,20] Mitochondrial-based enzyme activity was reduced, particularly the activity of 3-hydroxyacyl-CoA-dehydrogenase.[19,20] Capillary density per cross-sectional area was normal.

Of particular note, Drexler et al[21] measured volume density of mitochondria and surface density of mitochondrial cristae on a large group of patients and healthy control subjects: 57 patients with heart failure and 18 healthy control subjects. Both measures of mitochondrial characteristics were decreased in the patients with heart failure (Fig-

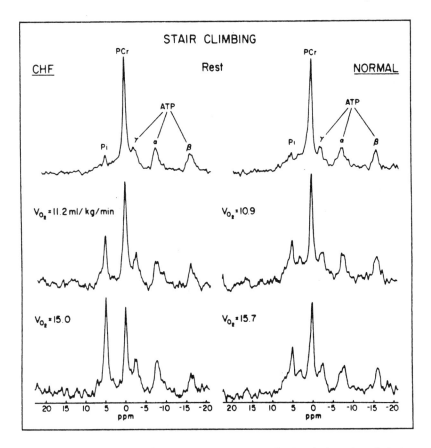

Figure 1: Nuclear magnetic resonance spectra obtained at rest and during plantarflexion in a patient with heart failure and a normal control subjects. TUP = plantarflexion (toe-up), CHF = heart failure, NORMAL = normal control subject, Pi = inorganic phosphate, Pcr = phosphocreatine, ATP = adenosine triphosphate, $\dot{V}O_2$ = oxygen consumption. (From Reference 34).

ure 2). They also note a significant relationship between volume density of mitochondria and peak exercise $\dot{V}O_2$ (r = 0.57), leading these investigators to postulate that muscle mitochondrial content is a key determinant of exercise performance in heart failure.

In further support of this hypothesis, they observed a significant correlation between changes in peak $\dot{V}O_2$ noted over a 4-month period of treatment and changes in mitochondrial volume density. It should be noted, however, that many of the patients in their study who had significant exercise limitation also had mitochondrial density levels clearly overlapping the normal range, raising some questions about the link between muscle changes and exercise performance.

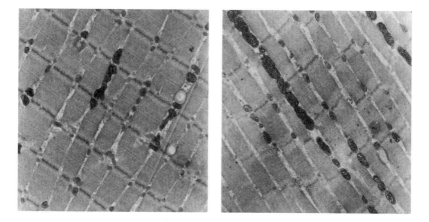

Figure 2: Electron micrographs of cytochrome-c oxidase in a patient with severe heart failure (left panel) and in a normal subject (right panel). Enzyme activity within the mitochondria (black) is reduced in heart failure. (From Reference 21).

Other skeletal muscle abnormalities described in heart failure include reduced total skeletal muscle mass[22] and reduced muscle endurance. In a series of studies using isokinetic knee extensions, Minotti et al[23–25] examined quadriceps strength and endurance in patients with heart failure. They observed normal strength, as measured by maximal developed tension. They note, however, that muscle endurance, as measured by the rate of decline in developed tension during repetitive knee extensions, was reduced in patients with heart failure when compared to normal control subjects. They also noted a striking correlation (r = 0.90) between peak exercise $\dot{V}O_2$ and isokinetic quadriceps endurance, suggesting a close relationship between muscle performance and maximal exercise performance.

To be certain that these changes were not simply a product of reduced muscle mass, Minotti et al[25] used magnetic resonance imaging to measure quadriceps cross-sectional area. They observed decreased muscle area in patients with heart failure, but normal maximal-force generated per cross-sectional area unit. Minotti et al suggest that this pattern of normal force development coupled with reduced muscle endurance could be caused by a reduction in type I fibers, the fibers most closely coupled to isometric and dynamic endurance in normal subjects.

Skeletal Muscle Abnormalities And Training

Why do skeletal muscle changes develop in patients with heart failure? A number of different mechanisms have been proposed to explain these changes, including increased tissue necrosis factor, elevated corticosteroid levels, and tissue underperfusion. However, the dominant culprit appears to be inactivity and deconditioning.

It has long been recognized that patients with heart failure frequently become inactive due to physician recommendations, fear of exercise, and exertional symptoms. However, the first direct evidence of a link between inactivity and skeletal muscle changes came from an elegant study by Minotti et al.[26] These investigators used phosphorus magnetic resonance spectroscopy to measure forearm metabolic responses to forearm exercise before and after 28 days of wrist flexion exercise. The nondominant arm was trained, while the dominant arm served as the control. Only five patients were studied, but even with this small population, the investigators were able to show that training improved forearm metabolism during exercise.

Since this initial study, a number of groups have confirmed that exercise training can improve peak exercise performance and muscle metabolic responses to exercise in patients with heart failure. Sullivan et al[27] enrolled 12 patients in a 6-month cardiac rehabilitation program. They observed a 23% increase in peak exercise $\dot{V}O_2$ and reduced muscle lactate release, but no change in leg blood flow when measured at comparable workloads; peak exercise leg flow increased.

Coats et al[28] enrolled 17 men in a randomized crossover trial of home exercise training using a stationary bicycle. Training increased peak exercise $\dot{V}O_2$ from 13.2 ± 0.9 to 15.6 ± 1.0 mL/min/kg, and decreased sympathetic activity, as measured by whole-body radiolabeled norepinephrine spillover. Interestingly, training reduced both minute ventilation and the slope relating minute ventilation to carbon dioxide production, supporting the concept that skeletal muscle influences ventilatory behavior in heart failure.

Adamopoulos et al[29] used phosphorus-31 nuclear magnetic resonance spectroscopy to study calf muscle metabolism in 12 patients undergoing 8 weeks of home-based bicycle exercise training. Patients were studied using a randomized crossover trial design. Training increased maximal oxygen consumption from 12.2 ± 1.3 to 14.1 ± 1.5 mL/min/kg, decreased calf phosphocreatine depletion, and attenuated calf acidification during exercise.

Hambrecht et al[30] enrolled 22 patients in a randomized trial of training versus normal activity. Percutaneous needle biopsy of the vastus lateralis muscle was performed at baseline and after 6 months of training. Training improved peak exercise $\dot{V}O_2$ by 31% and the anaerobic threshold by 23%. The total volume density of mitochondrial and volume density of cytochrome-c oxidase-positive mitochondrial increased by 19% and 41% respectively. Changes in volume density of cytochrome correlated with change in peak $\dot{V}O_2$, suggesting that improved maximal exercise performance was mediated by changes in skeletal muscle structure.

These findings have led to the general presumption that deconditioning is responsible for much of the exercise intolerance experienced by patients with heart failure. However, a more careful review of prior studies raises some concerns about this conclusion. Individual patient responses to training varied widely in nearly all studies, with significant improvements in peak exercise $\dot{V}O_2$ often due to substantial changes in a minority of patients. In fact, Barlow et al[31] studied 10 patients and found no significant increase in peak exercise $\dot{V}O_2$. Belardinelli et al[32] studied 55 patients and noted improvements in only a small subgroup.

One possible explanation for these findings is that the relative contribution of muscle underperfusion versus intrinsic muscle changes differs amongst patients. Specifically, it is possible that patients with severe muscle underperfusion are limited mainly by flow abnormalities, even when intrinsic muscle changes occur, whereas patients with preserved muscle perfusion are limited by muscle changes.

We recently sought to test this hypothesis by measuring hemodynamic responses to maximal treadmill exercise in 32 patients with chronic heart failure.[33] Patients were then enrolled in a standard 3-month cardiac rehabilitation program. The relationship between the response to rehabilitation and the hemodynamic response to exercise was then examined. Twenty-one patients had a normal cardiac output response to exercise. All 21 patients participated in the rehabilitation program without difficulty, and 9 (43%) responded to rehabilitation, as defined by a >10% increase in both peak exercise $\dot{V}O_2$ and the anaerobic threshold. Eleven patients had a reduced cardiac output response to exercise. Three of these patients discontinued rehabilitation due to severe exhaustion and only one qualified as a responder (9%; $P<.04$ versus preserved cardiac output).

These findings suggest that patients with heart failure and a normal cardiac output response to exercise frequently improve with exercise training. Patients with severe hemodynamic dysfunction during exercise usually do not improve with training, suggesting that they are primarily limited by circulatory factors.

Summary

Our understanding of exertional symptoms in heart failure has progressed considerably over the past decade. The traditional perception that all exertional symptoms in patients are due to pump dysfunction is no longer tenable. It is now clear that intrinsic muscle changes, possibly due to deconditioning, frequently occur in patients with heart failure, and that these muscle changes can be a target for therapeutic interventions.

However several key issues remain unresolved. The relative contributions of muscle underperfusion, lung dysfunction, and skeletal muscle abnormalities to exertional symptoms in heart failure still is unclear. The cause for blood flow, lung, and skeletal muscle abnormalities must be clarified. Finally, the role of exercise training in heart failure and the optimal training protocol is uncertain. Hopefully, ongoing research efforts will yield answers to these important questions.

References

1. Wilson JR, Martin JL, Schwartz D, Ferraro N. Exercise intolerance in patients with chronic heart failure: Role of impaired nutritive flow to skeletal muscle. *Circulation* 1984;69:1079–1087.
2. Weber K, Kinasewitz G, Janicki J, Fishman A. Oxygen utilization and ventilation during exercise in patients with chronic heart failure. *Circulation* 1982;65:1213–1223.
3. Franciosa JA, Ziesche S, Wilen M. Functional capacity of patients with chronic left ventricular failure. *Am J Med* 1979;67:460–466.
4. Liang C, Stewart DK, LeJemtel TH, et al. Characteristics of peak aerobic capacity in symptomatic and asymptomatic subjects with left ventricular dysfunction. *Am J Cardiol* 1992;69:1207–1211.
5. Sullivan MJ, Knight JD, Higginbotham MB, Cobb FR. Relation between central and peripheral hemodynamics during exercise in patients with chronic heart failure. *Circulation* 1989;80:769–781.
6. Hammond MD, Bauer KA, Sharp JT, Rocha RD. Respiratory muscle strength in congestive heart failure. *Chest* 1990;98:1091–1094.
7. McParland C, Krishnan B, Wang Y, Gallagher CG. Inspiratory muscle weakness and dyspnea in heart failure. *Am Rev Respir Dis* 1992;146:467–472.
8. Clark AL, Piepoli M, Coats AJ. Skeletal muscle and the control of ventilation on exercise: Evidence for metabolic receptors. *Eur J Clin Invest* 1995;25:299–305.
9. Wilson JR, Rayos G, Yeoh TK, Gothard P. Dissociation between peak exercise oxygen consumption and hemodynamic dysfunction in potential heart transplantation candidates. *J Am Coll Cardiol* 1995;26:429–435.
10. Wilson JR, Mancini DM, Dunkman WB. Exertional fatigue due to skeletal muscle dysfunction in patients with heart failure. *Circulation* 1993;87:470–475.
11. Wilson JR, Martin JL, Ferraro N, Weber KT. Effect of hydralazine on perfusion and metabolism in the leg during upright bicycle exercise in patients with heart failure. *Circulation* 1983;68:425–432.
12. Wilson JR, Martin JL, Ferraro N. Impaired skeletal muscle nutritive flow during exercise in patients wtih congestive heart failure: Role of cardiac pump dysfunction as determined by the effect of dobutamine. *Am J Cardiol* 1984;53:1308–1315.
13. Maskin CS, Kugler J, Sonnenblick EH, LeJemtel TH. Acute inotropic stimulation with dopamine in severe congestive heart failure: Beneficial hemodynamic effect at rest but not during maximal exercise. *Am J Cardiol* 1983;52:1028–1032.
14. Mancini DM, Wilson JR, Bolinger L, et al. In vivo magnetic resonance spectroscopy measurement of deoxymyoglobin during exercise in patients with heart failure. *Circulation* 1994;90:500–508.
15. Wilson JR, Fink L, Maris J, et al. Evaluation of energy metabolism in skeletal muscle of patients with heart failure with gated phosphorus-31 nuclear magnetic resonance. *Circulation* 1985;71:57–62.

16. Wiener DH, Fink LI, Maris J, et al. Abnormal skeletal muscle bioenergetics during exercise in heart failure: Role of reduced muscle blood flow. *Circulation* 1986;73:1127–1136.

17. Massie B, Conway M, Yonge R, et al. Skeletal muscle metabolism in patients with congestive heart failure: Relation to clinical severity and blood flow. *Circulation* 1987;76:1009–1019.

18. Massie BM, Conway M, Rajagopalan B, et al. Skeletal muscle metabolism during exercise under ischemic conditions in congestive heart failure. *Circulation* 1988;78:320–326.

19. Mancini DM, Coyle E, Coggan A, et al. Contribution of intrinsic skeletal muscle changes to 31P NMR skeletal muscle metabolic abnormalities in patients with chronic heart failure. *Circulation* 1989;80:1338–1346.

20. Sullivan MJ, Green HJ, Cobb FR. Skeletal muscle biochemistry and histology in ambulatory patients with long-term heart failure. *Circulation* 1990; 81:518–527.

21. Drexler H, Riede U, Munzel T, et al. Alterations of skeletal muscle in chronic heart failure. *Circulation* 1992;85:1751–1759.

22. Mancini DM, Walter G, Reichek N, et al. Contribution of skeletal muscle atrophy to exercise intolerance and altered muscle metabolism in heart failure. *Circulation* 1992;85:1364–1373.

23. Minotti JR, Christoph I, Oka R, et al. Impaired skeletal muscle function in patients with congestive heart failure. *J Clin Invest* 1991;88:2077–2082.

24. Minotti JR, Pillay P, Chang L, et al. Neurophysiological assessment of skeletal muscle fatigue in patients with congestive heart failure. *Circulation* 1992;86:903–908.

25. Minotti JR, Pillay P, Oka R, et al. Skeletal muscle size: Relationship to muscle function in heart failure. *J Appl Physiol* 1993;75:373–381.

26. Minotti JR, Johnson EC, Hudson TL, et al. Skeletal muscle response to exercise training in congestive heart failure. *J Clin Invest* 1990;86:751–758.

27. Sullivan MJ, Higginbotham MB, Cobb FR. Exercise training in patients with chronic heart failure delays ventilatory anaerobic threshold and improves submaximal exercise performance. *Circulation* 1989;79:324–329.

28. Coats AJS, Adamopoulos S, Radaelli A, et al. Controlled trial of physical training in chronic heart failure. *Circulation* 1992;85:2119–2131.

29. Adamopoulos S, Coats AJS, Brunotte F, et al. Physical training improves skeletal muscle metabolism in patients with chronic heart failure. *J Am Coll Cardiol* 1993;21:1101–1106.

30. Hambrecht R, Niebauer J, Fiehn E, et al. Physical training in patients with stable chronic heart failure: Effects on cardiorespiratory fitness and ultrastructural abnormalities of leg muscles. *J Am Coll Cardiol* 1995;25:1239–1249.

31. Barlow CW, Qayyum MS, Davey PP, et al. Effect of physical training on exercise-induced hyperkalemia in chronic heart failure. *Circulation* 1994;89: 1144–1152.

32. Belardinelli R, Georgious D, Cianci G, et al. Exercise training improves left ventricular diastolic filling in patients with dilated cardiomyopathy. *Circulation* 1995;91:2775–2784.

33. Wilson JR, Groves J, Rayos G. Circulatory status and response to cardiac rehabilitation in patients with heart failure. *Circulation* (in press).

34. Mancini DM, Ferraro N, Tuchler M, et al. Detection of abnormal calf muscle metabolism in patients with heart failure using phosphorus-31 nuclear magnetic resonance. *Am J Cardiol* 1988;62:1234–1240.

Chapter 17

Central and Peripheral Responses to Training After Cardiac Transplantation

John R. Stratton, MD

Introduction

Despite the marked improvements in symptomatology that typically occur following cardiac transplantation, cardiovascular function during exercise does not return to normal. In fact, the circulatory response to exercise is markedly abnormal despite the presence of a new heart. At least part of this persistent abnormality in exercise capacity and function might be due to inactivity/deconditioning, which precedes the transplantation, and it is reasonable to postulate that at least a portion of the abnormality might be reversed by exercise training. This chapter will review the abnormalities that occur in the response to exercise, post transplantation, and the available literature on the effects of exercise training following transplantation. From this review, it will be apparent that the physiology of the transplanted heart and the response to exercise are relatively well described; however, there is a paucity of solid scientific information on the effects of exercise training on the heart transplant recipient, and much work remains to be done in this area.

Exercise Responses Following Cardiac Transplantation

Resting Hemodynamics

One of the most striking changes, post transplantation, is the increase in resting heart rate, which is about 25% to 35% higher than nor-

Supported by the Medical Research Service of the Department of Veterans Affairs.

From: Balady GJ, Piña IL (eds). *Exercise and Heart Failure.* Armonk, NY: Futura Publishing Company, Inc.; ©1997.

mal at rest due to cardiac denervation. The resting tachycardia is associated with a 15% to 40% reduction in left ventricular end-diastolic volume and an 18% to 38% reduction in resting stroke volume index compared to normal.[1-5] Resting cardiac output is normal[1,5] or mildly reduced.[2,6] Resting ejection fraction has been normal in nearly all reported studies,[2,3,5–12] although Verani and colleagues[13] find a lower left ventricular ejection fraction in 35 post-transplant patients compared to only five controls, and Hartmann et al[7] report a significant reduction in resting left ventricular ejection fraction with time post-transplant. However, Hosenpud et al[11] find no drop in resting ejection fraction between 1 and 2 years in 20 patients, nor do Kao et al.[3] Although resting left ventricular systolic function is normal, right ventricular function, as measured by the ejection fraction, is reduced at rest and exercise.[8] Resting mean blood pressure is increased by ~10% to 15% compared to normals,[2,3] and resting systolic and diastolic blood pressures are elevated.[1,2]

Intracardiac pressures are elevated at rest. Pulmonary capillary wedge pressure at rest is elevated about 30% to 35% compared to normal,[2,3,6,14–16] and mean pulmonary pressure is similarly increased by about 40%.[2,3] Right atrial pressure tends to be elevated.[2,3,6,8] The most comprehensive hemodynamic studies of patients post transplantation are reported by Kao and colleagues in two groups of subjects studied either relatively early (1 month to 16 months)[2] or late (27 months to 70 months) following transplantation.[3] Their results comparing post-transplant patients and normal controls are summarized in Table 1 and Table 2 for resting and exercise values.

Exercise Performance And Hemodynamics

A reduction in peak oxygen consumption and in peak workload has been a uniform finding.[2,4,17–24] Patients post-transplant have a peak workload or peak oxygen consumption that is only 45% to 66% of normal age-matched controls. Furthermore, the abnormal maximal oxygen consumption, although it may improve mildly late following transplant, remains clearly abnormal indefinitely.[2,3,20,21,24,25] The magnitude of the deficit is relatively marked, as underlined by the fact that Stevenson et al[17] report that post-transplant patients did not differ from patients with advanced heart failure stabilized on optimal sustained medical therapy in regard to maximal exercise workload, maximal oxygen uptake, anaerobic threshold, or maximum oxygen pulse.

At maximal exercise, the peak heart rate in transplantation patients is reduced, being 20% to 30% lower than age-matched normal subjects.[2–5,20,23] Thus, the heart rate reserve, which is the increase in heart rate with exercise, is markedly reduced in patients post transplantation;

Table 1

Comparison of Supine Rest and Maximal Upright Hemodynamic Responses Expressed as the Percentage Difference in 30 Transplant Patients (3–16 months) versus 30 Age-Matched Controls

	Rest Supine		Maximal Upright Exercise	
	Transplant vs. Control	p Value	Transplant vs. Control	p Value
Heart rate	+32%	0.001	−30%	0.001
Cardiac index	−18%	0.01	−41%	0.001
Stroke volume index	−38%	0.001	−17%	0.001
End-diastolic volume index	−32%	0.001	−14%	0.05
End-systolic volume index	−24%	0.01	−11%	NS
Ejection fraction	−6%	NS	−1%	NS
Mean systemic blood pressure	+15%	0.001	−9%	0.01
Systemic vascular resistance index	+39%	0.01	+43%	0.001
Pulmonary capillary wedge pressure	+35%	0.01	+50%	0.01
Mean pulmonary artery pressure	+43%	0.001	+15%	0.05
Pulmonary vascular resistance index	+81%	0.001	+61%	0.001
Right atrial pressure	+26%	NS	+83%	0.05
Max workload (kpm)	NA	NA	−53%	0.01
VO_2 mL/kg/min	−16%	0.001	−46%	0.001
AVO_2D, vol%	+2%	NS	−24%	0.001

NS = not significant; NA = not applicable. From Reference 2.

it is only 20%, compared to a 119% increase in heart rate in normal subjects during exercise.[2] The stroke volume index at peak exercise is also reduced to about 15% to 20% lower than normal.[2-4] The reduced stroke volume at peak exercise is largely due to a decreased end-diastolic volume, which is about 15% to 20% lower than normal, since ejection fraction at peak exercise is either normal[2,3] or only mildly reduced.[4] The peak cardiac index is reduced by 30% to 45% compared to normal,[2-4] due largely to the reduced heart rate.

Intracardiac pressures at peak exercise are substantially elevated, with pulmonary capillary wedge pressure about 25% to 50% higher than normal, and mean right atrial pressure about 80% to 100% higher than normal at peak exercise.[2,3,8,10,14,23] Both right atrial pressure and pulmonary artery wedge pressure increase substantially more in trans-

Table 2

Comparison of the Percentage Change in Hemodynamic Values from Upright Rest to Upright Maximal Exercise in 30 Transplant Patients and 30 Age-Matched Controls

	Transplant Patients	Normal Controls	p Value
	Upright Maximal Exercise vs. Upright Rest	Upright Maximal Exercise vs. Upright Rest	For Absolute Change From Rest to Max Exercise in Transplant vs. Controls
Heart rate	+20%	+119%	0.001
Cardiac index	+84%	+197%	0.001
Stroke volume index	+51%	+34%	NS
End-diastolic volume index	+35%	+16%	0.05
End-systolic volume index	+9%	−11%	0.05
Ejection fraction	+13%	+16%	NS
Mean systemic blood pressure	+11%	+31%	0.001
Pulmonary capillary wedge pressure	+249%	+197%	0.01
Mean pulmonary artery pressure	+83%	+129%	NS
VO_2 mL/kg/min	+256%	+509%	0.001
AVO_2D, vol%	+76%	+122%	0.001

NS — not significant. From Reference 2.

plant patients than in normal controls, despite the substantially lower maximal workload. From upright rest to maximal upright exercise, the transplant group had a much lesser increase in heart rate than normal controls (+20% versus +119%), and a much lesser increase in cardiac index (+84% versus +197%), but there was no significant difference in the absolute increase in either stroke volume index or ejection fraction between transplant patients and normal controls (Table 2).[2]

In a study restricted to 13 long-term survivors of transplantation (2 years to 6 years), the rest and exercise hemodynamic profile remained markedly abnormal at rest and at peak exercise, confirming that the hemodynamic changes persist indefinitely.[3] Rudas and colleagues[26] note some improvement in right atrial and wedge pressures during exercise between 3 months and 12 months post transplantation. Hosenpud and colleagues[11] found no change in exercise pressures over time, nor even an increase in right atrial pressure between 1 and 2 years.

The majority of studies are in agreement that exercise systolic ventricular function, as assessed by the ejection fraction, is normal or near normal post transplantation,[2,3,12,27] although Hartmann[7,28] found a reduced exercise ejection fraction with time following transplant. More precise assessments of left ventricular contractile function done by Borow et al[29] indicate no impairment of contractility or contractile reserve as measured by left ventricular end-systolic pressure-dimension and stress-shortening relationships.

Diastolic Function

Significant diastolic dysfunction occurs following transplantation. Elevated left ventricular filling pressures at rest and during exercise post transplantation indicate reduced left ventricular compliance.[2,3,10,14] At rest, Kao et al[2] found a significantly elevated pulmonary capillary wedge pressure/end-diastolic volume index relationship. Moreover, during upright exercise the slope of this pressure/volume relationship was 250% higher in transplant patients compared to normal controls ($P<0.001$). Moreover, transplant patients had significantly less shortening in the time constant of left ventricular pressure decay during exercise compared to controls (-7% versus -19%).[28,30] In addition, myocardial stiffness is increased in patients post transplantation,[31] which appears related both to donor heart ischemic time and donor age. These studies provide evidence of diastolic relaxation abnormalities in patients post transplantation, which likely contribute importantly to the observed exercise limitations after transplantation. In normal subjects, increases in β-adrenergic tone regulate, in part, increases in diastolic filling with exercise.[32] It is likely that the autonomic denervation that occurs following transplantation contributes to the exercise diastolic function abnormalities. Whether these diastolic abnormalities can be ameliorated with exercise training, as can occur in older normal subjects,[33] remains to be determined.

Autonomic Nervous System/Cardiac Denervation

The surgical denervation that occurs with transplantation abolishes both vagal and sympathetic efferent control, and results in a loss of afferent signals from intracardiac receptors. Thus, autonomic nervous system function modulation of cardiac function during exercise, which typically accounts for a large part of the cardiovascular responses to dynamic exercise,[34] is lost. With complete denervation, there is an associated resting tachycardia due to the lack of vagal tone, and an abnormal control of the heart rate during exercise, with a slower increase in heart rate at the onset of exercise, since the increased heart rate depends on a rise in circulating catecholamines.[35] The maximal heart rate is markedly reduced, being only 70% to 80% of normal, likely largely due to the loss of direct efferent sympathetic innervation of the sinoatrial node.[36] The reduced maximal heart rate is the major cause of the reduction in maximal cardiac output, since the peak stroke volume is relatively less reduced in transplant patients.[2]

There has been evidence of limited sympathetic reinnervation in human orthotopic heart transplants,[37–40] but of relatively mild degree. Among patients with evidence of reinnervation, there was a significant, but still definitely subnormal, increase in left ventricular dP/dt, and a decrease in coronary sinus blood flow following stimulation of sympathetic neurons with tyramine, suggesting some functional significance of the reinnervation.[41] There has been no evidence of vagal reinnervation.[42] It is likely that reinnervation has minimal effects on exercise responses. Heart rate changes over time following transplantation are relatively minor and have been used both to support[7,43] or refute[20] the idea of functional reinnervation. Thus, available data are compatible with a limited sympathetic component of reinnervation, but no vagal reinnervation.

Following transplantation, resting norepinephrine levels are reduced at rest compared to the elevated levels that occur pretransplantation,[44,45] and are generally within the normal range or mildly increased,[36,46,47] as is plasma epinephrine.[36,47,48] Quigg et al[36] found that at peak exercise, peak levels of epinephrine and norepinephrine tended to be higher than in normal controls. Plasma norepinephrine was also significantly elevated during exercise in other studies.[46–49] There are no solid data regarding the effects of training in transplant patients on autonomic tone or sympathetic responsiveness.

Peripheral Changes

Abnormalities of the peripheral vessels and muscle persist after transplantation, due in part to deconditioning, abnormal neurohumoral abnormalities, drugs, or nonreversible defects present prior to transplant and associated with advanced heart failure. Braith and colleagues[50] found that a leg-strength deficit persisted for at least 18 months, and the magnitude of the leg-strength deficit correlated with the reduction in maximal oxygen consumption. They suggest that the decrement in peak oxygen consumption observed in heart transplant recipients was partially explicable by skeletal muscle weakness, and that training was important. Diminished respiratory muscle endurance has also been noted to persist after transplantation.[51]

Several peripheral limitations to exercise have been noted after transplantation. Kavanagh et al[1] report that lean mass was reduced a mean of 6 kg in 36 patients compared to normal subjects, and was likely due to deconditioning. The reduction in muscle mass undoubtedly played a major role in limiting maximal exercise performance.

Kao et al[2] note a 24% lower arteriovenous oxygen difference at maximal exercise in transplant patients compared to normals, suggesting an abnormality in peripheral oxygen utilization or oxygen transport. This finding is not confirmed by Fleg et al.[4] At submaximal exercise of 60 watts, Mettauer et al[52] note that heart transplant patients had much higher lactate levels than controls despite adequate oxygen transport, which they feel might be amenable to training. One group describes significant increases following transplantation in both oxidative and glycolytic enzymes in vastus lateralis biopsies done before transplantation, and 3 months and 18 months post transplantation, and an increase in Type IIa and IIb fiber type cross sectional area, but no change in the number of capillaries per fiber.[53,54] These results might represent spontaneous improvements after transplantation but might also be due to reversal of deconditioning effects.

Abnormalities of peripheral oxidative metabolism can also alter use of the oxygen transported to muscle. Using magnetic resonance spectroscopy, we found that the skeletal muscle metabolic responses to exercise remained abnormal for indefinite periods following transplantation.[55] During forearm exercise in a group studied early (<6 months) after transplantation, all of the changes noted in a pretransplant group persisted and were, if anything, somewhat worse. In a group studied late after transplantation (mean 15 months), there was a significant improvement in PCr resynthesis rate compared with the early-post-transplant group, and statistically-nonsignificant trends toward improvements in submaximal exercise pH and PCr/(PCr + Pi) ratio and V_{max}. However, compared with normal subjects, exercise duration and submaximal PCr/(PCr + Pi) were still reduced in the late-post-transplant group. Thus, despite successful heart transplantation, skeletal muscle abnormalities of advanced heart failure persisted for indefinite periods, although partial improvement occurred at late times. The persistent abnormalities may contribute to the reduced exercise capacity that is present in most patients after transplantation.

Peripheral vascular resistance, conductance, flow, and reactivity are all abnormal following transplantation,[56-60] but abnormalities improve with time.[56,61] In both cross sectional and longitudinal studies by Kubo et al,[61] heart transplantation is associated with a significant improvement in the forearm blood-flow responses to methacholine, an endothelium-dependent vasodilator, but not nitroprusside, providing evidence that endothelium-dependent dilation of the peripheral vasculature improves following transplantation.

Thus, various forms of evidence suggest that multiple peripheral abnormalities are important contributors to the reduced exercise tolerance following transplantation.

Possible Contributors to Exercise Dysfunction

Why is exercise tolerance reduced following heart transplantation? The reasons are likely multifactorial. Contributing factors include cardiac denervation, an important contributor to the lower maximum cardiac output, which is due in turn to the lower maximum heart rate and stroke volume. Other contributing factors include higher filling pressures, which are a reflection of diastolic dysfunction, chronically increased afterload, an abnormal atrial contribution to cardiac output,[62,63] deconditioning, residual abnormalities in the peripheral circulation and skeletal muscle oxidative metabolism, and possibly drug-induced changes, especially by cyclosporin[64] and prednisone. Ischemia due to occult or overt coronary disease, and subclinical or mild episodes of rejection, leading to myocardial fibrosis, may also impair cardiovascular performance. Moreover, abnormalities occurring as a result of the process of brain death of the donor,[65,66] and damage during organ-preservation may contribute. In addition, abnormal pulmonary gas exchange may possibly contribute to diminished peak oxygen consumption in some heart transplant recipients.[67] No factor individually explains the abnormalities; the dysfunction is seen relatively early prior to prolonged hypertension or multiple episodes of rejection. It is seen in patients with normal coronary angiograms, in patients without rejection, and it was seen prior to the introduction of cyclosporin. Thus, studies of "normal" cardiovascular function following transplant are confounded by several factors that might alter the function of the transplanted heart.[68]

Exercise Training Effects

Deconditioning due to inactivity is virtually uniform in patients early following heart transplantation, since long periods of inactivity typically precede cardiac surgery. Hall et al[69] provide quantitative evidence of muscle deconditioning in 12 post-transplantation patients. The increase in arterial potassium relative to energy expenditure (dK^+/W) was used as an index of deconditioning, since training in healthy individuals reduces the (dK^+/W) during exercise. The heart transplant patients had significantly higher (dK$^+$/W) compared to seven healthy controls (P<0.002), compatible with muscle deconditioning.

The literature regarding the effects of exercise training following cardiac transplantation is very sparse. There has been only a single randomized controlled trial of the effects of exercise training following cardiac transplantation, which is available only in abstract form.[70] The available trials have all used somewhat different training protocols, and there has been a relative paucity of endpoints studied in detail. In addition, there are almost no mechanistic data regarding training adaptations in post-transplant patients. The existing studies that have examined five or more subjects are reviewed in Table 3. Most available data are limited to the effects of training on peak workload or peak oxygen consumption in limited numbers of subjects.

The most comprehensive study to date is reported by Kavanagh and colleagues[1] in a 1988 study. They trained 36 orthotopic heart transplant recipients for a mean of 16 months beginning at a mean of 29 weeks postsurgery, using a walk/jog protocol at ~60% to 70% of VO$_{2max}$ five times weekly.[1] Patients progressed to an average distance of 24 km per week, at an average pace of 8.5 min/km. Among all patients, training was associated with a 33% increase in peak work, and a 19% increase in maximal oxygen consumption corrected for weight. Resting heart rate declined mildly by 4% (−4 bpm, P<0.05) and there were favorable 9% falls in both resting systolic and diastolic blood pressures. Peak heart rate increased by 10% (+13 bpm, P<0.001). Ventilatory anaerobic threshold increased by 24% (P<0.001). There was also a significant reduction in the rating of perceived exertion at any given power output following training. During submaximal exercise at two different workloads there were no changes in oxygen consumption, cardiac output, stroke volume, arteriovenous oxygen difference, or heart rate among all 36 subjects. Despite the training-induced changes in resting and exercise heart rates, resting heart rate remained higher and peak exercise heart rate lower than in normal subjects.

The Kavanagh study reports the only available data on the effects of training on cardiac volumes in patients following transplantation.[1] Somewhat surprisingly, there was no change in resting stroke volume, which typically increases significantly with training. In this trial, resting cardiac output and arteriovenous oxygen difference were also unchanged, as were submaximal exercise cardiac output and arteriovenous difference. There are no data available on the effects of training on peak stroke volume, cardiac output, or arteriovenous difference.

Among the eight most compliant subjects who walked/jogged >32 km/week at an average rate of 6.5 min/km (one of whom completed the Boston marathon), the increase in peak oxygen consumption was very substantial (+51%). The associated training changes also ap-

Table 3

Studies of Exercise Training Following Cardiac Transplantation

	Time and Type of Training					Results of Training						
Number Studied	Time post transplant	Length of training	Frequency and duration	Type of training	Peak Work	VO$_2$ Max mL/kg/min	Rest Heart Rate	Peak Heart Rate	Rest Systolic BP	Peak Systolic BP	Other Major Findings
Degre 1986 (74) 3 2 Controls	2.3 years	21 weeks	3×/week 30 min	Calisth-enics	+50% (p < .05)	40% (p = NS)		+10% (p = NS)		+21% (p = NS)	Submax VO$_2$ (−9%) and heart rate (−11%) reduced, both p = NS.
Savin 1983 (78) 5 7 Controls	?	16 weeks	≥5×/wk ≥30 min	Cycle at ≥75% peak heart rate	+44% (p < .05)	+17% (p < .05)	NSC	NSC			Submax heart rate decreased 11%.
Kavanagh 1988 (1) 36 No trained controls	7 ± 6 months	16 ± 7 months	5×/wk 45 min	Walk jog at 60% to 70% max VO$_2$ Average of 24 km/wk	+49% (p < .01)	+19% (p < .01)	−4% (p < .05)	+9% (p < .01)	−10% (p < .001)	NSC	Increased lean mass (+4%) and ventilatory threshold (+24%). Reduced rest (−10%) and peak diastolic BP (−9%). No change rest or submax stroke volume, cardiac index or AVD.

Kavanagh 1988 (1)	8 Highly motivated subjects	32 ± 17 weeks			Walk/jog ≥32 km/wk	+65% (p < .01)	+51% (p < .01)	−10% (p < .01)	+8% (p < .01)	NSC	NSC	Increased lean mass (+4%). Reduced rest diastolic BP (−14%). Increased peak ventilation (+17%).
Kavanagh 1989 (82)	10 Heterotopic transplants	70 ± 36 weeks		5×/wk 30–60 min	Walk/jog at 60% to 70% max VO_2	+33% (p < .01)	+18% (p < .01)	−4% (p < .01)	+6% (p = NS)	−8% (p < .05)	NSC	Peak ventilation increased 17%. Five controls had no significant change over time.
Keteyian 1991 (71)	12 Trained 5 Untrained controls	12–15 weeks	10 weeks	2–3×/week to Borg of 12–14	32 min aerobic exercise		+17%	+4% (p < .05)	+14% (p < .01)	NSC	NSC	
Keteyian 1990 (108)	19	12 ± 3 weeks	12 weeks	3×/week 24 sessions	32 min aerobic exercise		+17%	+4% (p < .05)	+8% (p < .05)			Lower perceived exertion at submax exercise.
Ehrman 1992 (72)	11	2.5 months	8–10 weeks	3×/week 9 ± 2 weeks	32 min aerobic exercise		+12%		+9% (p < .05)			Absolute VO_2 at ventilatory threshold decreased 13% (p < 0.05).

Table 3—continued

Studies of Exercise Training Following Cardiac Transplantation

		Time and Type of Training				Results of Training						
	Number Studied	Time post transplant training	Length of training	Frequency and duration	Type of training	Peak Work	VO$_2$ Max mL/kg/min	Rest Heart Rate	Peak Heart Rate	Rest Systolic BP	Peak Systolic BP	Other Major Findings
Mettauer 1995 (79)	13	10 ± 3 months	6 weeks	3×/week 45 min	Modified interval training	+16% (p < .05)	+9% (p < .05)					Reduced submax heart rate, norepi and lactate. Mitochondrial density but not capillary density tended to increase in vastus lateralis biopsies.
Saini 1995 (94)	7	10.6 months	6 weeks	3×/week 45 min	Modified interval training	+36% (p < .05)		−10% (p < .05)				No significant training change in rest/exercise osmolality, ANP levels, plasma renin activity, or aldosterone.
Kobashigawa (70)	11 13 Controls	4 weeks	5 months	20 sessions	Treadmill	Tm > C (p < .05)	Tm > C (p < .05)					
Sieurat 1986 (78)	8 Heterotopic		8 weeks			+35%				+26%		Decreased ventiltory equivalent for CO$_2$.
Niset 1988 (112)	62	4 days		5×/week	30 min	+34%	+33%		+11%		+18%	

AVD = arteriovenous oxygen difference; ANP = atrial natriuretic peptide; BP = blood pressure; NSC = no significant change; Tm = trained; C = control.

peared larger, with a 10% decline in resting heart rate and a significant decline in submaximal exercise heart rates that was not seen in the entire cohort. These data, although not controlled, offer evidence of significant training effects post transplantation.

Keteyian and colleagues[71] studied the cardiovascular effects of a much shorter training protocol of 10 weeks in heart transplant subjects starting at 12 weeks to 15 weeks post transplant; they also studied five nonexercising post-transplant controls. In the trained group, maximal oxygen uptake, corrected for weight, increased by 20% compared to a 4% increase in the untrained control transplant subjects.[71] There was also a significant 18 beat per minute $(+14\%)(P<0.05)$ increase in peak heart rate in the trained group compared to only a 6 beat per minute increase in controls. Maximum ventilation also significantly increased by 17%. In this study there was no decrease in resting heart rate and no decrease in resting systolic or diastolic blood pressure. There were no changes in peak exercise respiratory rate, respiratory exchange ratio, or ventilatory equivalents for O_2 or CO_2.

Ehrman, Keteyian and colleagues[72] examined the effects of training in 11 subjects on ventilatory threshold. Peak $\dot{V}O_2$ increased by 19%. The absolute $\dot{V}O_2$ at the ventilatory threshold increased by 12.5% $(P<0.05)$. The ventilatory threshold as a percentage of peak $\dot{V}O_2$ was unchanged. The mean rating of perceived exertion at the ventilatory threshold was 13.2 before training, and was unchanged by training.

Mettauer and Lonsdorfer and colleagues[73,74] describe seven transplant patients who underwent 6 weeks of training. During submaximal exercise at the same level before and after training, there was no change in stroke volume or cardiac index, but a significant decrease in heart rate (135 bpm to 121 bpm, $P<0.05$), lactate (5.7 to 4.1 mmol/L, $P<0.05$), and plasma norepinephrine (1712 to 1147 pg/mL, $P<0.05$).[73] No resting or maximal exercise data were presented, however.

In a preliminary report, Derman and colleagues[75] note a 23% increase in $\dot{V}O_{2max}$, a 32% increase in total work, and no change in resting ejection fraction after a 5-week training program in five subjects, begun 7 weeks post transplantation. Other small studies have also been published.[76–78]

In another preliminary report, Mettauer and colleagues[79] describe 13 patients who underwent training, beginning a mean of 10 months following transplantation. Peak work increased by 16% $(P<0.05)$ and $\dot{V}O_{2max}$ by 9% $(P<0.05)$. Submaximal heart rate declined by 7%, as did submaximal plasma norepinephrine and lactate, both compatible with a training effect. These are the only available data on the effects of training on catecholamines or lactate in patients following transplantation that we found.

The only randomized trial is reported in abstract form by Kobashigawa and colleagues.[70] They randomize 24 subjects 1 month post transplantation to a structured cardiac rehabilitation program (n = 11 subjects) or routine exercise at home (n = 13 subjects). The rehabilitation program involved a total of 20 sessions over 1 to 6 months post transplantation, and offered treadmill exercise and personalized exercise instruction. The patients in the rehabilitation group had a greater increase in peak workload from 1 to 6 months postoperatively ($+40\pm26$ watts versus $+12\pm17$ watts, $P<0.05$) and in peak $\dot{V}O_2$ ($+6.4\pm3.4$ mL/kg/mn versus 2.6 ± 2.6 mL/kg/min, $P<0.05$), as well as a greater improvement in the ventilatory efficiency, as indicated by a fall in the ventilatory equivalent for CO_2 (-14 ± 8 versus -5 ± 7, $P<0.05$). Thus, training was associated with a greater exercise capacity and ventilatory efficiency.

Niset[80] describes a cohort of 62 subjects who started at 4 days post transplantation and continued for an uncertain duration. The training program is not well described. At 1 year, the $\dot{V}O_{2max}$ had increased by 33%, and the peak heart rate by 11%.

There have been two exercise training studies of patients with heterotopic transplants.[81,82] In heterotopic transplantation, the new heart is attached to the diseased heart, which is not removed as it is in orthotopic transplantation. Heterotopic transplants comprise less than 1% of all transplants. Sieurat and colleagues[81] report eight patients and Kavanagh and colleagues[82] report 10 patients. In the study by Sieurat, peak workload increased by 35% and peak heart rate increased by 26%. In the study by Kavanagh, peak workload increased by 33%, $\dot{V}O_{2max}$ increased by 18%, resting heart rate decreased by 4%, and resting systolic pressure decreased by 8% (all $P<0.05$ compared to pre-training). Peak heart rate increased by 6%, which was not statistically significant.[82] These changes were quite similar to those seen in their larger study of patients following orthotopic transplantation. Based on these small studies, there are no apparent major differences in the training responses between heterotopic and orthotopic transplant patients.

Heart Rate

The reduction in resting and submaximal heart rates has been a fairly consistent finding of the available training studies. Kavanagh found that those who attained the greatest training level had the greatest reductions in rest and submaximal heart rates. The reduced heart rate at submaximal exercise may be due to a decrease in serum norepinephrine,[83-85] or downregulation in cardiac β-receptor sensitivity, changes known to occur with training in nontransplant populations. Data in humans regarding the effects of exercise training on β-adrenergic responsiveness in nontransplant subjects are limited and conflicting.[86] There are no data detailing either the response of plasma catecholamine levels or catecholamine responsiveness pre- and post-training in transplant patients.

An increase in peak heart rate has been found in most, but not all, studies as a result of training following cardiac transplantation. The increase in peak heart rate likely in part accounts for the increase in maximal oxygen consumption, unlike in normal subjects, where peak heart rate is unchanged by training. Kavanagh attributes this increase to a strengthening of the leg muscles, as evidenced in part by the increase in lean mass.[1,87] He postulates that the increased leg strength allowed a longer exercise duration to a higher power output, which in turn lead to a greater increase in plasma catecholamines, in turn increasing the heart rate. There are no adequate data to support or refute this possibility.

Stroke Volume and Cardiac Output

Whether maximal stroke volume or cardiac output improves is unknown with certainty. In normal young and old subjects, both peak stroke volume and cardiac index improve with training.[88] The increase in peak heart rate and $\dot{V}O_{2max}$ are both compatible with an increase in peak cardiac output in transplant patients, but definitive data are surprisingly lacking.

The Superfit

Despite the clear-cut abnormalities that persist following transplantation, training allows some highly-motivated cardiac transplant recipients to achieve relatively remarkable performances. DeSmet and colleagues[89,90] describe a subject who completed a 20 km run in 146 minutes, 9 months after surgery. Douglas[91] describes a subject who completed a triathlon (1.5 km swimming, 40 km cycling, and 10 km running) in 4 hours and 12 minutes. Kavanagh[92] describes a patient who completed the 42 km Boston Marathon in under 6 hours, 15 months post transplantation, after training for 12 months.

Peripheral Effects of Training in Transplant Patients

In congestive heart failure, skeletal muscle abnormalities, which may be intrinsic, contribute importantly to exercise intolerance.[93] The same abnormalities may persist post transplantation.[55] To a degree, the effects of congestive heart failure on skeletal muscle can be reversed by exercise training.[94–96] However, whether exercise training can improve the peripheral abnormalities that occur following transplantation has not been studied in detail.

In a preliminary report, Mettauer et al[79] assess the peripheral effects of a 6-week training program in 13 subjects a mean of 10 months post transplant. On serial vastus lateralis biopsies, there was no significant change in ultrastructural capillary density, but there was a tendency for an increase in mitochondrial density ($+17\%$, P = NS), mostly because of a subsarcolemmal mitochondrial density increase ($+60\%$, $P<0.05$). Both maximal power ($+16\%$) and peak $\dot{V}O_2$ ($+9\%$) increased significantly ($P<0.05$).

Derman and colleagues,[75] in a preliminary report, examined changes in skeletal muscle pathology and exercise performance in five subjects before and after a 5-month exercise program begun 7 weeks post transplantation. Using a skeletal muscle pathology score, transplant patients were significantly different from five healthy controls prior to training (12.5 versus 1.6 arbitrary units, $P<0.05$). With training, the skeletal muscle pathology score improved from 12.5 to 5.8 ($P<0.05$). This study suggests that skeletal muscle structure and function improve with 5 months of training. However, it is unclear whether training or transplantation itself was responsible, since there was no untrained transplant control group. The changes noted by Brussieres-Chafe and colleagues[53,54] in oxidative and glycolytic enzymes and fiber type may well have been in part due to reconditioning.

In the study by Kavanagh and colleagues[1] of 36 patients trained for a mean of 16 months, the lean tissue mass increased by 3.5% ($P<0.001$). Lean mass remained lower than in age-matched controls, however. Arteriovenous oxygen difference at submaximal exercise was unchanged with training in their study.

Endocrine Responses

A variety of endocrine responses were studied before and after exercise training, by Saini and colleagues,[97] in seven transplant patients and seven controls. Training (6 weeks) increased maximal tolerated power by 36% ($P<0.05$). Osmolality and hormonal responses were serially measured during exercise and recovery. Following training in the transplant patients, there were no significant changes in any of the rest or exercise assays, including osmolality, circulating atrial natriuretic peptide, plasma renin activity, plasma aldosterone, and plasma arginine vasopressin. There was a more rapid postexercise recovery decline in plasma renin activity following training, and a nonsignificant tendency toward a decline in resting plasma renin activity. Overall, these results show very minor changes in the measured hormones. To our knowledge, the only data regarding the effects of training on plasma catecholamines in patients following transplantation are reported in abstract form only by Mettauer and colleagues.[73,79] In 15 subjects, they report a 35% reduction in submaximal exercise plasma norepinephrine levels. Resting and peak exercise values are not reported.

Other Possible Training Effects

In nontransplantation populations, there are data that exercise training may ameliorate some of the adverse effects of long-term corticosteroid use. An exercise program in rats significantly retarded glucocorticoid-induced muscle atrophy.[98–100] Training prevented muscle mass loss by 25% to 60%, and significantly increased citrate synthase activity, a marker of training.[98,99] In addition, training is known to prevent bone mass loss,[101] another side effect of steroid use. Arterial hypertension occurs in a very high proportion of patients treated with cyclosporin.[102–104] It is possible that this may be ameliorated by training in transplant patients.

There are very limited data regarding the potential beneficial effects of training in regard to psychosocial variables after transplant. In a nonrandomized trial, Kavanagh preliminarily reports that training in 39 males is associated in a significant reduction in depression and anxiety.[8] Shepard[105] feels that training facilitates the correction of postoperative psychological disturbances without supporting data.

Summary and Conclusions

In summary, there is evidence that exercise training post transplantation increases maximal oxygen uptake and peak work, increases peak heart rate, increases maximal minute ventilation, increases lean mass, and reduces ratings of perceived exertion at the same workload. There is possible evidence that submaximal heart rate and resting heart rate are lowered and that skeletal muscle pathology may be improved. There is conflicting evidence in regard to whether training lowers blood pressure either at rest or with exercise.

All of the available training data must be interpreted with some caution, due to the lack of randomized well-controlled trials. The possibility for spontaneous recovery post transplantation is probably great, and there may have been physician or self-selection to the exercise programs that may have influenced the results in a positive direction. In the absence of well-controlled trials it is difficult to ascertain the extent to which the reported training effects are due to spontaneous recovery of function, or potentially due to physician or self-selection into exercise programs.[106]

Although physical capacity is improved post transplantation, heart transplant recipients still have major reductions in maximal work capacity compatible with the detrained state. At the present state of knowledge, it is difficult to dissect out the portion of changes that are due to detraining versus other causes.

There is a large gap in our knowledge of the effects of training following transplantation. Remaining questions include the precise nature of training adaptations and the relative contributions of peripheral and central mechanisms. Additional questions include the effects of training on lipids, blood pressure, fibrinolytic function, and immune function; whether the peripheral skeletal muscle defects can be reversed completely; training effects on adrenergic tone and responsiveness; whether cardiac dilatation occurs; whether maximal stroke volume and cardiac output can be improved; whether exercise ventricular function can be improved; whether diastolic function can be improved; and whether training can be cost-effective in improving outcomes such as quality of life, occurrence of complications, or cost of care. Thus, much important work remains to be done.

References

1. Kavanagh T, Yacoub MH, Mertens DJ, et al. Cardiorespiratory responses to exercise training after orthotopic cardiac transplantation. *Circulation* 1988; 77:162–171.
2. Kao AC, Van TPr, Shaeffer MGS, et al. Central and peripheral limitations to upright exercise in untrained cardiac transplant recipients. *Circulation* 1994;89:2605–2615.
3. Kao AC, Van TPr, Shaeffer MGS, et al. Allograft diastolic dysfunction and chronotropic incompetence limit cardiac output response to exercise two to six years after heart transplantation. *J Heart Lung Transplant* 1995;14:11–22.
4. Fleg J, O'Connor F, Kassper E, et al. Long-term effects of cardiac transplantation on cardiovascular performance during dynamic exercise (abstract). *Circulation* 1995;92:I467.
5. Pflugfelder PW, Purves PD, McKenzie FN, Kostuk WJ. Cardiac dynamics during supine exercise in cyclosporine-treated orthotopic heart transplant recipients: Assessment by radionuclide angiography. *J Am Coll Cardiol* 1987;10:336–341.
6. Greenberg ML, Uretsky BF, Reddy PS, et al. Long-term hemodynamic follow-up of cardiac transplant patients treated with cyclosporine and prednisone. *Circulation* 1985;71:487–494.
7. Hartmann A, Maul FD, Huth A, et al. Serial evaluation of left ventricular function by radionuclide ventriculography at rest and during exercise after orthotopic heart transplantation. *Eur J Nucl Med* 1993;20:146–150.
8. Burger W, Hartmann A, Herholz C, et al. Right ventricular volumes and hemodynamics after successful orthotopic heart transplantation. A compari-

son to coronary artery disease using thermodilution. *Int J Cardiol* 1992;37: 155–163.

9. Younis LT, Melin JA, Schoevaerdts JC, et al. Left ventricular systolic function and diastolic filling at rest and during upright exercise after orthotopic heart transplantation: Comparison with young and aged normal subjects. *J Heart Transplant* 1990;9:683–692.

10. Hosenpud JD, Morton MJ, Wilson RA, et al. Abnormal exercise hemodynamics in cardiac allograft recipients 1 year after cardiac transplantation: Relation to preload reserve. *Circulation* 1989;80:525–532.

11. Hosenpud JD, Pantely GA, Morton MJ, et al. Lack of progressive "restrictive" physiology after heart transplantation despite intervening episodes of allograft rejection: Comparison of serial rest and exercise hemodynamics one and two years after transplantation. *J Heart Transplant* 1990;9:119–123.

12. Reid CJ, Yacoub MH. Determinants of left ventricular function one year after cardiac transplantation. *Br Heart J* 1988;59:397–402.

13. Verani MS, Nishimura S, Mahmarian JJ, et al. Cardiac function after orthotopic heart transplantation: Response to postural changes, exercise, and beta-adrenergic blockade. *J Heart Lung Transplant* 1994;3:181–193.

14. Pflugfelder PW, McKenzie FN, Kostuk WJ. Hemodynamic profiles at rest and during supine exercise after orthotopic cardiac transplantation. *Am J Cardiol* 1988;61:1328–1333.

15. Pflugfelder PW, Purves PD, Menkis AH, et al. Rest and exercise left ventricular ejection and filling characteristics following orthotopic cardiac transplantation. *Can J Cardiol* 1989;5:161–167.

16. Frist WH, Stinson EB, Oyer PE, et al. Long-term hemodynamic results after cardiac transplantation. *J Thorac Cardiovasc Surg* 1987;94:685–693.

17. Stevenson LW, Sietsema K, Tillisch JH, et al. Exercise capacity for survivors of cardiac transplantation or sustained medical therapy for stable heart failure. *Circulation* 1990;81:78–85.

18. Cerretelli P, Grassi B, Colombini A, et al. Gas exchange and metabolic transients in heart transplant recipients. *Respir Physiol* 1988;74:355–371.

19. Cerretelli P, Marconi C, Meyer M, et al. Gas exchange kinetics in heart transplant recipients. *Chest* 1992;101(suppl):199S–205S.

20. Mandak JS, Aaronson KD, Mancini DM. Serial assessment of exercise capacity after heart transplantation. *J Heart Lung Transplant* 1995;14:468–478.

21. Cohen-Solal A, Laperche T, Page E. Cardiovascular adaptations during exercise after heart transplantation. *Heart Failure* 1994;April/May:89–96.

22. Sigmund M, Beck FJ, Silny J, et al. Cardiopulmonary exercise capacity before and after heart transplantation. *Z Kardiol* 1994;3:97–102.

23. Martin TW, Gaucher J, Pupa LE, Seaworth JF. Response to upright exercise after cardiac transplantation. *Clin Cardiol* 1994;17:292–300.

24. Degre SG. Are cardiac transplant recipients still suffering cardiac failure? [editorial]. *Acta Cardiol* 1993;48:1–9.

25. Labovitz AJ, Drimmer AM, McBride LR, et al. Exercise capacity during the first year after cardiac transplantation. *Am J Cardiol* 1989;64:642–645.

26. Rudas L, Pflugfelder PW, McKenzie FN, et al. Normalization of upright exercise hemodynamics and improved exercise capacity one year after orthotopic cardiac transplantation. *Am J Cardiol* 1992;69:1336–1339.

27. Teo KK, Yusuf S, Wittes J, et al. Preserved left ventricular function during supine exercise in patients after orthotopic cardiac transplantation. *Eur Heart J* 1992;13:321–329.

28. Hartmann A, Klepzig H, Standke R, et al. Multiparametric analysis using

radionuclide ventriculography in the assessment of left ventricular function following heart transplantation. *Nuklearmedizin* 1991;30:1–6.

29. Borow KM, Neumann A, Arensman FW, Yacoub MH: Left ventricular contractility and contractile reserve in humans after cardiac transplantation. *Circulation* 1985;71:866–872.

30. Paulus WJ, Bronzwaer JG, Felice H, et al. Deficient acceleration of left ventricular relaxation during exercise after heart transplantation. *Circulation* 1992;86:1175–1185.

31. Hausdorf G, Banner NR, Mitchell A, et al. Diastolic function after cardiac and heart-lung transplantation. *Br Heart J* 1989;62:123–132.

32. Stratton JR, Levy WC, Schwartz RS, et al. Beta-adrenergic effects on left ventricular filling: Influence of aging and exercise training. *J Appl Physiol* 1994;77:2522–2529.

33. Levy WC, Cerqueira MD, Abrass IB, et al. Endurance exercise training augments diastolic filling at rest and during exercise in older and young healthy men. *Circulation* 1993;88:116–126.

34. Stratton JR, Pfeifer MA, Halter JB. The hemodynamic effects of sympathetic stimulation combined with parasympathetic blockade in man. *Circulation* 1987;75:922–929.

35. Perini R, Orizio C, Gamba A, Veicsteinas A. Kinetics of heart rate and catecholamines during exercise in humans: The effect of heart denervation. *Eur J Appl Physiol* 1993;66:500–506.

36. Quigg RJ, Rocco MB, Gauthier DF, et al. Mechanism of the attenuated peak heart rate response to exercise after orthotopic cardiac transplantation. *J Am Coll Cardiol* 1989;14:338–344.

37. Wilson RF, Christensen BV, Olivari MT, et al. Evidence for structural sympathetic reinnervation after orthotopic cardiac transplantation in humans. *Circulation* 1991;83:1210–1220.

38. Kaye DM, Esler M, Kingwell B, et al. Functional and neurochemical evidence for partial cardiac sympathetic reinnervation after cardiac transplantation in humans. *Circulation* 1993;88:1110–1118.

39. Bernardi L, Bianchini B, Spadacini G, et al. Demonstrable cardiac reinnervation after human heart transplantation by carotid baroreflex modulation of RR interval. *Circulation* 1995;92:2895–2903.

40. Rundquist B, Eisenhofer G, Dakak NA, et al. Cardiac noradrenergic function one year following cardiac transplantation. *Blood Press* 1993;2:252–261.

41. Burke MN, McGinn AL, Homans DC, et al. Evidence for functional sympathetic reinnervation of left ventricle and coronary arteries after orthotopic cardiac transplantation in humans [see comments]. *Circulation* 1995; 91:72–78.

42. Morgan HNJ, Kenny RA, Scott CD, et al. Vasodepressor reactions after orthotopic cardiac transplantation: Relationship to reinnervation status. *Clin Auton Res* 1994;4:125–129.

43. Rudas L, Pflugfelder PW, Menkis AH, et al. Evolution of heart rate responsiveness after orthotopic cardiac transplantation. *Am J Cardiol* 1991;68: 232–236.

44. Olivari MT, Levine TB, Ring WS, et al. Normalization of sympathetic nervous system function after orthotopic cardiac transplant in man. *Circulation* 1987;76:V62–V64.

45. Levine TB, Olivari MT, Cohn JN. Effects of orthotopic heart transplantation on sympathetic control mechanisms in congestive heart failure. *Am J Cardiol* 1986;58:1035–1040.

46. Banner NR, Patel N, Cox AP, et al. Altered sympathoadrenal response to dynamic exercise in cardiac transplant recipients. *Cardiovasc Res* 1989;23: 965–972.

47. Braith RW, Wood CE, Limacher MC, et al. Abnormal neuroendocrine responses during exercise in heart transplant recipients. *Circulation* 1992;86: 1453–63.

48. Mettauer B, Lampert E, Lonsdorfer J, et al. Cardiorespiratory and neurohormonal response to incremental maximal exercise in patients with denervated transplanted hearts. *Transplant Proc* 1991;23:1178–1181.

49. Perrault H, Melin B, Jimenez C, et al. Fluid-regulating and sympathoadrenal hormonal responses to peak exercise following cardiac transplantation. *J Appl Physiol* 1994;76:230–235.

50. Braith RW, Limacher MC, Leggett SH, Pollock ML. Skeletal muscle strength in heart transplant recipients. *J Heart Lung Transplant* 1993;12:1018–1023.

51. Mancini DM, LaManca JJ, Donchez LJ, et al. Diminished respiratory muscle endurance persists after cardiac transplantation. *Am J Cardiol* 1995;75:418–421.

52. Mettauer B, Lampert E, Lonsdorfer J, et al. Evidence for peripheral muscular limitation during exertion after heart transplantation (abstract). *Circulation* 1992;86:I400.

53. Bussieres-Chafe LM, Pflugfelder PW, Taylor AW, et al. Morphologic changes in peripheral skeletal muscle after cardiac transplantation (abstract). *Circulation* 1993;88:I145.

54. Bussieres-Chafe LM, Pflugfelder PW, Taylor AW, et al. Skeletal muscle oxidative capacity increases after cardiac transplantation (abstract). *Circulation* 1993; 88:I145.

55. Stratton JR, Kemp GJ, Daly RC, et al. Effects of cardiac transplantation on bioenergetic abnormalities of skeletal muscle in congestive heart failure. *Circulation* 1994;89:1624–1631.

56. Sinoway LI, Minotti JR, Davis D, et al. Delayed reversal of impaired vasodilation in congestive heart failure after heart transplantation. *Am J Cardiol* 1988;61:1076–1079.

57. Petrasko M, Horak J, Prerovsky I. Progression of venoconstriction in patients after heart transplantation during exercise. *Int J Cardiol* 1994;44:243–250.

58. Morgan BJ, DeBoer LW, Pease MO, et al. Forearm vascular resistance increases during static exercise in heart transplant recipients. *J Appl Physiol* 1991;71:2224–2230.

59. Haywood GA, Counihan PJ, Sneddon JF, et al. Increased renal and forearm vasoconstriction in response to exercise after heart transplantation. *Br Heart J* 1993;70:247–251.

60. Rueckert P, Lillis D, Slane P, et al. Partial restoration of calf vascular conductance pattern and improvement in exercise capacity following heart transplantation (abstract). *Circulation* 1995;92:I209–I210.

61. Kubo SH, Rector TS, Bank AJ, et al. Effects of cardiac transplantation on endothelium-dependent dilation of the peripheral vasculature in congestive heart failure. *Am J Cardiol* 1993;71:88–93.

62. Freimark D, Silverman JM, Aleksic I, et al. Atrial emptying with orthotopic heart transplantation using bicaval and pulmonary venous anastomoses: A magnetic resonance imaging study. *J Am Coll Cardiol* 1995;25:932–936.

63. Spes CH, Schnaack SD, Theisen K, Angermann CE. Cardiac function during graded bicycle exercise: Doppler-echocardiographic findings in normal subjects and heart transplant recipients. *Z Kardiol* 1993;82:324–331.

64. Siostrzonek P, Teufelsbauer H, Kreiner G, et al. Relief of diastolic cardiac

dysfunction after cyclosporine withdrawal in a cardiac transplant recipient. *Eur Heart J* 1993;14:859–861.

65. DePasquale NP, Burch GE. How normal is the donor heart? *Am Heart J* 1969;77:719–720.

66. Banner NR, Yacoub MH. Physiology of the orthotopic cardiac transplant recipient. *Semin Thorac Cardiovasc Surg* 1990;2:259–270.

67. Braith RW, Limacher MC, Mills RMJ, et al. Exercise-induced hypoxemia in heart transplant recipients. *J Am Coll Cardiol* 1993;22:768–776.

68. Young JB, Winters WLJ, Bourge R, Uretsky BF. 24th Bethesda Conference: Cardiac transplantation. Task Force 4: Function of the heart transplant recipient. *J Am Coll Cardiol* 1993;22:31–41.

69. Hall MJ, Snell GI, Side EA, et al. Exercise, potassium, and muscle deconditioning post-thoracic organ transplantation. *J Appl Physiol* 1994;77:2784–2790.

70. Kobashigawa J, Leaf D, Gleeson M, et al. Benefit of cardiac rehabilitation in heart transplant patients: A randomized trial (abstract). *J Heart Lung Transplant* 1994;13:S77.

71. Keteyian S, Shepard R, Ehrman J, et al. Cardiovascular responses of heart transplant patients to exercise training. *J Appl Physiol* 1991;70:2627–2631.

72. Ehrman J, Keteyian S, Fedel F, et al. Ventilatory threshold after exercsie training in orthotopic heart transplant recipients. *J Cardiopulmonary Rehabil* 1992;12:126–130.

73. Mettauer B, Lampert E, Schnedecker B, et al. A short endurance training program increases the physical fitness of heart transplant recipients. *Science and Sports* 1993;8:25–26.

74. Lonsdorfer J, Lampert E, Mettauer B, et al. Physical fitness after cardiac transplantation: A proposal for an endurance training program and its assessment. *Science and Sports* 1992;7:39–44.

75. Derman E, Selley K, Emms M, et al. Exercise performance and skeletal muscle pathology improves after cardiac transplantation and exercise training (abstract). *Eur Heart J* 1993;14(suppl):2358.

76. Squires R, Arthur P, Gau G, et al. Exercise after cardiac transplantation: A report of two cases. *J Cardiopulmonary Rehabil* 1983;3:570–574.

77. Degre S, Niset G, Desmet JM, et al. Effects of physical training on the denervated human heart after orthotopic cardiac transplantation. *Ann Cardiol Angeiol Paris* 1986;35:147–149.

78. Savin W, Gordon E, Green S, et al. Comparison of exercise training effects in cardiac denervated and innervated humans (abstract). *J Am Coll Cardiol* 1983;1:722.

79. Mettauer B, Lampert E, Hoppeler H, et al. Short term endurance training increases the muscular aerobic capacity in heart transplant patients (abstract). *J Am Coll Cardiol* 1995;25:236A–237A.

80. Niset GL, Piret AA, Delbarre N, et al. Functional non-invasive cardio-respiratory evaluation a month and a year after orthotopic heart transplantation. *Ann Cardiol Angeiol Paris* 1988;37:9–12.

81. Sieurat P, Roquebrune JP, Grinneiser D, et al. Monitoring and rehabilitation of heterotopic cardiac transplantation patients during the period of convalescence. *Arch Mal Coeur Vaiss* 1986;79:210–216.

82. Kavanagh T, Yacoub MH, Mertens DJ, et al. Exercise rehabilitation after heterotopic cardiac transplantation. *J Cardiopulmonary Rehabil* 1989;9:303–310.

83. Cousineau D, Ferguson RJ, deChamplain J, et al. Catecholamines in coronary sinus during exercise in man before and after training. *J Appl Physiol* 1977;43:801–806.

84. Winder WW, Hickson RC, Hagberg JM. Training-induced changes in hormonal and metabolic responses to submaximal exercise. *J Appl Physiol* 1979;46:766–771.
85. Hartley LH, Mason JW, Hogan RP, et al. Multiple hormonal responses to prolonged exercise in relation to physical training. *J Appl Physiol* 1972;33: 607–610.
86. Stratton JR, Cerqueira MD, Schwartz RS, et al. Differences in cardiovascular responses to isoproterenol in relation to age and exercise training in healthy men. *Circulation* 1992;86:504–512.
87. Kavanagh T. Exercise training in patients after heart transplantation. *Herz* 1991;16:243–250.
88. Stratton JR, Levy WC, Cerqueira MD, et al. Cardiovascular responses to exercise: Effects of aging and exercise training in healthy men. *Circulation* 1994;89:1648–1655.
89. DeSmet JM, Niset G, Degre S, Primo G. Jogging after heart transplantation (letter). *N Engl J Med* 1983;309:1521–1522.
90. Niset G, Poortmans JR, Leclercq R, et al. Metabolic implications during a 20-km run after heart transplantation. *Int J Sports Med* 1985;6:340–343.
91. Douglas PS, Sigler A, O'Toole ML, Hiller WD. Endurance exercise in the presence of heart disease. *Chest* 1989;95:697–699.
92. Kavanagh T, Yacoub MH, Campbell RB, Mertens DJ. Marathon running after cardiac transplantation: A case history. *J Cardiopulmonary Rehabil* 1986;6:16–20.
93. Wilson JR. Exercise intolerance in heart failure: Importance of skeletal muscle (editorial; comment). *Circulation* 1995;91:559–561.
94. Adamopoulos S, Coats A, Brunotte F, et al. Physical training improves skeletal muscle metabolism in patients with chronic heart failure. *J Am Coll Cardiol* 1993;21:1101–1106.
95. Minotti JR, Johnson EC, Hudson TL, et al. Skeletal muscle response to exercise training in congestive heart failure. *J Clin Invest* 1990;86:751–758.
96. Stratton JR, Dunn JF, Adamopoulos S, et al. Training partially reverses skeletal muscle metabolic abnormalities during exercise in heart failure. *J Appl Physiol* 1994;76:1575–1582.
97. Saini J, Geny B, Brandenberger G, et al. Training effects on the hydromineral endocrine responses of cardiac transplant patients. *Eur J Appl Physiol* 1995;70:226–233.
98. Falduto MT, Czerwinski SM, Hickson RC. Glucocorticoid-induced muscle atrophy prevention by exercise in fast-twitch fibers. *J Appl Physiol* 1990;69:1058–1062.
99. Czerwinski SM, Kurowski TG, O'Neill TM, Hickson RC. Initiating regular exercise protects against muscle atrophy from glucocorticoids. *J Appl Physiol* 1987;63:1504–1510.
100. Hickson RC, Czerwinski SM, Falduto MT, Young AP. Glucocorticoid antagonism by exercise and androgenic-anabolic steroids. *Med Sci Sports Exerc* 1990;22:331–340.
101. Schoutens A, Laurent E, Poortmans JR. Effects of inactivity and exercise on bone. *Sports Med* 1989;7:71–81.
102. Olivari MT, Antolick A, Ring WS. Arterial hypertension in heart transplant recipients treated with triple-drug immunosuppressive therapy. *J Heart Transplant* 1989;8:34–39.
103. Shimizu K, McGrath BP. Sympathetic dysfunction in heart failure. *Baillieres Clin Endocrinol Metab* 1993;7:439–463.

104. Cavero PG, Sudhir K, Galli F, et al. Effect of orthotopic cardiac transplantation on peripheral vascular function in congestive heart failure: Influence of cyclosporine therapy. *Am Heart J* 1994;127:1581–1587.
105. Shephard RJ. Responses to acute exercise and training after cardiac transplantation: A review. *Can J Sport Sci* 1991;16:9–22.
106. Shephard RJ. Responses of the cardiac transplant patient to exercise and training. *Exerc Sport Sci Rev* 1992;11:S237–S240.

The Exercise Training Program

Chapter 18

Screening and Evaluation of Patients for Exercise Training

Gerald F. Fletcher, MD and
Victor M. Fernandez, BS

Screening and Evaluation For Exercise Training

The screening and evaluation process of patients who have left ventricular dysfunction or who have undergone cardiac transplantation is similar to, though more detailed than that of other patients who are entering a cardiac rehabilitation-exercise training program.[1]

The discussion to follow will address basic fundamental components regarding the evaluation of patients with left ventricular dysfunction for cardiac exercise training. Importance of the referral data and information on the patient prior to evaluation will be addressed. A very complete history and physical examination followed by an in-depth evaluation of drugs and pharmacological agents used by the patient will be considered. This will be followed by a discussion of co-morbid states that may exist in such patients, and then by special studies and laboratory evaluation. Finally, the importance of exercise testing will be emphasized as the final step in preparation of such patients for exercise training (Table 1).

Referral Data

Patients with left ventricular dysfunction who are referred for exercise training must have had a complete medical evaluation, and the referral data must be available for review. These data include, but are not limited to, the specific evaluation of left ventricular function[2] and etiol-

From: Balady GJ, Piña IL (eds). *Exercise and Heart Failure*. Armonk, NY: Futura Publishing Company, Inc.; ©1997.

Table 1

Fundamental Components in the Evaluation of Subjects
With Left Ventricular Dysfunction for Exercise Training

Referral Data

History and physical examination
Drugs and pharmacological agents
Comorbid states
Special studies and laboratory
Exercise testing

ogy of the heart failure, and information on the structural and myocardial function of these patients. With regard to left ventricular function, nuclear studies such as thallium and sestamibi testing, radionuclide wall motion studies, and echocardiographic studies with or without contrast must be available for review. Positron emission tomography (PET) to assess the viability and metabolism of the myocardium is a newer technology and though infrequently used, may be of great benefit, if available.

The level of left ventricular function in these patients is usually in the range of 25% to 35% of left ventricular ejection fraction (LVEF). This level of LVEF may be associated with multiple problems in exercise training, such as arrhythmias and pulmonary congestion. Knowledge of the coronary anatomy and the previous procedures that have been done on a given patient, such as angioplasty, stents, bypass surgery, and the degree of success or failure of these interventions is vastly important. Knowledge of the ventricular function based on follow-up studies after interventions, compared to studies before, are also important data to have available.

In the event of valvular heart disease such as aortic or mitral disease, the status of the valvular function is important. Many patients referred to programs have mitral valve regurgitation with or without repair or intervention. They can usually be exercise trained more easily than those with aortic valvular disease. Aortic valvular disease, particularly aortic stenosis, is often a subtle entity, particularly in the older population and in those who have heart failure. These patients may have associated coronary artery disease or may have had coronary bypass surgery and are slowly developing significant aortic valve stenosis. This condition must be evaluated in the context of the patient's left ventricular function and the status of the coronary artery disease intervention. Aortic regurgitation, although more often clinically significant than mitral regurgitation, is a clinical state often present in patients with heart failure. These patients can usually be exercise trained with safety as long as their medical therapy is optimal.

Knowledge of technologies used, such as pacemakers, internal defibrillators, and other interventions, is important. The precise data on all of the aforementioned is necessary from the patient's referral source or from physicians who may have been involved over time in the care of the patient. Assimilation of these data and proper interpretation by the exercise training health professional staff, especially the physician in charge, is vital.

History and Physical Examination

The next step in the evaluation of the patient is the in-depth history and physical examination. The history will often incorporate much of the previous data on ventricular function, status of interventions, and complete information on medical therapy. The history must also include the attitude of the patient regarding exercise, the patient's previous exercise history, and whether or not the patient has had "athletism" as a part of his or her life prior to cardiac intervention. An in-depth history is important to procure knowledge of cardiovascular risk factors, obtain detailed past medical history and family history, and provide an opportunity for the patient and his or her spouse to discuss issues regarding his or her current state of health and health management.

The physical examination by the physician may be done with the aide of a nurse or physician extender. Blood pressure should be checked in both the standing and supine positions in order to assess postural hypotensive changes. Evaluation of the precordium for changes in left ventricular dynamics by inspection and palpation is of vast importance. Frequently, a hypokinetic or dyskinetic area of myocardial infarction may be the only clue to the persistence of left ventricular dysfunction. Atrial and ventricular gallop movements may also be seen and felt. This, incorporated with careful auscultation using both bell and diaphragm of the stethoscope are important. Subtle murmurs of aortic stenosis or aortic regurgitation may often be detected in certain patients, particularly the elderly, and detection can only be done by careful auscultation. Often, the echocardiogram will report trivial amounts of valvular regurgitation, which in a clinical examination are really of no significant impact; careful examination will clarify these issues. Careful auscultation for gallop rhythm—S_4 sound versus S_3 sound—is of importance. This is particularly noteworthy following exercise testing. Neck examination for evidence of jugular venous distention and increased venous pressure, with careful observation for waves of tricuspid regurgitation can be very helpful in an evaluation. In many patients, rhythm may be determined by careful observation of the atrial A wave in the neck. Evaluation of the carotid arteries by palpation and auscultation is of benefit as well. Alteration in the arterial pulse contour may suggest certain valvular disease, ie, an accentuated anacrotic notch (aortic stenosis) or a rapid upstroke (aortic or mitral regurgitation). Examination of the lungs, by percussion, for dullness, to suggest presence or absence of atelectasis or pleural fluid, and by auscultation, to determine presence or absence of pulmonary congestion, must be done. Abdominal examination to assess for an enlarged liver secondary to heart failure and also to evaluate the abdominal aorta for aneurysmal changes must be included. Examination of the peripheral pulses, particularly the femoral posterior tibials and dorsalis pedis, is important to evaluate for peripheral vascular disease. Often in patients with coronary artery disease, the atherosclerotic process is diffuse and carotid disease as well as peripheral vascular disease may be present. The presence or absence of pedal edema must be recorded.

The aforementioned physical examination findings are important with regard to evaluation of the patient for consideration of medication changes. It is also important to refer back to the physician for further management of the disease and/or to record progress, as these findings change in the exercise program.

Drugs and Pharmacological Agents

An in-depth review of drugs and pharmacological agents is next in importance. These may include digitalis preparations, nitrates, calcium blockers, β-blockers, angiotensin converting enzyme (ACE) inhibitors, and various types of diuretics. In addition, lipid-lowering agents, particularly the statin drugs (reductase inhibitors), antioxidants and in women particularly, estrogen-hormonal replacement may have been prescribed. Anticoagulants and antiplatelet agents should be addressed, specifically salicylates and warfarin drugs. The "pharmacological armamentarium" that many of these patients experience is quite complicated and must be addressed by the cardiac rehabilitation specialists as these patients are enrolled into the cardiac rehabilitation/exercise program. At times, patients have been seen by several physicians, and drugs that are not compatible, and may even be harmful, may have been prescribed. It is the role of the rehabilitation exercise screening to assess these drugs, dosages, times of consumption, and side effects. During the exercise program with an improved training effect, loss of weight, and with other changes, drug dosages and time of administration may need to be changed. This is best done on a regular basis by the rehabilitation team in concert with nurses and the medical director. Often, the patient's performance in the exercise training program is influenced by drugs and their metabolites. This should be considered, as one often finds that drugs are administered in doses that are too great or at times that are inconvenient for exercise.

Comorbid States

Comorbid states should be evaluated in detail, and assessment made of the potential impact on the training process.

Body Weight

The body weight of a patient in heart failure or with left ventricular dysfunction is of great concern. The greater the body weight, the more circulatory demands on an already compromised left ventricle. Dietary guidelines of calorie, fat, and cholesterol intake to control body weight are, therefore, immensely important.

Diabetes Mellitus

Diabetes mellitus is another prevalent condition, and is often seen in patients with left ventricular dysfunction. Diabetic cardiomyopathy has been described, and even in the presence of other types of cardiovascular disease such as coronary artery or valvular disease, the status of the diabetic state is of great importance. Control of hyperglycemia and hypoglycemia is important; the latter in particular during an exercise training program. Doses of insulin or oral hypoglycemic agents may have to be changed—an important component of the healthcare professional's role with these patients.[3-6]

Chronic Obstructive Pulmonary Disease

Chronic obstructive pulmonary disease is frequently seen in patients with left ventricular dysfunction. This state of lung compromise adds to the already decompensated cardiopulmonary status of these patients. Proper "pulmonary toilet" and medications administered under the care of a specialist are also of importance.

Peripheral Vascular Disease

Peripheral vascular disease may, in itself, be a limiting factor and impair the physical training of patients with left ventricular dysfunction. Atherosclerosis involves many vessels of the body in patients with coronary disease and ischemic cardiomyopathy, and can be improved with weight loss and regular exercise. These also tend to improve the peripheral arterial disease state.[7–9]

Special Studies and Laboratory Data

Next in the patient's evaluation are special studies and laboratory data acquired either prior to evaluation for the program or done during the time of evaluation. First and foremost is the 12-lead electrocardiogram (ECG). This is specifically helpful for the detection of arrhythmias, patterns of myocardial infarction, ventricular hypertrophy, bundle branch block conduction, and alteration of ST segments. A recent ECG should be available on entry to an exercise program. Chest x-rays (P-A and lateral views) are important and should be taken appropriately at entry. Review of the chest x-ray can detail pleural effusion and subtle signs of heart failure. In addition to the aforementioned, blood and urine studies are important. The status of the patient's red cell count, renal perfusion based on creatinine studies, and the status of the serum electrolytes (particularly the serum potassium level) are very important. Many patients with compromised left ventricles will be taking diuretics and must have blood potassium levels monitored. Chronic anemia is at times seen in heart failure, and when corrected, can improve the performance of such individuals.

Exercise Testing

Exercise testing has been considered in detail in Section IV of this book. However, it must be emphasized here that after all of the aforementioned data are collected, the exercise test is the most important basis on which to enter a patient into exercise training.[10] Testing should be done on a comfortable system adapted to the patient, preferably using a motorized treadmill or a bicycle ergometer. Emphasis should be placed on hemodynamics, heart rate and rhythm changes, ECG changes, and symptoms. The attainment of appropriate heart rate and systolic and diastolic blood pressure responses to exercise testing are very important in the screening process. Prognostic information can also be obtained by exercise testing.[11–13] Oxygen consumption studies are important, but are not necessary although they can provide more information with regard to the level of physical conditioning, initially and on follow-up testing.[14,15]

A pilot study of serial exercise testing in the setting of left ventricular dysfunction was done in 10 subjects to explore and evaluate testing methodology and assess results of testing in a sedentary cohort.

Patient Population

Ten male subjects ranging in age from 48–67 years ($\bar{x}$ 58), and receiving maintenance treatment for heart failure were studied. Heart failure was secondary to coronary heart disease in eight subjects; hypertensive heart and valvular heart disease in one, and coronary heart disease and cardiomyopathy in another. All showed evidence of severe left ventricular dysfunction (19% to 32% $\bar{x}$25) LVEF. Pulmonary disease was excluded by history, physical examination, and chest x-ray. No subject had experienced a myocardial infarction within 6 weeks nor did he or she have any mental or physical limitation, other than heart failure, that would impair performance of the exercise test. Subjects were also excluded from exercise testing if exercise capacity was severely limited because of mental, physical, or medical problems other than heart failure.

Protocol

Written informed consent was obtained from each subject. A modified progressive protocol (Table 2) that increases the estimated oxygen uptake by one metabolic equivalent (MET: 3.5 mL/kg of oxygen consumed per minute per stage) and is similar to the Modified Naughton Exercise Protocol was used. The grade was changed at every stage, thereby minimizing fatigue. The subjects were required to make weekly follow-up visits. Symptoms and signs of heart failure and New York Heart Association Functional Class[1a] were determined at every visit. Exercise testing and gas exchange determinations were performed at

Table 2

Graded Exercise Test Modified Progressive Protocol

Stage	Speed (mph)	Grade (%)	Duration (min)	Total Time Elapsed (min)
1	1.5	0.0	2	2
2	2.0	3.5	2	4
3	2.0	7.0	2	6
4	2.0	10.5	2	8
5	3.0	7.5	2	10
6	3.0	10.0	2	12
7	3.0	12.5	2	14
8	3.0	15.0	2	16
9	3.4	14.0	2	18

mph = miles per hour.

weeks 2, 4, 5, 6, 8, and 10. To establish an exercise intensity, at the end of each stage subjects were asked to rate their perceived exertion using the Borg Scale[16] and were encouraged to progress to their point of exhaustion. Other endpoints were: impaired blood pressure response, significant ECG S-T segment changes, and high-grade arrhythmias. A physician was in attendance for all testing. ECG was monitored continuously, as were vital signs at the end of each stage. Oxygen consumption and carbon dioxide production were measured continuously with a gas consumption analysis mixing chamber system.

Results

Study-entry laboratory results (hematology, chemistry, and urinary) were unremarkable and no clinically noteworthy changes were observed in follow-up tests. Throughout the serial-exercise testing period subjects were able to exercise for an average duration of 496 seconds per test without complications (Table 3). The reason most often cited for terminating exercise was fatigue and dyspnea.

One subject died 8 days after his last clinical visit. He collapsed while performing recreational activity and was resuscitated and defibrillated several times before admittance to a hospital intensive care unit. He was further treated for recurrent arrhythmias, but again experienced cardiovascular-pulmonary arrest and was not resuscitated.

Table 3

Baseline Exercise Testing and Left Ventricular Ejection Fraction Data in 10 Subjects with Left Ventricular Dysfunction

PT	ETT (seconds)	VO_2 max (mL/kg/min)	RER	EF (%)
1	467	17.66	1.16	19
2	328	12.23	1.13	21
3	478	18.80	1.03	30
4	288	19.70	0.94	28
5	442	16.80	1.18	23
6	490	19.00	0.91	32
7	517	19.50	1.08	25
8	714	25.40	1.06	26
9	682	27.60	1.01	22
10	558	16.10		28
Mean	496	19.28	1.06	25

PT = patient; ETT = exercise test time; VO_2 max = maximal oxygen consumption; RER = respiratory exchange ratio; EF = ejection fraction.

Summary

In summary, the screening and evaluation for exercise training of subjects with left ventricular dysfunction is a systematic process that includes obtaining previous data to determine details of the disease process and the manifestations of the disease, learning the patient's current history and physical examination, drug status and comorbid conditions, performing laboratory work, and most importantly, exercise testing. In the 10 subjects herein described and others reported, exercise testing was proven safe and efficacious[10] with carefully done protocols and proper supervision. Studies also reveal that subjects with left ventricular dysfunction can achieve a training effect with exercise rehabilitation.[17] The effect may be even greater with high-intensity training and this should be considered when appropriate.[18]

References

1. Fletcher GF, Balady G, Froelicher VF, et al. Exercise standards: A statement for healthcare professionals from the American Heart Association. Writing Group *Circulation* 1995;91:580–615.
1a. The Criteria Committee of the New York Heart Association, Inc. *Diseases of the Heart and Blood Vessels: Nomenclature and Criteria for Diagnosis. Sixth Edition;* Boston: Little Brown; 1964.
2. Hetherington M, Haennel R, Teo KK, Kappagoda T. Importance of considering ventricular function when prescribing exercise after acute myocardial infarction. *Am J Cardiol* 1986;58:891–895.
3. Devlin JT, Hirshman M, Horton ED, Horton ES. Enhanced peripheral and splanchnic insulin sensitivity in NIDDM men after single bout of exercise. *Diabetes* 1987;36:434–439.
4. Holloszy JO, Schultz J, Kusnierkiewicz J, et al. Effects of exercise on glucose tolerance and insulin resistance: Brief review and some preliminary results. *Acta Med Scand* 1986;711(suppl):55–65.
5. Kemmer FW, Tacken M, Berger M. Mechanism of exercise-induced hypoglycemia during sulfonylurea treatment. *Diabetes* 1987;36:1178–1182.
6. King DS, Dalsky GP, Clutter WE, et al. Effects of exercise and lack of exercise on insulin sensitivity and responsiveness. *J Appl Physiol* 1988;64:1942–1946.
7. Hiatt WR, Regensteiner JG, Hargarten ME. Benefit of exercise conditioning for patients with peripheral arterial disease. *Circulation* 1990;81:602–609.
8. Lundgren F, Dahllof AG, Schersten T, et al. Muscle enzyme adaptation in patients with peripheral arterial insufficiency: Spontaneous adaptation, effect of different treatments and consequences on walking performance. *Clin Sci (Colch)* 1989;77:485–493.
9. Lundgren F, Dahllof AG, Lundholm K, et al. Intermittent claudication: Surgical reconstruction or physical training? A prospective randomized trial of treatment efficiency. *Ann Surg* 1989;209:346–355.
10. Tristani FE, Hughes CV, Archibald DG, et al. Safety of graded symptom-limited exercise testing in patients with congestive heart failure. *Circulation* 1987;76:V154–V158.

11. Bobbio M, Detrano R, Schmid JJ, et al. Exercise-induced ST depression and ST/heart rate index to predict triple-vessel or left main coronary disease: A multicenter analysis. *J Am Coll Cardiol* 1992;19:11–18.
12. Dubach P, Froelicher VF, Klein J, et al. Exercise-induced hypotension in a male population. Criteria, causes, and prognosis. *Circulation* 1988;78:1380–1387.
13. Lee TH, Cook EF, Goldman L. Prospective evaluation of a clinical and exercise-test model for the prediction of left main coronary artery disease. *Med Decis Making* 1986;6:136–144.
14. Cohn JN. Quantitative exercise testing for the cardiac patient: The value of monitoring gas exchange: Introduction. *Circulation* 1987;76(suppl VI):VI-1–VI-2.
15. Morris CK, Myers J, Froelicher VF, et al. Nomogram based on metabolic equivalents and age for assessing aerobic exercise capacity in men. *J Am Coll Cardiol* 1993;22:175–182.
16. Borg GA. Psychophysical bases of perceived exertion. *Med Sci Sports Exerc* 1982;14:377–381.
17. Sullivan MJ, Higginbotham MB, Cobb FR. Exercise training in patients with chronic heart failure delays ventilatory anaerobic threshold and improves submaximal exercise performance. *Circulation* 1989;79:324–329.
18. Oberman A, Fletcher GF, Lee J, et al. Efficacy of high-intensity exercise training on left ventricular ejection fraction in men with coronary artery disease (the Training Level Comparison Study). *Am J Cardiol* 1995;76:643–647.

Chapter 19

Training Methods and Monitoring of Heart Failure Patients

Barbara J. Fletcher, BSN, RN, MN and Sandra Dunbar, RN, DSN

Current clinical guidelines for cardiac rehabilitation programs classify patients with left ventricular ejection fraction ≤30%, complex ventricular arrhythmias, and a flat or decreasing systolic blood pressure with exercise, as high risk individuals.[1] Exercise training for patients with depressed left ventricular ejection fraction (LVEF) must be individualized with regard to prescription, for length of monitoring and progression of activity. Generally, from 6 to 12 sessions of continuous ECG monitoring are adequate. However, if after this initial monitoring period, the patient is not considered clinically stable for his or her cardiac condition, more monitoring may be indicated. Some, but not all, patients with depressed LV function are capable of gradually progressing their activity to 85% of their testing capacity. Each patient should begin their exercise program at about 50% of capacity and progress to a maintenance level of 60% to 85%. It must be noted the maintenance level may be altered as the patient's clinical condition changes.

The recent *Clinical Practice Guidelines for Cardiac Rehabilitation* recommends exercise training for patients with heart failure and/or LV dysfunction to enhance functional and symptomatic improvement, but cautions a potential likelihood of adverse events.[2] This recommendation is based on data from five randomized control trials,[3-7] three nonrandomized control trials, and four observational reports. The five randomized control trials supported significant improvement in functional capacity, decreases in submaximal heart rate and rate pressure product, decreases in symptoms, and increases in maximal oxygen consumption and exer-

From: Balady GJ, Piña IL (eds). *Exercise and Heart Failure.* Armonk, NY: Futura Publishing Company, Inc.; ©1997.

cise duration. One[3] of the these studies reported a significant improvement in LVEF in the exercise group. These studies are limited by small numbers, and include mostly young male subjects with coronary artery disease as a major etiology of LV dysfunction. However, the predominant message, in addition to improvement in functional capacity, was that there was no correlation of improvement in this functional capacity compared with improvement in LVEF. It is this relationship of exercise training and change in LVEF that this chapter will address.

The five randomized, controlled studies aforementioned were predominantly done with lower extremity exercise training protocols[3-7] and a total duration of exercise training ranging from 800 minutes[4,5] to greater than 1800 minutes.[3,6,7] The one study reflecting positive change in LVEF[3] incorporated some arm exercise and included 1800 minutes of exercise training (Table 1). Three additional studies demonstrating improvement in LVEF with exercise training included upper extremity exercise and/or were greater than 1800 minutes of exercise training (Table 1).[8-10] In one study,[8] the exercise training protocol included both the use of an arm crank and a rowing machine for a mean duration of 1620 minutes, and demonstrated a significant between-group improvement in resting EF ($P<.05$), with the exercise group increasing EF (56% to 59%) and the usual care group decreasing EF (56% to 54%). At 1 year, the Training Level Comparison Trial (TLC)[9] showed that high intensity exercise training improved the change from rest to peak exercise LVEF in coronary artery disease subjects with normal LVEF at the outset, 6.20% to 6.73% compared to a decrease in LVEF in a similar group exercising at low intensity ($P<.05$). A trend towards improvement in LVEF was also seen in subjects randomized to high-intensity exercise training but with depressed LVEF at the outset. This study was of long duration (1 year) and included some upper extremity exercise. In addition to the TLC, the Physically Disabled/Coronary Artery Disease Study (PD/CAD) demonstrated a 10% ($P<.001$) increase in change in rest to peak exercise LVEF. This randomized experimental trial included men with coronary artery disease who had a concomitant physical disability requiring use of a wheelchair for daily activities. In this study, all subjects were randomized to exercise, trained only with upper extremities for a duration of 6 months, and were compared to the control group receiving usual and customary care.[10] Thus, data relating to exercise training and LVEF from these three studies,[8-10] and one other[3] raise important questions regarding the potential beneficial effect of added afterload in upper-extremity exercise training.

Based on this question of the added benefit of upper extremity exercise training in patients with depressed LVEF, we further examined subsets of two of the aforementioned studies, TLC[9] and PD/CAD.[10] TLC consisted of a total sample of 200 subjects prospectively randomized to 24 months of exercise training three times a week, with subjects randomized

Table 1

Exercise Training Studies Supporting Improvement in LVEF

Author/Year	Groups Training (N)	Groups Control (N)	Length of Training (Minutes)	Mode of Training	Change in LVEF
Grodzinski, Jetté, et al,[3] 1987	53	46	1800	Lower extremity Some swimming	▲ rest → peak Ex Gp 4.5% (p < .05) Control Gp − 2.0%
Ben-Are, Rothbaum, et al,[8] 1989	60	68	1080–2160 $\bar{x}$ 1620	Variety of stationary equipment, included rowing machine and arm crank	▲ rest EF Ex Gp 56% → 59% Control Gp 56% → 54% p < .05 between groups
Oberman, Fletcher, et al.,[9] 1995	111	89	7020	Walk/jog Arm-leg cycle Ergometer	▲ rest → peak Ex Gp 6.2% → 6.7% Control Gp 6.6% → 6.0% P < .05 between groups
Fletcher, Dunbar, et al,[10] 1994	41	47	2600	Upper extremity only	▲ rest → peak Ex Gp −1.2% → 8.8% (p = 0.01) Control Gp 4% → 6% (p = NS)

LVEF = left ventricular ejection fraction.

Table 2

Training Level Comparison
Exercise Prescription Baseline

EF 30%   Randomized: 85% Exercise Training

NAME:

RANDOMIZATION: X   HIGH _____ LOW

MONITOR: 04 _____ LEVEL: 9   SESSION: 9

EVALUATION 1 TM/02/DATA: MAX VO$_2$ 20.92 m/kg/min MAX METS   5.98

WEIGHT:LB   144   DIAGNOSIS: Anterior MI

Target HR Range	91–101 → HIGH:	Use HRs at 50-85% Vo$_2$ MAX ± bpm
Target MET Range	1.8–5.0 → HIGH:	30-85% MAX METS

PRE-EXERCISE   BP   122/82
              HR   60

METS	DEVICE	EXER Rx/ADJUST	HR	RPE	ARRHYTHMIAS	COMMENTS
2.0	Calisthenics	5 min	72	12	1 PVC	
4.9	Air Dyne	15 min / 1.5 resis	97	15	Frequent PVCs	
2.9	Arm Ergometer	7 min / 50 rpm / 1 BEL	96	15	1 vent couplet	
5.0	Treadmill	15 min / 4.1 mph / 0 grade	98	15	2 PVCs	

---

42   TOTAL MINUTES   POST-   BP 140/80

                           EXERCISE   HR 97

ADDITIONAL COMMENTS: Patient stable; will terminate continuous ECG monitoring

INITIALS OF EXERCISE SPECIALIST: _____ INITIALS OF M.D.: _____

to 50% $\dot{V}O_{2max}$ exercise training (low intensity) or 85% $\dot{V}O_{2max}$ exercise training (high intensity). This exercise protocol predominantly trained lower extremities, but did not incorporate a stationary bicycle ergometer, which exercise trains both arms and legs. In addition to the arm-leg bicycle ergometer, subjects participated in a walk/jog program consisting of 45 to 60 minutes, three times per week, at their prescribed intensity.

Table 3

Training Level Comparison
Exercise Prescription *3 months*

EF 30%   Randomized: 85% Exercise Training

NAME:

EXERCISE PRESCRIPTION

TARGET HR RANGE   103   to   113
         10 s Count   17   to   19

EXERCISE INTENSITY   MAX METS: 8.2

TRAINING MET LEVEL (80% to 85%)   6.6 to 7.0

METS:

6.5 Walk: 30 minutes @ 1 : 41 min/lap FOR 18 laps
X Jog: ____ minutes @ ___ : ___ min/lap FOR ____ laps
6.9 Airdyne: 15 minutes @ 2.25 workload

The subpopulation of TLC selected for this discussion consisted of those patients with LVEF $\leq 50\%$ (N = 67 of 200) at the outset. Thirty of 67 patients were prospectively randomized to exercise training at low intensity, versus 37 randomized to high intensity exercise training. It is of note that all subjects with depressed LVEF could safely exercise at their prescribed intensity, whether high or low, for the duration of the study, and continuous ECG monitoring was terminated for all subjects between 6 and 12 sessions.

Exercise prescriptions for both groups were derived from each previous exercise test, which included measured oxygen consumption. Metabolic levels were then calculated and the exercise prescription adjusted according to the randomized category. Arrhythmias noted during exercise tended to be not unique to the randomization, but unique to the individual patient. Patients were able to progress and to achieve their exercise prescription without complications, whether randomized to 50% $\dot{V}O_{2max}$ exercise training, or 85% $\dot{V}O_{2max}$ exercise training. An example of baseline and 3-month, 85% $\dot{V}O_{2max}$ exercise prescription are seen in Table 2 and Table 3.

Results of the subset with subjects of $\leq 50\%$ LVEF at baseline are noted in Table 4, with regard to change in rest and peak ejection fraction

Table 4

Results: Training Level Comparison Study
Ejection Fraction Results for Baseline LVEF ≤50% Groups

x̄ Rest EF% (SE)(Range)   (N = 67)

Exercise Gp	Baseline	6 Months
50% VO$_2$ Max (N = 30)	40.23 (1.42)(22.0–49.0)	44.00 (1.85)(28.0–64.0)*
85% VO$_2$ Max (N = 37)	42.03 (.088)(29.0–49.0)	46.16 (1.14)(3.1.0–61.0)*

x̄ Peak EF% (SE)(Range)

50% VO$_2$ Max	43.29 (1.79)(24.0–56.0)	48.83 (2.29)(28.0–68.0)*
85% VO$_2$ Max	45.49 (1.33)(31.0–63.0)	50.87 (1.62)(35.0–72.0)*

*$P < .001$ within groups; N = number; Gp = group.
LVEF = left ventricular ejection fraction.

at baseline and 6 months, for both low and high exercise groups. There was a significant increase within groups, both for rest and peak LVEF at 6 months. However, since considerable intersubject variation exists, one should consider these results only a trend towards demonstrating an improved LVEF, whether randomized low-intensity or high-intensity, with lower and upper extremity exercise training for a duration of 3500 minutes. There were no significant differences in baseline to 6 months in rest or peak heart rate and systolic blood pressure.

The PD/CAD[10] study sample consisted of 72 male subjects, all with coronary artery disease and an accompanying physical disability requiring use of a wheelchair. All underwent baseline exercise testing prior to randomization to home exercise or to a control group for 6 months. There were 57 subjects with LVEF greater than 50% in this study, thus leaving a subset of 15 subjects with LVEF of ≤50%. Of these 15, eight were randomized to home exercise for 6 months and seven were randomized to control for 6 months.

Subjects in the home-exercise group were given wheelchair ramps that transformed their wheelchairs into stationary wheelchair ergometers. Exercise training consisted of "free wheeling" the stationery wheelchair with upper extremities for 20 minutes a day, five times per week. The control group, also wheelchair bound, followed routine physician orders. The results of this subgroup (Table 5) of the PD/CAD study showed a significant increase in rest LVEF at 6 months in the home-exercise group ($P<.01$) and peak exercise LVEF at 6 months ($P<.05$ within and between groups).

Table 5

Results: Physically Disabled/Coronary Artery Diseases Study

Ejection Fraction Results for Baseline
LVEF ≤50% Groups
(N = 15)

	Baseline	6 Months
x̄ Rest EF% (SD)(Range)		
Home exercise	44.6 (4.93)(36.0–50.0)	57.8 (10.22)(47.0–79.0)*
(N = 8)		
Control	40.0 (6.76)(26.0–48.0)	46.4 (14.35)(27.0–64.0)
(N= 7)		
x̄ Peak EF% (SD)(Range)		
Home exercise	50.1 (9.39)(38.0–62.0)	60.9 (8.34)(52.0–77.0)†
Control	53.8 (7.69)(38.0–60.0)	46.8 (12.93)(37.0–69.0)

*$P < .01$ (Within group)

†$P < .05$ (Within and between groups).

Summary

In summary, methods and monitoring of exercise training in patients with depressed LVEF, are similar to methods and monitoring of patients with normal LVEF. The progression may be slower and require additional ECG monitoring. Limited data do support improved LVEF with exercise training in patients with LV dysfunction, especially in those studies incorporating upper-extremity exercise training as part of the protocol and/or duration of ≥1800 minutes of exercise training. Substantial data support additional benefits of exercise training as well as safety of exercise training in this same subset of patients. The exact type of exercise program that will be most beneficial with regard to modality and intensity of exercise training in subjects with LV dysfunction remains to be seen. Until further studies are available, it is realistic to recommend upper-extremity exercise training as part of the exercise prescription in subjects with depressed LVEF.

References

1. *Guidelines for Cardiac Rehabilitation Programs, American Association of Cardiopulmonary Rehabilitation, 2nd Edition.* Champaign, Il: Human Kinetics; 1995.
2. *Cardiac Rehabilitation as Secondary Prevention, Clinical Practice Guidelines,* #17. AACPR. Publication #96–0673, October 1995.
3. Grodzinski E, Jetté M, Blümchen G, et al. Effects of a four-week training

program on left ventricular function as assessed by radionuclide ventriculography. *J Cardiopulmonary Rehabil* 1987;7:517–524.

4. Coats AJS, Adamopaulos S, Meyer TE, et al. Medical science: Effects of physical training in chronic heart failure. *Lancet* 1990;335:63–66.

5. Meyer TE, Casadei B, Coats AJS, et al. Angiotensin-converting enzyme inhibition and physical training in heart failure. *J Int Med* 991;230:407–413.

6. Giannuzzi P, Tavazzi L, Temporelli PL, et al. Long-term physical training and left ventricular remodeling after anterior myocardial infarction: Results of the Exercise in Anterior Myocardial Infarction (EAMI) Trial. *J Am Coll Cardiol* 1993;22:1821–1829.

7. Giannuzzi P, Temporelli PL, Tavazzi L, et al. EAMI-Exercise training in anterior myocardial infarction: An ongoing multicenter randomized study: Preliminary results on left ventricular function and remodeling. *Chest* 1992;101:315–321.

8. Ben-Are E, Rothbaum DA, Linnemeir TA, et al. Benefits of a monitored rehabilitation program versus physician care after emergency percutaneous transluminal coronary angioplasty: Follow-up of risk factors and rate of restenosis. *J Cardiovascular Pulm Rehab* 1989;7:281–285.

9. Oberman A, Fletcher GF, Lee JY, et al. Efficacy of high-intensity exercise training on left ventricular ejection fraction in men with coronary artery disease. (The Training Level Comparison Study). *Am J Cardiol* 1995;76:643–647.

10. Fletcher BJ, Dunbar SB, Felmer JM, et al. Exercise testing and training in physically disabled men with clinical evidence of coronary artery disease. *Am J Cardiol* 1994;73:170–174.

Chapter 20

Training Methods and Monitoring of Cardiac Transplant Patients

Ileana L. Piña, MD

Patients who have undergone cardiac transplantation pose a challenge to the cardiac rehabilitation team. Not only have many of these patients been hospitalized repeatedly and for prolonged periods, leading to marked deconditioning, but they are also often cachectic and malnourished. Cardiac transplantation offers these patients a new source of central cardiovascular blood flow. The periphery, however, remains the same or perhaps worse due to anesthesia and further prolonged bed rest added to steroid use. In addition, after transplantation, the state of denervation does not allow the heart rate to be used as a measure of work intensity. Hence, the rehabilitation team must rely on clinical judgment and on perceived level of exertion to guide exercise therapy.

Pre-Transplantation

Ideally, transplant candidates should initiate exercise as soon as they undergo evaluation, if at all possible. The program should include aerobic training as well as resistive exercise. Aerobic training has been shown to be safe in heart failure patients.[1,2] Resistive training, however, is not as well studied in this population. If a program is instituted pretransplantation, the patient will be familiar with exercise modes such as range of motion, and be able to reinitiate these with minimal re-education shortly after transplantation. Moreover, if in a better conditioned state pretransplant, the few days of intubation and inactivity will do little to reverse this level of conditioning.

For those patients who become dependent on inotropic therapy and are listed as Status I, the same type of program can be instituted

From: Balady GJ, Piña IL (eds). *Exercise and Heart Failure.* Armonk, NY: Futura Publishing Company, Inc.; ©1997.

in the hospital. A set routine consisting of bicycle, treadmill, upper body ergometry, and free weights can be carried out safely in the controlled intensive care setting. Walking can often dissipate boredom and add to the patient's functional capacity. The exercise intensity may have to be determined by patient symptomatology, rather than by heart rate or rating of perceived exertion (RPE). We recommend exercise as an adjunct to pharmacological therapy during the entire waiting period for Status II patients. The recently published Agency for Health Care Policy and Research (AHCPR) Guidelines on Cardiac Rehabilitation recommends exercise training both prior to and after transplantation.[3]

Post Transplantation

Post transplantation, while chest tubes and pacer wires are present, exercise consists mainly of passive and active range of motion accompanied by incentive spirometry to facilitate pulmonary toilet. Sitting in a chair follows soon thereafter, when leg raising and hip girdle exercises become useful as a preparation to transfer weight from sitting to standing. Once the patient is able to stand, ambulation ensues, initially in the patient room, then progressing to the ward. It is assumed at this point that the patient is on telemetry monitoring. Intensity continues to be assessed by RPE, more commonly using the Borg Scale. Prior to discharge, if no rejections are experienced, the patient may be able to exercise on a stationary bicycle ergometer and/or treadmill. It is our preference to perform a predischarge cardiopulmonary exercise test to better define an exercise prescription for an outpatient program. The rehabilitation team should not be surprised to find a peak $\dot{V}O_2$ that is very similar to the value pretransplantation, demonstrating the importance of the deconditioned periphery. The impact of corticosteroids on the exercise response has not been well studied to date in cardiac transplant recipients.

The exercise prescription post transplantation includes all the essentials of intensity, duration, frequency, and progression. The receiving rehabilitation programs should also be given specific exercise modalities such as resistive training, after the first 6 weeks post transplantation. The RPE at the anaerobic threshold serves to prescribe intensity, since as noted above, the heart rate will not be commensurate of effort. The anaerobic threshold or ventilatory threshold has been shown to correlate with the lactate threshold in transplant recipients.[4] Warm up and cool down are essential, with a minimum of 20 minutes at the prescribed intensity. Exercises should be performed in a monitored setting three times per week for 6 to 8 weeks. A walking program is recommended for alternate days. An extension of this timetable is often necessary to take into account early episodes of rejection or infection that may preclude exercise for several days at a time.

The results of an exercise program will depend highly on the motivation of the individual, and are presented in detail in Chapter 18. Kavanagh and colleagues[5] show a significant difference in the VO_{2max} achieved in the more compliant patients after transplantation. Table 1 compares the hemodynamic responses before and after training in a group of moderately compliant (n = 28) and highly compliant (n = 8) patients, after a 2-year walk-jog program. In the more compliant group, the resting heart rate decreased by a greater amount and the VO_2 also increased significantly higher than in the moderately compliant group. In both groups, however, the amount of work achieved increased, as did the peak double product achieved at similar effort levels, as measured by RER and RPE.

Table 2 illustrates the hemodynamic response of a group of 21 cardiac transplant recipients who underwent the rehabilitation program at Temple University Medical Center, which consists of training at or near the ventilatory threshold with aerobic interval modalities for at least 20 minutes, two to three times per week. Upper-body ergometry was used, as well as small free weights of 2 to 5 lbs. Warm-up and cool down consisted of stretching and range-of-motion activity for 5 to 10 minutes. Patients were tested while free of rejection. The duration of exercise, as well as the peak VO_2, improved significantly with similar level of effort. The improvement in the ventilatory threshold mirrored the peak VO_2. Neither the peak exercise heart rate nor the blood pressure changed. The O_2 pulse, as an indirect measurement of stroke volume also improved.

Table 1

Rehabilitation PostCardiac Transplantation

	Pre-training Moderately Compliant	Post-training Moderately Compliant	Pre-training Highly Compliant	Post-training Highly Compliant
Rest HR (bpm)	100	99	117	106
Peak HR (bpm)	133	146	146	158
Rest SBP (mm Hg)	139	125	132	126
Peak SBP (mm Hg)	182	174	165	175
VO$_2$ Max (cc/min/kg)	21.8	24.5	21.3	32.3

HR = heart rate; SBP = systolic blood pressure. Adapted from Reference 5.

Table 2

Cardiopulmonary Testing in Cardiac Transplant Recipients
Before and After Cardiac Rehabilitation

	Pre-rehab	Post-rehab
Heart rate (bpm)	119 ± 27	127 ± 24
Peak BP (mm Hg)	$144 \pm 29/77 \pm 13$	$139 \pm 26/75 \pm 12$
Peak VO_2 (cc/min/kg)	17.1 ± 5.3	$23.0 \pm 8.8*$
Peak RER	1.1 ± 0.12	1.07 ± 0.0
Duration	11.0 ± 4.6	$15.7 \pm 6.0*$
O_2 pulse	10.5 ± 3.6	$13.6 \pm 5.4*$
VT	12.5 ± 6.1	$17.8 \pm 7.2*$
(cc/min/kg)	(n = 13)	(n = 18)

BP = blood pressure; RER = respiratory exchange ratio (VCO_2/VO_2); Duration = time
on treadmill in minutes; O_2 pulse = VO_2/hr; VT = ventilatory threshold.

References

1. Giannuzzi P, Temporelli PL, Tavazzi L, et al. EAMI-exercise training in anterior myocardial infarction: An ongoing multicenter randomized study: Preliminary results on left ventricular function and remodeling. *Chest* 1002;101(suppl 5):315S–321S.
2. Giannuzzi P, Tavazzi L, Temporelli PL, et al. Long-term physical training and left ventricular remodeling after anterior myocardial infarction: Results of the Exercise in Anterior Myocardial Infarction (EAMI) Trial. *J Am Coll Cardiol* 1993;22:1821–1829.
3. Wenger NK, Froelicher ES, Smith LK, et al. *Cardiac Rehabilitation, Clinical Practice Guideline, No. 17.* US Department of Health and Human Services, Public Health Service, Agency for Health Care Policy and Research, National Heart, Lung, and Blood Institute, AHCPR Publication No. 96–0672, Rockville, MD:1995.
4. Brubaker PH, Berry MJ, Brozena SC, et al. Relationship of lactate and ventilatory thresholds in cardiac transplant patients. *Med Sci Sports Exerc* 1993;191–196.
5. Kavanagh T, Yacoub MH, Mertens DJ, et al. Cardiorespiratory responses to exercise training after orthotopic cardiac transplantation. *Circulation* 1988; 77,1:162–171.

Chapter 21

Costs and Reimbursement Issues for Exercise Training Programs

Suzanne K. White, MN, RN, FAAN, FCCM, CNAA

The American health care system is under scrutiny. Total medical expenses continue to climb each year. An estimated $900 billion, 13.4 % of the GNP, was spent in 1993 on health care. Cardiovascular disease, in particular, is expensive and estimated to cost $151.3 billion in 1996[1]. To combat these expenditures, many believe that managed care is our future. It is predicted by the year 2000, managed care will overwhelmingly predominate. Basically, managed care integrates payment for care with delivery of care, with the primary objective to provide the enrollee with the best care at the least cost. If managed care health plans are to be successful, they must keep people healthy and out of the hospital. With national attention focused on rising health care costs, the government and medical insurers are demanding justification of the economic benefits of medical therapies. Cardiac therapies such as cardiac rehabilitation (exercise training, risk factor modification, education, and counseling) are being questioned as to cost effectiveness. Does this therapy keep patients healthier and out of the hospital? This chapter will address the costs and reimbursement of exercise training in patients with heart failure and after cardiac transplantation.

Heart failure places an enormous burden on society, consuming more than $10 billion in health care expenditures each year. It is estimated that over 4 million Americans currently have heart failure, and that it is the only cardiovascular disorder that is increasing in prevalence. Heart failure is the most common discharge diagnosis for Medicare patients who are hospitalized, and the fourth most common discharge diagnosis for all hospitalized patients in the United States.[2] Additionally, about 2300 heart transplants were performed in 1993. Almost 80% will

From: Balady GJ, Piña IL (eds). *Exercise and Heart Failure*. Armonk, NY: Futura Publishing Company, Inc.; ©1997.

survive more than 2 years. An average transplant costs about $100,000 plus an annual drug cost of $15,000, representing an expense of about $265 million for the transplants in 1993.[1] Application of cardiac rehabilitation services to patients with heart failure and after cardiac transplantation has gained increasing recognition and acceptance, as its benefits and safety are documented.[3]

Potential Benefits of Cardiac Rehabilitation in Patients with Heart Failure and Cardiac Transplantation

Most studies of exercise training in patients with heart failure and moderate-to-severe left ventricular dysfunction do not demonstrate deterioration in left ventricular function. In fact, most studies document improvement in functional capacity and symptoms. Some limitations of these studies include small numbers, with predominately younger male populations and coronary disease as the major cause of heart failure. Peripheral (skeletal muscle) adaptations appear to create the favorable training effect in exercise tolerance. Exercise training augments the symptomatic and functional benefits of angiotensin-converting enzyme (ACE) inhibitor therapy. Low-to-moderate intensity exercise and home-exercise programs provide benefit, but adverse events may occur in this high-risk patient group. In summary, cardiac rehabilitation training is recommended to attain functional and symptomatic improvement.[3]

Cardiac transplantation is a relatively recent surgical therapy, particularly as related to the use of exercise training as an intervention. Limited studies demonstrate improvement in exercise capacity in these medically-complex and often debilitated patients, pretransplant. Pretransplant strength training may enhance preoperative status and operative recovery. The effects of exercise training post transplant requires further study.[3]

Basic Economic Terms

In economics, a distinction is typically made between the concept of costs and that of charges. *Costs* reflects what a hospital actually spends to provide goods or services. *Charges* are what a hospital bills a patient or the patient's insurer for goods or services. While an assessment of actual costs is very beneficial to insurance companies, it is unlikely that hospitals will actively pursue cost studies or make actual costs available to third-party payers.[4] Therefore, any discussion of the costs of cardiac rehabilitation really concerns patient charges. Thus, costs and charges will be used interchangeably. Increasingly insurers—especially public insurers (Government—Medicare, Medicaid)—desire discounts. They do not want to pay full-billed charges. Another significant term is *reimbursement*, or what an insurer pays for goods or services.[4] Today reimbursement reflects neither costs nor charges, but rather some dollar amount, possibly negotiated between the insurer and health care facility.

There are two large categories of payers in the United States: (1) Public (Government—Medicare, Medicaid) and (2) Private (insurance companies).

Cost-Benefit Data

Although cost-benefit data are limited, studies show that comprehensive cardiac rehabilitation programs reduce hospitalization rates, lessen the need for cardiac medications, and increase the rates of return to work.[5-10] Although none of these studies provide comprehensive economic analysis, the costs of cardiac rehabilitation must be considered in view of the benefits.[2] Through review of the literature and a survey of major facilities throughout the United States, some costs and benefits will be presented in this chapter. No studies were found, that specifically addressed the cost-benefit of cardiac rehabilitation in patients with heart failure or cardiac transplantation. Limited studies have shown some clinical benefits of cardiac rehabilitation in these patients, as discussed previously. Therefore, the costs of cardiac rehabilitation programs in general are relevant and will be reviewed.

Average participation charges of cardiac rehabilitation programs vary based on the model chosen, the provider, the region of the country, and patient status. In 1991, program charges in the United States ranged from $1080 to $3600 (unpublished data, Linda Hall, 1992) for a 3-month program. In 1988, a survey of 1100 cardiac centers calculated a mean charge of $1305 for a standard 36-session, 3-month program of supervised exercise and risk factor modification,[14] along with $200 to $250 for a baseline exercise tolerance test. Costs for long-term Phase III programs are significantly lower than for Phase II programs, and are generally in the range of $400 to $750 per year.[8] In 1993, Bittner and Oberman[12] report that in a typical program with 30 sessions in 12 weeks (80% compliance) and an average cost of $40 per session, the estimated annual cost of cardiac rehabilitation is $1200 per participant or $120 million for each 100,000 participants. The cost-benefit of cardiac rehabilitation may occur by favorably changing the course of atherosclerotic disease or by changing patient behavior such that inpatient health care is minimized and work productivity is maximized.[5]

According to Ades, Huang, and Weaver, participation in a 3-month outpatient cardiac rehabilitation program was associated with a significantly decreased cost for cardiac readmissions in 580 patients after their coronary events. Over a 21-month follow-up period, per capita hospital admission billing was $739 lower in the cardiac rehabilitation patients ($P = 0.022$).[5] Two Swedish trials of cardiac rehabilitation in coronary bypass patients[13] and myocardial infarction patients[7] further support lowered health care costs following cardiac rehabilitation. In the initial study of 147 coronary bypass patients, readmissions to the hospital were reduced by 62% over a 1-year period in the outpatient cardiac rehabilitation group. A subsequent 5-year study compared comprehensive cardiac rehabilitation with routine care in 305 nonselected postmyocardial infarction patients. The average hospital length of stay was reduced from 16.1 days to 10.7 days in the intervention group. The authors conclude that the actual costs of the rehabilitation program were balanced over a 5-year follow-up period by the decrease in readmissions for cardiovascular diseases. Also, rehabilitated patients returned to work more frequently and had decreased costs due to sick leave, resulting in an overall 5-year cost savings of $12,250 (U.S. dollars) per patient.

In a randomized trial of 8 weeks of comprehensive cardiac rehabilitation, 6 weeks following a myocardial infarction, each patient was estimated to gain 0.052 quality-adjusted life years. This is similar to the cost-effectiveness of medical interventions such as coronary artery bypass surgery for left main coronary artery disease and more cost-effective than interventions such as captopril for hypertension, or lovastatin for hypercholesterolemia.[10] In another randomized study, an occupational work evaluation was the primary intervention in patients who were working prior to myocardial infarction. Patients were given instructions about exercise and other interventions to be performed at home with nurse follow-up. At the 6-month follow-up, an earlier return to work in the intervention patients resulted in an average increase in earned salary of $2100 per patient. Additionally, intervention patients had an average decrease in outpatient medical care costs of $500 per patient.[14] Finally, a nonrandomized trial of 190 patients, 65 years of age or older, following myocardial infarction described effects of a nurse-managed educational program of 4 months duration and low-intensity exercise training of 8 weeks duration. This resulted in significantly lower rates of rehospitalization ($P<.04$) and days of rehospitalization ($P = .05$) in the intervention group compared to the control group at 3 months. Additionally, significantly fewer emergency department visits occurred in the intervention patients within 1 year ($P = .005$). No financial data were reported, but this difference is likely to result in substantial savings.[15]

Participation charges in a survey of 10 cardiac rehabilitation programs across the United States range from $47 to $80 per session or $1692 to $2880 for 12 weeks in Phase II. Charges for long-term Phase III programs are much lower than Phase II, and are generally in the range of $34 to $115 per month or $408 to $1380, annually. Exercise stress test costs vary from $250 to $350. The differences in models of cardiac rehabilitation and costs make it difficult to compare across institutional programs.

Reimbursement of Services

Lack of support from third-party payers may limit the access of many patients to cardiac rehabilitation services, even though studies have shown clinical benefit of these services. Medicare generally covers 80% of the defined payment if criteria are met. Coverage is considered reasonable and necessary only for patients with a clear medical need, who are referred by their attending physician and (1) have a documented diagnosis of acute myocardial infarction within the preceding 12 months; or (2) have had coronary bypass surgery; and/or (3) have stable angina pectoris.[16] Currently nonischemic dilated cardiomyopathy is not considered a reimbursible diagnosis for cardiac rehabilitation under Medicare.

Cardiac rehabilitation programs may be provided by either the outpatient department of a hospital or in a physician-directed clinic. Coverage for either program is subject to the following conditions:[16]

- The facility must meet the definition of a hospital outpatient department or a physician-directed clinic, ie, a physician is on the premises and available to perform medical duties at all times the facility is open, and each patient is under the care of a hospital or clinic physician.
- The facility must have available for immediate use all the necessary cardiopulmonary emergency diagnostic and therapeutic life-saving equipment accepted by the medical community as medically necessary, eg, oxygen, cardiopulmonary resuscitation equipment, or defibrillator.
- The program must be conducted in an area set aside for the exclusive use of the program while it is in session.
- The program must be staffed by the personnel necessary to conduct the program safely and effectively, who are trained in both basic and advanced life-support techniques and in exercise therapy for coronary disease. Services of nonphysician personnel must be furnished under the direct supervision of

a physician. Direct supervision means that a physician must be in the exercise program area and immediately available and accessible for an emergency at all times the exercise program is conducted. It does not require that a physician be physically present in the exercise room itself, provided that the contractor does not determine that the physician is too remote from the patients' exercise area to be considered immediately available and accessible.

- The nonphysician personnel must be employees of either the physician, hospital, or clinic conducting the program and their services are "incident-to a physician's professional services."

A prospective candidate for a cardiac rehabilitation program must be evaluated for his or her suitability to participate. A valuable diagnostic test for this purpose is the exercise test. The program need not necessarily include an exercise test, but may accept one performed by the patient's attending physician. Exercise testing performed in the outpatient department of a hospital or in a physician-directed clinic may be covered when reasonable and necessary for one or more of the following[16]: (1) Evaluation of chest pain, especially atypical chest pain; (2) Development of exercise prescriptions for patients with known cardiac disease; and/or (3) Pre-and postoperative evaluation of patients undergoing coronary artery bypass procedures.

ECG rhythm strips (and other ECG monitoring) constitute an important and necessary procedure that should be done periodically while a cardiac patient is engaged in a patient-controlled exercise program.[16] Services provided in connection with a cardiac rehabilitation exercise program may be considered reasonable and necessary for up to 36 sessions, usually three sessions a week in a single 12-week period. Coverage for continued participation in cardiac exercise programs beyond 12 weeks is allowed only on a case-by-case basis with exit criteria taken into consideration.[16]

Although firm exit criteria for terminating the therapeutic outpatient exercise treatment and rehabilitation program have not been established, the following guidelines have been identified as acceptable:[16]

- The patient has achieved a stable level of exercise tolerance without ischemia or dysrhythmia.
- Symptoms of angina or dyspnea are stable at the patient's maximum exercise level.
- Patient's *resting* blood pressure and heart rate are within normal limits.
- The stress test is not *positive* during exercise. (A *positive* test

in this context implies an ECG with a junctional depression of 2mm or more associated with slowly rising, horizontal, or down sloping ST segment).

Medicaid generally will not pay for any follow-up after a transplant or for Phase III. Medicaid will pay for Phase II if it is medically necessary and not related to a transplant. Commercial carriers usually pay a percentage of Phase II and Phase III. This percentage ranges from 50% to 80%. Some Blue Cross plans will pay for Phase II as long as it is medically necessary. Some Blue Cross plans will pay for Phase III and some will not. Managed care plans' coverage ranges from 30% to 50% for Phase III. Each individual's insurance plan must be reviewed to determine if cardiac rehabilitation is covered.

Suggestions for Proactive Entry into Managed Care

As managed care and HMOs assume a greater role in health care delivery, the role of cardiac rehabilitation will be different than it has been in a fee-for-service system. Cardiac rehabilitation will almost certainly be an integral part of managed care. It is important that managers and leaders in cardiac rehabilitation become fluent in the language of managed care, and knowledgeable about its structure. These managers and leaders must be proactive and help design the role of cardiac rehabilitation in a managed care environment. Hall[17] makes the following suggestions for proactive entry into managed care:

1.   Cost-out the specific patient care activities involved in the cardiac rehabilitation program: How much does it cost to apply one unit of service and what is the revenue for the service? How does this compare to the closest competitors?
2.   Measure outcomes of applied services to determine the following: Change over time (3, 6, and 12 months) in risk factors, rehospitalizations, return to work, and psychosocial outcomes. Of particular interest is money saved from reduction in medications, rehospitalizations, physician office visits, and return to work.

In July, 1994 the Social Security Administration redefined its cardiovascular guidelines for determining disability. A heart transplant is considered a life-improving treatment, and disability is only granted for 1 year post-transplant. This presents quite a different picture from previous years, when having a heart transplant granted one a "permanent" type of disability. Disability has always been subject to reevaluation, but a much lower priority was set for review following heart transplantation. Many heart transplant recipients who have been out of the job force for a long time are unable to return to their previous occupation or lack the skills to reenter the job force successfully. Studies across the nation are reporting the unemployment rate for recipients at a minimum of 83%. This demonstrates a crucial need for substantial rehabilitation services if the transplant is to be considered completely successful.

3. Start to work with the managed care department that is designing the managed care models. Be ready with several plans to accomplish excellent outcomes within a managed care model.
4. Review cardiac rehabilitation department services, personnel, and procedures. Look at every aspect and ask the following: Is the best possible outcome achieved using the fewest resources? Compare cardiac rehabilitation services from the closest competitor in the geographic area.

Additionally, recent studies have explored new approaches to deliver cardiac rehabilitation services with the goals of increasing availability and decreasing costs, while preserving efficacy and safety. The future of cardiac rehabilitation will continue to include these discussions of alternate approaches to delivery such as transtelephonic services and other means of home-based rehabilitation. These alternate approaches have the potential to provide cardiac rehabilitation services to low- and moderate-risk patients, who comprise the majority of patients with stable coronary disease. The feasibility, safety, efficacy, and economic impart of these alternate approaches have yet to be established in large numbers of patients with stable coronary disease, particularly elderly patients, those with ventricular dysfunction, and other patients of higher risk status.[3]

Recommendations for Further Scientific Studies

The following recommendations for further scientific studies related to this chapter are noted in the *Cardiac Rehabilitation Clinical Practice Guidelines*.[3] The broad scope of cardiac rehabilitation highlights many issues that require further study.

- Evaluation of cost-effectiveness and cost outcomes resulting from the delivery of various models of cardiac rehabilitation services.
- Evaluation of outcomes of exercise rehabilitation, with and

without supervision and with and without ECG monitoring and surveillance, in patients from higher-risk groups, including those with heart failure, elderly patients, and those with complex cardiovascular disease.

- Evaluation of the safety and efficacy of strength training in higher-risk populations such as elderly patients, women, unfit cardiac patients, and others at moderate-to-high cardiovascular risk.
- Prospective evaluation of the safety and benefit of exercise rehabilitation in patients with compensated heart failure and impaired ventricular systolic function.
- Development of optimal education and counseling strategies for cost-effective coronary risk reduction.
- Evaluation of the effects of cardiac rehabilitation on rates of return to work, specifically targeting vocational rehabilitation counseling as a cardiac rehabilitation service.

The probability that rehabilitation may have a significant effect on secondary prevention, reduced disability, increased productivity, improved quality of life, and associated influences on heath care costs should encourage government, the insurance industry, private health care agencies, and academic institutions to foster and support research in these areas.

Conclusions

Cardiac rehabilitation services are widely underused despite their proven benefits. The costs and reimbursement of these services remain variable, based on the provider, the patient's status, the region, and the payer. Studies that reveal cost-benefit data are limited. Future studies should include an evaluation of supervised cardiac rehabilitation programs, office-managed care, and supervised home programs, with regard to improvements in functional capacity, modification of risk factors, long-term compliance, rehospitalization, quality of life, and medical costs incurred. Productivity should be gauged not only in rates of return to remunerative work, but also by the attainment of self-sufficiency and independence in persons disabled by cardiac illness. The effect on subsequent need for support from employed family members, homemaker services, or other costly social support systems should be considered. In this context, the establishment of a national cardiac rehabilitation database for the analysis of data collected in the daily delivery of cardiac rehabilitation services among urban, suburban, and rural populations may provide considerable useful information, and serve as an important scientific and clinical frame of reference.[18]

The *Cardiac Rehabilitation Clinical Practice Guidelines* will serve as a guide for clinical decision-making regarding the cost-effectiveness of cardiac rehabilitation services, and hopefully will influence the costs and reimbursement of these services in the future.

References

1. American Heart Association: *Heart and Stroke Facts: 1996 Statistical Supplement*. Dallas: AHA, 1995.
2. U.S. Department of Health and Human Services: *Heart Failure: Evaluation and Care of Patients with Left-Ventricular Systolic Dysfunction*. Rockville, MD: AHCPR; 1994.
3. U.S. Department of Health and Human Services: *Cardiac Rehabilitation Clinical Practice Guidelines*. Rockville, MD: AHCPR; 1995.
4. Evans RW. Organ transplantation costs, insurance coverage, and reimbursement. In Terasaki P ed: *Clinical Transplants*. Los Angelos: UCLA Tissue Typing Laboratory; 1990.
5. Ades PA, Huang D, Waver SO. Cardiac rehabilitation participation predicts lower rehospitalization costs. *Am Heart J* 1992;123(pt 1):916–921.
6. Hedback B, Perk J. Five-year results of a comprehensive rehabilitation programme after myocardial infarction. *Eur Heart J* 1987;8:234–242.
7. Levin LA, Perk J, Hedback B. Cardiac rehabilitation: A cost analysis. *J Int Med* 1991;230:427–434.
8. Shephard RJ. Exercise in secondary and tertiary rehabilitation. *J Cardiopulm Rehab* 1989;9:188–194.
9. Ades PA. Decreased medical costs after cardiac rehabilitation. A case of universal reimbursement. *J Cardiopulm Rehab* 1993;13:75–77.
10. Oldridge N, Furlong W, Feeny D, et al. Economic evaluation of cardiac rehabilitation soon after acute myocardial infarction. *Am J Cardiol* 1993;72:154–161.
11. Byl N, Reed P, Franklin B, Gordon S. Cost of Phase II cardiac rehabilitation: Implications regarding ECG-monitoring practices. (abstract) *Circulation* 1988;78(suppl II):II-136.
12. Bittner V, Oberman A. Efficacy studies in coronary rehabilitation. *Cardiol Clin* 1993;11:333–347.
13. Perk J, Hedback B, Engvall J. Effects of cardiac rehabilitation after coronary artery bypass grafting on readmission, return to work, and physical fitness: A case-control study. *Scand J Soc Med* 1990;18:45–51.
14. Picard MH, Dennis C, Schwartz RG, et al. Cost-benefit analysis of early return to work after uncomplicated acute myocardial infarction. *Am J Cardiol* 1989;63:1308–1314.
15. Bondestam E, Breikss A, Hartford M. Effects of early rehabilitation on consumption of medical care during the first year after acute myocardial infarction in patients > 65 years of age. *Am J Cardiol* 1995;75:767–771.
16. AMA Current Procedural Terminology Book. *Cardiac Rehabilitation Services*. CPT Codes 93797 and 93798. 1993.
17. Hall L. The future of health care implications for cardiac and pulmonary rehabilitation. *J Cardiopulm Rehab* 1994;14:228–231.
18. American Heart Association: *Cardiac Rehabilitation Programs, Medical/Scientific Statement*. Dallas: AHA, 1994.

Index